Functional Anatomy of Yoga

A Guide for Practitioners and Teachers

David Keil

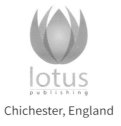

lotus
publishing

Chichester, England

First published in 2014, and redesigned in 2017 by
Lotus Publishing
Apple Tree Cottage, Inlands Road, Nutbourne, Chichester, PO18 8RJ

Anatomical Illustrations Amanda Williams and Emily Evans
Photographs Jose Caban
Text Design Medlar Publishing Solutions Pvt Ltd., India
Cover Design Paula Morrison
Printed and Bound in India by Replika Press

MEDICAL DISCLAIMER: The following information is intended for general information purposes only. Individuals should always see their health care provider before administering any suggestions made in this book. Any application of the material set forth in the following pages is at the reader's discretion and is his or her sole responsibility.

British Library Cataloguing-in-Publication Data
A CIP record for this book is available from the British Library
ISBN 978 1 905367 46 7

CONTENTS

ACKNOWLEDGMENTS

There are many people who have been a part of making this book possible. First and foremost is my wife who has put up with me quitting the task, picking it up again, and all the complaining that happened until I finally got it done. Secondly, is my publisher, who is extremely patient, and put up with me going way over the deadline. Third, is my final editor Eryn Kirkwood, who did a fantastic job of helping me convey the subject clearly.

The book wouldn't be in your hands right now if a series of events hadn't happened in just the right order at just the right time.

I must say a very special thanks to Iris Burman and the staff that supported me at Educating Hands School of Massage in Miami, Florida. Without their support, guidance and ultimately tossing me into the deep end to start teaching, I would not have honed my skills as a teacher. It was also at Educating Hands that I met my first mentor in bodywork, Nick Chitty. His guidance, friendship, and mentoring propelled my work to the next level.

My very first anatomy workshop for yoga students would not have happened if not for Karen Schachter who in 2000 asked me to teach a group of her friends at a local yoga studio. My very first hosts were Ryan Spielman and Marisa Gallardo at Yoga Grove in Miami, Florida.

The real work of understanding my anatomy was through the practice of yoga. For that I had to meet John Scott and his wife Lucy Scott in 2001. If I had not met them I would never have made it to Mysore, India. It was there that I met Sri K. Pattabhi Jois and his grandson Sri R. Sharath. It was John and Lucy's guidance of my practice and the discipline that I found in Mysore that pushed me deeper into my own practice. This depth and focus helped me to understand my anatomy, especially as it related to yoga.

Beyond that, there have been countless studios that have warmly welcomed me to be part of their teacher training programs and present anatomy to their students. All of them have helped to get this book into your hands as well. Without the questions, comments, or looks of utter confusion from these students, I would not have refined my teaching. After all, we always grow through relationship. With great thanks to all of these students, I appreciate your feedback and interactions.

Last, but certainly not least, is the assistance from everyone here at Yoganatomy.com. A very special thank you to, Christine Wiese, Amy Dolan, Aaron Segall, and Guy Andefors.

FOREWORD

In 2001 David arrived at our yoga studio in Penzance, Cornwall, UK, to work with Lucy and myself, in developing his Ashtanga Vinyasa yoga practice. David had been practicing *asana* (yoga postures) for some time, but it was obvious that he was not breathing or using *bandha* (subtle body controls) correctly or efficiently; he needed to refine his relationship and the balance between *sthira* (steady, still, and firm foundation) and *sukha* (good space). For the *yogin* (one who practices yoga), understanding *sthira and sukha* deepens the understanding of the relationship between posture, gravity, and breath and for the anatomist who practices *asana*, discovering *sthira* and *sukha* will bring understanding of the structure, function, breath and movement of the human body to a whole new level.

When we met David so many years ago, his immense understanding of anatomy and experience gained from teaching and working in the field of massage was also evident. He presented a short yoga anatomy workshop at our studio for local and visiting students who were practicing with Lucy and I. His animated delivery emphasized how remarkable the human body is. At the end of the evening, a local doctor who was participating said that in all her years of medical training and anatomy classes, this one session with David brought the body alive for her. Lucy, also an experienced body worker and massage therapist, was so impressed that she went straight to David and invited him to teach the anatomy for our yoga teacher trainings.

That evening was the beginning of a mutual journey of growth, with Lucy, David, and myself together exploring, discovering, having insights, and gaining first hand a new appreciation for this amazing body we inhabit. This journey with David will continue for years to come, and I'm sure this will be the first of many books he will write.

The information in this book has not come from researching other books but from deep exploration on the yoga mat. David does not reduce the body to mere parts. For practical reasons, the work is divided into chapters, but at all times, David maintains a wider perception, holding the body as a unified living, breathing, moving organism. He takes anatomy to a whole new level.

As with other anatomy texts, David references body parts with anatomical words and descriptions; however, he goes further. Using his own experience with yoga *asana*, putting his own body into the many gravity-defying structures, he creates an understanding for you, the reader, in everyday language. This book is a bridge across the gap between the professional academic and the self-exploring yoga student. You, too, will gain a personal understanding and insight by taking David's gems of wisdom to your yoga mat, and through your own personal practical exploration, will connect all separated parts into one whole functioning and breathing body, alive steady in *asana – sthira/sukha*.

It is an honor and a pleasure to write a foreword to this exploratory journey into the functioning of the physical body. When I read through David's draft, I could hear his voice, the complexity yet simplicity of the presentation. It felt as though I was present in one of his workshops, eager to be led by David through the practical anatomical exercise on the yoga mat. This book is a journey of deep exploration that will enhance each individual's understanding of what it really means to inhabit a body that not only stands in anatomical neutral, *samasthitih*, but also moves with the breath to create *asana*. A body that "shape shifts" towards the postural understanding of our bodies, tension free, relaxed, still, and steady—gracefully moving in space, mastering the relationship of posture, breath, and gravity.

—Enjoy

John Scott

INTRODUCTION

My idea for this book grew as I traveled around the world teaching anatomy to prospective yoga teachers. Usually I serve as an adjunct faculty in a teacher training program, offering the minimum amount of anatomy training required to certify new teachers. Twelve hours is barely an introduction to this wonderfully complicated body of ours. My hope is that this book offers a more complete exploration of the human body in a context that is both accessible and exciting.

As I teach, I sometimes question whether those on the sincere path of a yogi really need to know anatomy. By this I mean, if you're practicing yoga for the ultimate intention of self-knowledge and not just jumping around on a mat, how much anatomy do you really need to know? The truth is if we adhere to the definition of yoga offered in Patanjali's sutras, yoga is the cessation of the fluctuations of the mind. It is detaching from all of the voices (and their stories) in our head long enough to realize our true self.

So what does this have to do with anatomy? Well, honestly, not much. Most of us do not have the wherewithal to simply sit down, quiet our mind, and enter into a state of yoga. So what are we to do? What is our vehicle for accessing this state? How do we find our way there? The answer is simple: through our very own research laboratory—the body.

Hatha Yoga was born to accommodate those of us who can't just sit down and quiet our mind. *Asana* (a.k.a., jumping around on our mat) is the vehicle with which we begin to purify the body (*annamayakosha*). The *asanas* touch us on all levels. At the most basic level, they increase our flexibility and strength. More subtly, they purify our tissues, and even more subtly, they affect the energetic system that supports and sustains our tissues. Finally, when all the moving and jumping is done, the *asanas* bring us to a state where we might sit comfortably and quietly without our mind being distracted by our body. This "jumping around" on the mat is also our vehicle for studying the body in a deep and kinesthetic way. This is where anatomy intersects *asana*.

If you have practiced *asana* consistently for 10 years or more for at least one hour each day, it is certain that you know the workings of your body quite well. You may not have the technical anatomical names or understandings, but your kinesthetic knowledge is a very real and powerful way to know the body. This is knowledge that cannot be learned from a book.

Unfortunately, many people today are teaching yoga before they have practiced for even one year. In general, if you haven't done the exploration in your own body, it will be harder to lead someone through an exploration of theirs. But every teacher and student must start somewhere. For those of you who have not dedicated the time to exploring your body deeply on a daily basis, it is crucial for you to understand anatomy and the wide variety of differences in individual anatomy. Keep in mind, however, that at some point you must do the self-inquiry.

If you are reading this book to learn what your students should or shouldn't do with this or that condition or pain, the answer is, "There is no answer." Oh yes, I am serious. If you think these conditions can be boiled down, categorized, systematized, and then spat back, you will never be a great teacher. I assume that each teacher wants to be the best they can be, and for that, you need to practice and study for years. You need to think, inquire, and be open to possibilities!

You might have gathered that the information in this book is not the final answer to any particular situation or problem. You're right: it isn't. But you *will* find explanations that may fit what you observe in class. I try to provide these in a way that helps you understand the bigger picture that always goes along with the little picture expressing itself in your class. I provide broad anatomical explanations that might be applied to any individual in your class.

After reading this book, you will be filled with information that inspires you to think critically. You will have the tools to hypothesize what's going on in a student's (or in your own) body and what to do about it. I want you to be a thinker. Question everything you read and hear (including what I say), not for the sake of

questioning, but for a deeper comprehension. And finally, I want you to understand what you will learn by practicing.

In teaching anatomy, I seek to strike a balance between simplicity and honoring the complexity of the human body. Most of the questions I receive from students are the "why and what" questions: "Why can't I do this *asana*?" "What is restricting me in this pose?" "What do you do if you have knee pain?" "What poses should I avoid with this condition?" These are practical questions.

The aim of this book is to be as practical as possible. At the same time, I offer many possibilities and perspectives. I don't do this to confuse you, but to keep you aware of the myriad possibilities; filtering through many possibilities is the reality of a yoga teacher. When I make suggestions to my students about their problems, conditions, and restrictions, I offer a working hypothesis. In other words, I make an educated guess at what may be causing the concern and what might help to alleviate or improve the situation. I have to be willing to change my hypothesis based on the student's feedback or what I observe the student doing as we move forward.

If there is an inherent problem with studying anatomy, it is that we divide the body into pieces and parts in order to talk about it. There is no other way I can think of to approach the information. The downside of this is that we then think of the body as being distinct parts that are somehow assembled together.

We need to remember that our body started its formation with yoga. The literal translation of the word is "yoking" or "joining." It is when the sperm meets the egg that the first physical yoking begins in our own body. From this point, a single cell is formed. From that single cell, every bone, muscle, organ, piece, and part has formed out of cell division. The body did not name its own parts. That's something we humans have done. So, as the body functions as a whole (rather than as an assembly of individual parts), we need to approach it as a whole.

There is a similar issue in approaching yoga from an anatomical perspective. While it is hoped that any serious student will study all of yoga's eight limbs, because this is an anatomy book, we deal exclusively with only one limb—*asana*. Most yoga students today enter the path of yoga via *asana*. This is neither good nor bad. *Asana* is a great way to engage with the whole of yoga. Yoga does not care how we interact with it. That we are interacting with it on any level suggests it will lead us through the whole of the practice over time.

As practitioners, it is important that we do not get stuck in *asana*. It's definitely possible. There is a lifetime of work to do in fully understanding and experiencing these postures, and studying anatomy can add to this natural emphasis on the physical. It is not my intention to get you stuck in your thinking mind or your body. As you read, I hope you will take this information and experience it for yourself, thereby merging your intellect with your physicality.

As you read, allow your understanding of what anatomy means to expand. Begin to explore your body as an integrated whole. As you practice, experience *asanas* not as individual postures but as elements that are related to one another in the context of a greater whole.

In summary, this book will encourage you to explore your understanding of anatomy via the personal laboratory that is your own body. As a result, you will become a more mindful practitioner and a better teacher. If I do my job well, you will be inspired to continue your study of anatomy, your practice, and yourself well beyond the pages of this book.

Namasté,

David Keil

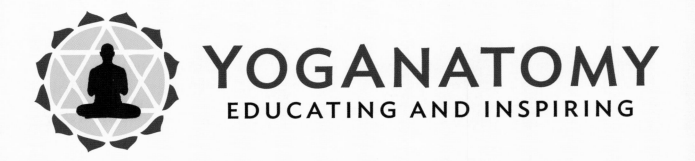
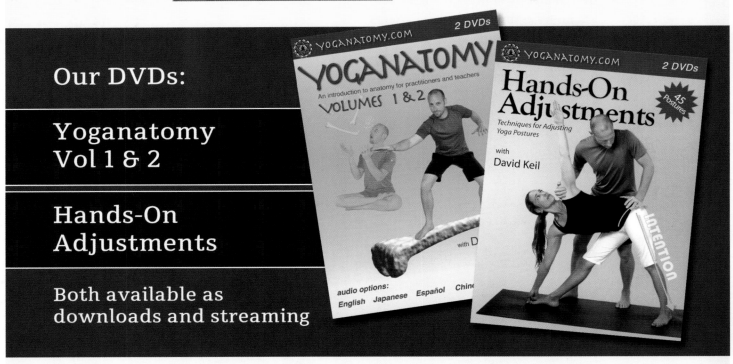

Part I

Functional Anatomy

CONVERGING HISTORIES

From the moment of our birth, our bodies are affected by the lives we live. There is a convergence of information and energy that comes together inside of us. Circumstances, decisions, accidents, and intentions all influence who we are. They form us as certainly as we were physically formed in our mother's womb. It is impossible to separate a person from their life experiences.

I call these life experiences or influences "Converging Histories." These histories comprise a wide array of informational energies that are absorbed by our system. Every event in our life, from watching a movie to riding a bicycle or practicing yoga, has an influence on our being. All of these events have a certain energetic, physical, and emotional quality that impact and become part of our physical body.

Our converging histories make us exactly who we are in this moment. Some of these histories happened to us; we had no conscious control over them. Some of them we chose; we consciously added them to our life experiences. Every moment that we live, we choose experiences, activities, and relationships that become part of our own sea of converging histories. They become part of us.

The first and most basic of these histories is common to us all. It is the history of human evolution. What has human evolution done to our bodies? Imagine for a moment that it is billions of years ago and we are quadrupeds. Our center of gravity as four-legged creatures is in a different place. Our feet and hands are also different. Thus when we evolve to bipedalism, our bodies have to change. As two-legged creatures, the relationship of muscle to bone must shift.

As two-legged creatures, walking is our main mode of transportation. Therefore, we have developed strong lower bodies designed to propel us forward. Along with this development, our upper half has evolved as well. We are quite good at interacting with things in front of us. We grab, pull, and manipulate the tangible world as perceived by our eyes, nose, and mouth. Due to the incredible mobility of our hands, we're better able to protect our front and our more vulnerable underside.

Our fantastic "new" appendages have made using tools and playing the piano possible. And our hands have helped further the development of our brain. Yes, our ability to pick things up, manipulate objects, and create new things with our hands has fed our brain massive amounts of information, which has in turn led to the human consciousness and intelligence we now know.[1] Our upper limbs are also useful in their coordination with the lower half. We use our arms to help move the body while running and to maintain balance in difficult situations. (Can anyone say *Utthita Hasta Padangusthasana?*)

Our genetic history is another piece of our converging histories. From the vast pool of possibilities, we have been born to two parents, each with their own genetic make-up. Out of this genetic mixing pot come our eye color, foot size, and shape of the arches in the feet (or lack thereof). Our height and weight predispositions, the length of our torso relative to our arms, and so on, also come out of the mix. On a physiological level, our parental genetic history predisposes us to certain diseases or illnesses. The implications of genetic history are far-reaching.

Somewhat related to genetics is the history I refer to as "Learned Parental Behavior." This is a scary one for some of us. It can be distressing to wake up one morning and realize that we are turning into our parents, which we swore we would never do. It's hard to escape the powerful imprints left by our parents during the formative years.

On a physical level, we learn how to walk by watching and mirroring the way our parents walk. We talk, make expressions, and have similar body language as our parents. This is only natural. Our parents are the first place we saw any of these things happening.

In addition, we adopt ways of thinking, ways of being, and patterns of thought from the input and influence of our parents. Even our mental attitudes derive in part from our learned parental history. The implications are deep. Perhaps this is one way to explain why millions of people are in therapy trying to eradicate the "negative" influence of their parents. In no way should we pass judgment on Mom and Dad. They did the best they could. It is our work to recognize the traits and behaviors that stem from our learned parental history and then determine which to maintain and which to discard.

The fourth and fifth converging histories I've identified are physical ones. Our "Activities History" comprises all the physical activities we have learned over the years. Perhaps we played sports such as baseball, football, or soccer. Or maybe we spent time dancing, horseback riding, or practicing martial arts. All of these activities create patterns of movement in our bodies and help forge relationships between the brain, the senses, and our motor skills. The degree of refinement we develop in our activities and how long we participate in them helps to determine the strength of the patterns developed.

I was exposed to yoga very early in life by my pre-school teacher, Mrs. Elphenbein. We did yoga a few times a week on our little rugs. I don't fully know the degree to which this impacted my body or mind. But I have to believe these formative experiences played a role in my later desire to study Tai Chi Chuan and yoga.

I also did judo for a short time and played baseball for a number of years. I played catcher, which definitely left a physical imprint on me. I had to squat for long periods of time, which lengthened or built certain muscles in my lower body and likely impacted my posture. Some, like me, have done many activities in their lives while others have participated in just a few. Either way, they all have an influence on how our body develops and the patterns that we acquire.

We also need to consider our "Injury History." Sometimes our injuries are the result of our activities and sports. Sometimes they are the result of accidents, such as falling out of a tree and breaking an arm, stepping off a curb and twisting an ankle, or even getting hit by a car. No matter the cause, all injuries have an influence on our patterns, and we might not be aware of what these are. Perhaps the position of our sacrum or pelvis is changed in a fall. Or maybe the healing of a broken bone causes one leg to become slightly longer. We must become aware of the far-reaching effects of our injury history as we come to know and understand our body.

When I was nine years old I broke my femur (thigh bone). I was playing soccer at the time. I kicked a soccer ball at the exact same moment that my neighbor (a boy at least twice my size) kicked the ball in the opposite direction. The impact of our simultaneous kicks completely broke my femur. Is it any wonder that this leg is a bit twisted, a bit longer, and definitely harder to get behind my head? Even the food we ate as children or the amount of beer we drank in college can influence our bodies and what they are capable of. Thus we also have a "Nutritional History" that influences who we are right now.

Finally we have what is perhaps a larger and more profound history that can impact who we are, what injuries we have had, and how our body moves. It influences the very essence of our being. I call this our "Spiritual History." Within this history are some very large questions about who we are, what we believe, and how we live. Our spiritual beliefs not only inform our inner well-being, but can impact our physical body as well.

Since we are talking about yoga, we should also consider whether there is an influence from past lives. What about personal karma or *samskaras* and their effect on our physical body? Is it possible we did yoga in a past life? If so, how is it influencing our practice of *asana* today?

There is just one more history worth mentioning: our "Mental/Emotional History." Our emotional history plays a part in shaping how we view the world and ourselves. These influences can come from our parents, embarrassing or proud moments, and even our injuries. As a teacher, I see this in students all the time. By watching the way they approach their practice or deal with their aches and pains, I can tell a lot about their history. An injury that happened years ago can keep a student from even trying a given posture.

For example, I met a student who had an injury to his hip joint about 15 years before I met him. Pins were placed inside temporarily to keep the cartilage against the end of the bone so that it could heal. From that point on, he had assumed there was some boney deformation that prevented him from adducting his hip joint or bringing his femur to his chest.

His approach to practice was one of caution (a good thing). By the time I met him he had basically given up on a regular practice because it was causing more trouble than good, and most teachers were baffled by the condition of his hip. I could see how strong the beliefs were, the connection to the old injury, and the assumptions that were turned into fact. A number of postures were just not going to happen with all of these beliefs and stories in place.

To be honest, I didn't know what the truth was, but neither did the student. With three days of practice and a lot of trust, we got his femur to his chest and his hip joint did adduct. Slowly but surely, the beliefs and emotions stored within the body were being released—often showing up in the form of hopeful and joyful tears; disbelief and recognition of stories that were wrong and as stuck as the hip itself were dissolving.

It doesn't matter how you divide or categorize the "histories"; I could have done it differently. What is important is that you see how each one of them ultimately ties together to create our state of being in any given moment.

When we look at a student, we are seeing the product of these converging histories. Beginning to observe what shows up (inside and out) in the moment is the best way to see someone. Learning to see beyond the body is part of learning to teach yoga. As we become able to see beyond the body, we become better able to see our students as they are in the moment. But we need to keep in mind that sometimes (perhaps in a large class situation) individuality is lost and everyone is given the same instruction for the same pose, despite their individual differences.

So, how do we treat each student as an individual? Each pose has its basic principles and guidelines. For instance, everyone should rotate their thigh outward or inward and engage this or that in a given pose, right? How do we layer these fundamentals with our consideration of who a particular student is right now, in this moment? And how can we move our students from where they are now to where we think they should be in a way that suits them? How many of these histories are you able to see when you watch your students practice? Should students do (or not do) certain postures on the basis of their personal histories? How do these histories fit into a student's development in the practice of *asana* as well as the larger picture of yoga? These are just a few things to consider. Let's leave it at this: It is enough that you begin to look for these pieces of the puzzle in your students. It is enough that you try to see beyond the body.

IT IS ALL ONE

Now that you have a taste for how hard it really is to see the whole person, perhaps you can sense the difficulty in teaching anatomy in a way that emphasizes how well-integrated the body actually is. As it is easy to lapse into our old mindset of seeing the body without taking into account the person alongside their life experiences, it is quite natural to disregard the interconnection of all of our parts. We tend to think of our sore shoulder, tight hip, or flexible spine as separate issues with little to no correlation. And when taking a subject as broad and complex as anatomy, it is helpful (and perhaps necessary) to divide it into pieces for easier comprehension. This certainly has value. The problem arises if we forget to put these pieces back together or don't make an effort to understand how they interrelate to create the whole.

It is common for us to think of a muscle as one piece, a bone as another piece, and connective tissue as yet another piece of the body. And it doesn't help our cause that we can actually replace a knee, hip, or shoulder. The miracle of modern medicine reinforces this idea of our being distinct pieces—and replaceable pieces at that! Although it is true that we can replace certain broken parts, this is not the way we were created, manufactured in a plant using nuts and bolts. Far from it.

Our beginnings and, therefore, the beginning of all of our "parts" is much more magical and integrated than that. If we start from the very beginning, there were two parts: one sperm and one egg. That miraculous act of fertilization initiated the amazing process of formation. We developed from that point on. One cell split into two cells, which split into four cells, which split into eight, and so on. This is our true beginning, one cell dividing into many until those cells began to specialize and eventually comprise all of our parts. Although the crux of my message is the integration of the body, that information has to be given in pieces. However, we must always step back and look at the individual part in relationship to everything that surrounds it.

THE BASICS OF
FUNCTIONAL ANATOMY

CONNECTIVE TISSUE

It is fitting that we begin our exploration of anatomy with the tissue that exemplifies the interconnected nature of all of our "parts"— the connective tissue. The very structure of connective tissue compels us to acknowledge that the slightest and most subtle change in one area of the body necessarily has an impact on the whole. A small movement in the big toe is like a fly landing on a spider web. When the fly hits the web, vibrations are sent through the web all the way to the other end, where the spider sits and waits. A small movement of the big toe affects the foot, ankle, and conceivably even the position of the pelvis. The toe is connected to all of these parts by a web of connective tissues.

Perhaps you have never heard of connective tissue. It can be difficult to visualize, but the fact is that the following parts of your body are *all* connective tissue:

- Bones
- Cartilage
- Muscles
- Fascia
- Tendons
- Ligaments
- Scar tissue

How is connective tissue important to yoga? It is a key component of our flexibility. Other components help to determine flexibility as well, including the muscles, skeletal system, and nervous system, which tell the muscles what to do, and we will discuss these components in depth. But for now we will explore connective tissue.

So, what is this stuff? Connective tissues are comprised of two proteins, collagen and elastin. Collagen is known for its strength. Elastin, as you may have guessed from its name, is elastic; it's the more pliable and resilient stuff. Put them together in varying proportions and densities

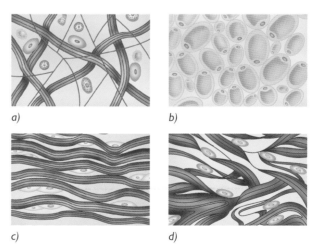

a)   b)

c)   d)

Figure 1.1: *The structure of the different types of connective tissue; a) loose connective tissue (areolar), b) loose connective tissue (adipose), c) dense regular connective tissue, d) dense irregular connective tissue.*

and you get the amazing array of connective tissues we find throughout the body.

Ligaments and Tendons

The denser and stronger the tissue, the more collagen is involved. Ligaments and tendons are made up of a higher proportion of collagen fibers (relative to elastin) and their fibers are tightly packed together. They are very strong. In fact, it is often said that ligaments and tendons have a tensile strength equal to steel cable of the same size. This is what makes them ideal tissues to accomplish their different functions.

Ligaments allow for and restrict movement in different directions. They are always situated around the junction between two bones. In other words, you find ligaments at joints or articulations. Because their collagen proteins are packed together so densely, they don't have a direct blood supply. There is no artery that burrows its way deep into the core of a ligament. The sheath of tissue encasing the ligament delivers the necessary nutrients for function and healing. This lack of blood supply is one of the main reasons ligaments do not normally heal when torn.

Tendons are similar to ligaments but perform a different function. Tendons are actually the ends of muscles that attach to the bones. They connect muscles to bones and allow the muscle to contract and move the bone at a joint in a particular way. Both are made of similar proportions of collagen and elastin and therefore have similar strengths.

Fascia

There are three main divisions of fascia in the body. Superficial fascia lies just under the skin and contains the fat cells that help maintain body temperature at the surface. Visceral fascia surrounds and suspends the organs, not just in the gut but also in the heart and lungs.

The last is the type we're most interested in: the deep fascia, which surrounds all of the muscles. You can think of the fascial system as a body glove or stocking. The stocking is not only on the surface, but also wraps around deeper structures such as muscles, arteries, veins, and bones. Each of these structures has their own layer of connective tissue. Each muscle, artery, vein, and bone is joined to one another through even more connective tissue. The spider web is an excellent analogy. All of these attachments

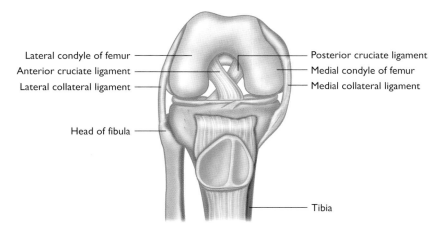

Lateral condyle of femur
Anterior cruciate ligament
Lateral collateral ligament
Head of fibula
Posterior cruciate ligament
Medial condyle of femur
Medial collateral ligament
Tibia

Figure 1.2: *Ligaments are like straps that bind the end of two bones together, stabilizing, allowing or restricting movement in different directions.*

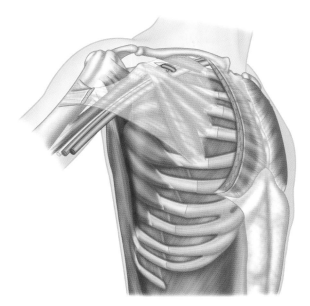

Figure 1.3: *Fascial sheath.*

create a web of tissue that wraps around one structure and then heads off to wrap around another structure and another and so on. The entire body is actually connected by this ubiquitous web of connective tissue. There is an abundance of connective tissue fully integrated into our muscles. It surrounds the muscles on a cellular, fascicle (bundle of cells), and overall muscle-belly level.

To maintain our integrated point of view, remember that we use the separate terms, muscle and fascia, to describe two parts of a single unit. To think of them as separate is not realistic or beneficial to our understanding of the body in a truly integrated way. Think of it like a peanut butter and jelly sandwich. You have peanut butter on one piece of bread and jelly on the other. Once you put those two pieces of bread together, you have the sandwich. You can talk about the peanut butter and the jelly as individual parts of the sandwich, but it's impossible to separate them. Similarly, talking about a muscle or fascia as if they are two things that can be separated is not realistic. Therefore, we can use more sophisticated language and

refer to muscles as myofascia. "Myo" refers to muscle and well, the rest is obvious—fascia.

The integration does not stop here. Because the tendons, ligaments, and tissue wrapping the bones are all connective tissue, the interaction and integration are fantastic. There is no obvious end to a tendon as it weaves its way into the connective tissue layer around the bone. Nor is there any obvious starting or stopping point to ligaments as they weave into bone tissue. When you see a picture of a knee with many tendons, ligaments, and the joint capsule all coming together, it is difficult to see obvious divisions between structures. All of these connective tissue combinations make possible the amazing display of movement we find not only in yoga but in other disciplines like dance, biking, and skiing, as well.

When connective tissue is freer, bones and posture shift into a more optimal position. By releasing long-held tensional patterns, the body and the mind are more at ease. Yoga is a great way of manipulating these tissues. By using the strength of some muscles to lengthen others, or by using the ground or gravity as resistance, we can actively lengthen our connective tissues. As a result, we can realign our own skeleton.

Integrating into the Muscular System

Let's take a closer look at the muscular system. First, let me ask you a question: What do you think muscle is made of? If you're struggling to come up with an answer, let's take it from another angle. What happens when you pull or tear a muscle, for example, your hamstring? What do you think that means, literally? It probably means you tore some muscle fibers, right?

Okay, let's say you tore a muscle fiber. What is a muscle fiber? If you look at the construction of a muscle, you find two types of proteins (actin and myosin) sitting in a long row. These proteins are waiting for the nervous system to send a signal to release calcium and cause these two types of protein to become attracted to one another like magnets. This is the basis for muscular contraction—the introduction of calcium molecules to two proteins that cause them to become attracted to one another.

Let's come back to what you find when you look at the structure of a muscle. What is it that holds these proteins in a row and allows them to contract in a particular direction? Connective tissue. In this case, we could be more specific and say *fascia*. At this layer of a muscle, a group of fibers are joined together to make a muscle cell. These muscle cells are like the pieces of pulp in a citrus fruit, each of which has its own layer of skin. In the muscle fibers, the "skin" is a layer of fascia surrounding them called the endomysium.

When you take a group of these muscle cells, bundle them together and wrap them with another layer of fascia, called the perimysium, you get what we call a fascicle. This is like the wedge in a citrus fruit, which is a group of pieces of pulp. Finally, you have the muscle itself, which is a bundle of fascicles surrounded with yet another layer of fascia called the epimysium. This last layer of fascia is like the peel of our citrus fruit.

Now back to our original question. What is a muscle made of? Layers and wrappings of fascia around proteins. So, really, muscles are made of connective tissue. Therefore, when you tear a hamstring, you are actually tearing connective tissue.

The integrated perspective that we're developing gives us a more complex and dynamic understanding of movement. We now know that contractions are not simply a row of proteins getting closer together and shortening the muscle. We know that each contraction intimately involves the fascial tissue surrounding those proteins. The health of the fascia is one factor that can impede

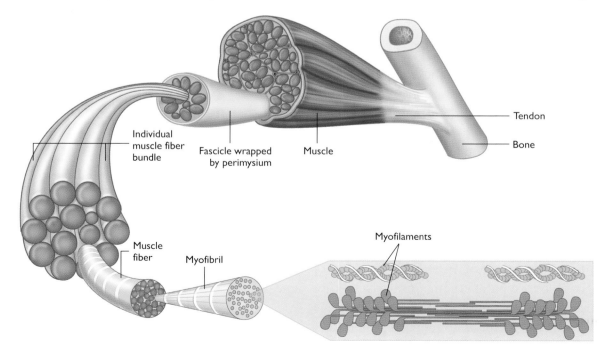

Figure 1.4: *Image of muscle layers with connective tissue.*

muscle function. The fascia and muscle together comprise one unit. When you are talking about lengthening a muscle in an *asana*, you are also talking about lengthening the fascia that's surrounding it. Our muscles and fascia are inseparable.

There are other ways in which the fascia can get "hung-up" and stuck together. The fascia separates and divides all of the muscles from one another. By its very nature, separating them is also a way of connecting them together, because the fascia is simply making divisions within the whole. It is possible that where these "individual" muscles are separated from one another they get stuck together.

This can happen as a result of too much movement, not enough movement, or an injury. For instance, moving too much could include lifting weights. Connective tissue has the ability to respond to stress that is placed on it locally. When lifting weights, the connective tissue has to adapt and change to the increased strength in the muscles. It does this by laying down new fibers of connective tissue and becoming denser, so that it can deal with the new amount of strength in that tissue.

Not enough movement means that the muscle begins to atrophy and weaken. In this case, the connective tissue is not pressed to stretch and shorten in any meaningful way. It consequently tightens up, along with the muscle that is no longer at optimal health.

An injury can also cause changes in the connective tissue. When scar tissue is created, it can change the amount of tension in an area of fascia. This can cause it to be glued together with the adjacent layer of fascia of the next muscle. This means a loss of independence of those two separate muscles. The two layers of fascia that sit there can no longer move easily relative to one another.

The hamstrings are a common example of this occurring due to overuse and not as a result of scar tissue. The hamstrings contract hundreds of times a day, even just in walking. It's common for these muscles to be tight on the average person. Some of that has to do with the amount of walking, sitting, and even sports activities that lead to generally tight hamstrings as they contract over and over again.

As a result, these three individual muscles can easily become "glued" to one another over time. When we say *glued together* we mean that the layers of connective tissue that separate and divide them also connect them together. If they become stuck together, they cannot function independently to their best capacity. Nevertheless, we don't require fine motor skills when using our hamstrings; they're built for power. So we won't necessarily notice how stuck together they could be, that is, until we try to stretch them. Then we wonder how our hamstrings got so tight! Part of it is simply muscular use and how that relates to the nervous system and tension. The other part is how the connective tissue has responded to stimulation: one way is by making the hamstrings grow together, reducing the individualization of these three muscles.

If this same level of stickiness happened in smaller muscles, such as those that move our fingers, we could have a problem. Fine motor skills would become difficult, since we need more individualization of the muscles that move our fingers than we do in our hamstrings to move the knee and hip joints.

FUNCTIONS OF THE MUSCULAR SYSTEM

There are technically four basic functions of the muscular system. They are movement, production of heat, guarding entrances to the body, and maintaining posture. Relative to yoga, we will focus on how the muscular system relates to movement.

Many aspects of the muscular system can be helpful to our overall understanding of movement. First and foremost is location and function of the various muscles in our body. It is not the intention of this book to teach the location and function of every single muscle in the body, but we will look at some specifically. I also want to help you understand concepts and principles that you can apply to any muscle to better understand its function. We will talk about various types of muscle contractions. We will even explore how gravity and body position affect which muscles work in different situations.

Finally, weaving its way into the muscular system is the nervous system, which tells the muscles what to do and how much tension to have.

It is easy to get lost in oversimplification within the muscular system. I hope, rather, to expand your knowledge of the muscular system and move you away from a false notion of separation. This will further enhance your understanding of the beauty and dynamics of this complex system.

Muscle Names

Knowing the names of the muscles will provide valuable information about their function, location, size, shape, or number of parts.

Rather than shutting off your brain when you see a complicated anatomical term, think about what it means.

Let's consider a few examples. Take the adductor longus, a muscle in the thigh. What do we know about this muscle based only on its name? Well, it functions as an adductor, that is, it pulls the associated body part towards the center of the body. What does longus mean? Naturally it means *long*. The adductor longus is the longest of the adductor muscles.

Similarly, we learn a lot about the biceps brachii (a muscle in the arm) from its name. "Bi" means two. "Ceps" refers to divisions or, as we sometimes say, "heads" of a muscle. Brachii refers to the upper arm, sometimes called the brachium. The biceps is a two-headed muscle located on the upper arm. Now the trapezius. This is a large muscle shaped like a trapezoid on our back. So it is named for its shape. This is also true of the rhomboids, which are located on the upper back.

You might have noticed another similarity between anatomy and yoga. In the same way that *asanas* are named based on their shape, how they mimic animals, or the quality of the posture, muscles are also named for a reason; those I have mentioned are only a few. This should give you a sense of how to consider muscle names with an eye to learning about their function and other important information.

Understanding Muscle Function

We often see muscle function taught based on points of origin, insertion, and action. For instance, the biceps brachii originates on the coracoid process of the scapula and the supraglenoid tubercle of the scapula. It inserts on the large bump called the radial tuberosity.

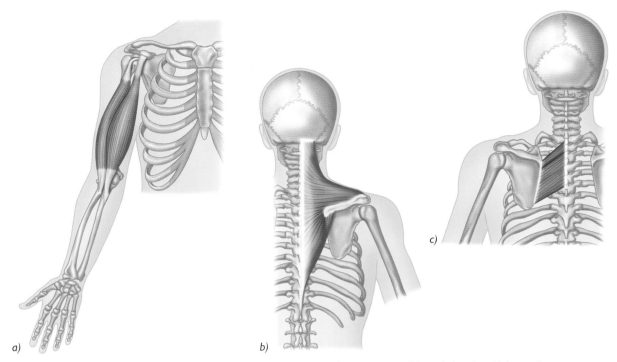

Figure 1.5: *Note the division of the biceps (a), as well as the shapes of the trapezius (b), and rhomboid (c) muscles.*

Its action is to rotate the forearm so that the palm is facing up (supination) and to bend the elbow (flexion). When thinking of muscle function this way, the origin is considered the more stable of the two bones and the insertion the more moveable. When the muscle contracts, the insertion moves towards the origin and the elbow and forearm supinate and/or flex.

However, when we discuss the origin, insertion, and action of a muscle, we are referring to it from the "anatomical position." Anatomical position looks like yoga's *Tadasana*, with the person standing erect, palms of the hands facing forward. All references to movements of flexion, extension, abduction, adduction, and rotation begin and end at the anatomical position. Although this isn't a surprise, it is potentially problematic. For instance, what if I am not initiating a movement from the anatomical position? (In real life, after all, we rarely find ourselves beginning each movement from here.) What if I'm in a backbend, or lying on the floor, or upside down in a forearm

balance? Does this change the way the muscles function? The answer to that question is *yes*.

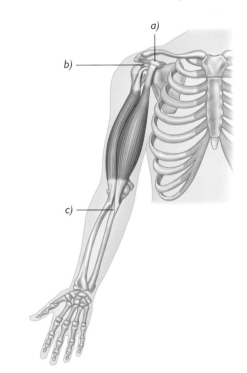

Figure 1.6: *Biceps brachii – the three elements: a) coracoid process, b) supraglenoid tubercle, c) radial tuberosity. Imagine how the forearm is moved relative to the more stable shoulder girdle.*

In addition, separating the muscles into the compartments of origin, insertion, and action leads us to believe that they function independently of each other. This oversimplification of the overall system further disconnects us from the beautiful integration of bodily tissues and perhaps even the overall experience of a pose.

The truth is there is normally one muscle that is the strongest in a particular action, but that doesn't mean it's the only one working. I don't think that one muscle ever works alone. If we focused on and isolated it, then yes, theoretically we could make just one muscle work, but that is not how we function in real life situations. Although it is true that the muscles attach at particular points on the skeletal system (the origin and insertion), it is better to look at the attachments more objectively; we shouldn't assume that the attachment that is considered to be stable (origin) cannot become the attachment that moves (normally the insertion).

Wouldn't it be more open-minded to look at the two ends of a muscle as attachment points? Neither point is always the origin or the insertion. They can switch, depending on the situation we find ourselves in. There are examples of what is normally considered to be the origin moving towards the insertion based on how we position ourselves or on which bones are stabilized during the muscular contraction.

For example, in *Laghuvajrasana* the quadriceps muscle changes its normal origin and insertion. Normally the quadriceps contract and straighten (extend) the knee by moving the lower leg (the tibia) at the knee joint. In this posture, movement is still happening at the knee joint. However, instead of the lower leg (normally the insertion) moving, as it would

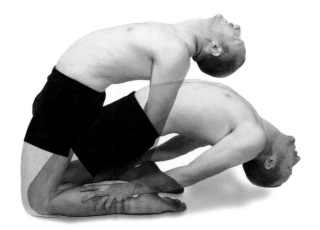

Figure 1.7: *The movement is happening at the knee joint, but the tibia is fixed.*

do if we were standing in anatomical position, the pelvis and femur (normally the origin) move towards the lower leg at the knee joint.

Look at Figure 1.7. Notice how my lower leg is on the floor. It can't move anywhere in this position. It would somehow have to move into the floor for that to happen. As I lean back into the posture, my femur, pelvis, and spine barely move relative to one another. They are stabilized. You will also notice that the only joint that changes significantly is the knee joint. But it's not the lower leg that's moving. In this posture, the upper leg and the rest of my body actually move around the knee joint.

After being in the pose, I have to engage my quadriceps (and of course stabilize the pelvis with abdominal strength) in order to come back to the starting position. In the action of coming up, contracting the quadriceps creates the movement at the knee joint. But in this instance, instead of the tibia moving as it normally does in extension of the knee, we move the rest of our body around the knee joint, effectively switching the commonly accepted origin and insertion of the muscle. There are other examples of this, but the takeaway is much more important: muscles contract. If they are going to create movement, one of the two ends will have to move towards the other (or both towards one another). The one that is more stable will not move. This way of understanding muscle function allows us to describe movement more realistically than using only the idea of origin, insertion, and action.

Muscular Contractions

Let's go a little deeper to look beyond the function of the muscle to the contraction itself. When a muscle contracts, not all the cells of that muscle are needed. The body determines how many cells to use based on past experience and current proprioceptive information gathered by the nervous system. This information takes into account things like weight, resistance, and strength of tissues. It would be terribly inefficient if every cell were required to lift objects regardless of their weight. When a cell within a muscle contracts, it contracts only until it uses up its energy, or adenosine triphosphate (ATP). Thus the body uses fewer cells in your biceps muscle to lift a pencil than it does when lifting a 20-pound weight.

If you do repetitions with that 20-pound weight, or just continue to hold it statically, eventually you will exhaust all the cells in the muscles involved. At that point, you will have exhausted all of the energy (ATP) in that muscle(s). Before that point, the mind/body knew to shift the responsibility from one cell to the next based on which cells still had energy to expend on the task at hand. In this way there is a constant shifting of cells contracting within a muscle. The cell contracts and uses up its ATP while another muscle cell begins its contraction. This process continues as each muscle cell rests for a moment and rebuilds its level of ATP.

We don't normally observe this shift happening, but if you hold something for long enough, you will see shaking occur in the muscle being used. That is the observable space between one cell contracting (using up its ATP) and a new cell contracting in order to take over the task. Muscles can shake for another reason that we see more commonly in yoga classes: tension. Tension occurs when one muscle tries to take us in one direction, say the quadriceps and other hip flexors in a standing forward bend, while the opposing muscles, in this case the hamstrings, resist the work of the quadriceps. The tensional struggle between the two creates shaking in the muscles.

Types of Contractions

In addition to the ability to recruit muscles when more energy is required, muscles can also engage in different ways. A muscle contracts on a cellular level the same way all the time. In fact, all a muscle cell can really do is receive a stimulus from the nervous system and contract. If the stimulus is taken away, it stops contracting. The most basic contraction is called a "tonic contraction." This is the continual low-level muscular contraction that maintains our basic awake-but-resting posture. If we were to "pass out," the tone created by the tonic contractions of our muscles would be lost and we would fall to the floor in a heap.

There are other types of contractions worth mentioning: isometric, isotonic concentric, and isotonic-eccentric. I want to explain these so that you have a larger picture of the capabilities of the muscular system and how it is used.

An isometric (iso = same, metric = length) contraction is one where the muscle contracts (the tone changes) but the overall length doesn't change. The two ends of the muscle do not move towards one another in this type of contraction. For example, if you were to do High Plank Pose (the top of a push-up) and stay there for about one minute, several muscles would contract to keep you in that position, even though none of your bones are moving. All of these muscles would be isometrically contracting. There is a change in tension but no movement and thus no change in the overall length of the muscle.

In isotonic (iso = same; tonic = tone or tension) contractions, the "tone" of the muscle stays the same. What changes is the length (metric changes). In isotonic contractions, either less distance or more distance is created between the two ends of the muscle. Basically, the bones are moving closer to one another (meaning that the overall length of the muscle is getting shorter), or the bones are moving further away from one another (the overall length of the muscle is getting longer). Both of these scenarios can happen during a muscular contraction. (If the idea of a muscle getting longer while it is contracting confuses you, read on.)

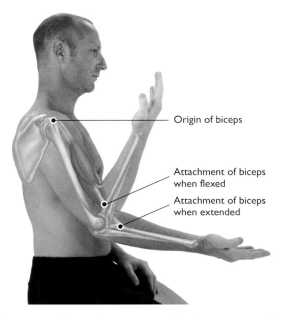

Origin of biceps

Attachment of biceps when flexed

Attachment of biceps when extended

Figure 1.8: *The attachment point of the biceps moves closer as the elbow flexes.*

The first of two types of isotonic contractions is an isotonic concentric contraction. In this instance, the ends of the muscle get closer together during the contraction. Most people are familiar with their biceps muscle, so we'll use this in our example. To keep it simple, the biceps attaches onto the proximal (upper) end of the radius in the forearm and above it attaches to two places in the shoulder. For measuring purposes, let's just say the attachment is the top front of the shoulder. Imagine that you are doing a dumbbell curl with a 20-pound weight. If you start with a straight elbow and begin to flex the elbow with the weight in it, the distance between the forearm bone and the shoulder is reduced. Therefore, the muscle is getting shorter. It is obviously contracting. You can feel it in your arm as it works to curl that 20 pounds.

In the second type of isotonic contraction, the muscle's overall length increases with the contraction. We call this an isotonic eccentric contraction. Using the biceps example again, imagine your arm at the top of the curl position (flexed elbow). Slowly begin to lower the 20-pound weight. If we agreed that the distance was getting shorter upon flexion, then it must be getting longer as the elbow extends or straightens. The distance between the bones and attachment points of the biceps is increasing. Now, because we slowly lowered it down, the biceps muscle was working to lower the weight. Had we just relaxed the muscle, the weight would have plummeted to our side, perhaps falling out of our hand. Many of you might have assumed that the triceps brachii would be responsible for bringing the arm back down and extending it. We will look at that idea in a moment.

It can be difficult for students to imagine a muscle getting longer while it contracts. It seems contradictory. But really we do this all

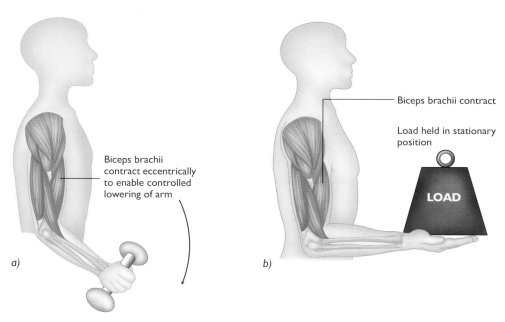

Figure 1.9: *a) eccentric contraction; b) isometric contraction.*

the time. For instance, walking and running require the hamstrings to contract and elongate (isotonic eccentric) to prevent too long of a step. What do you think prevents your leg from flying up in the air as you walk or run? It is the coordinated interplay of concentric and eccentric contractions of opposing muscles that makes fine motor skills possible.

Activities such as typing, playing piano, and guitar are good examples of this coordinated interplay. This is most apparent in our hands and the countless activities we depend on them for. But even larger coordinated movements such as walking, dance, gymnastics, *Surya Namaskara*, and yoga in general depend on the coordinated interplay of concentric and eccentric muscular contractions!

Again, by mentioning the various types of contractions I hope to enhance your understanding of the muscular system. After all, *asanas* are physically static. You don't move very much once you are in a pose. However,

these anatomical movement principles are used in the many transitions between postures.

The transition into *Uttanasana* (standing forward bend) is an example of an eccentric contraction within a yoga pose. *Uttanasana* requires that we lengthen the hamstrings. Now, you could just flop right over and grab your feet or touch the floor, or you could make your way down slowly, in a controlled way, folding at the hip joints. The hamstrings attach distally (at their bottom) just below the knee and proximally (at their top) at the sit bones. When we fold forward the hamstrings must allow the pelvis to rotate around the head of the femur. If we do this with control, the hamstrings will get longer while tension is maintained in the process. This is, by definition, eccentric contraction of the hamstrings.

By the way, the opposite action happens on the way up. The hamstrings bring the pelvis back around the head of the femur. They shorten and contract at the same time, doing a concentric contraction.

Neuromuscular Principles

How the nervous system controls muscles in different situations is fascinating. Not all of these relate directly to yoga, but the principle of opposing muscles is definitely worth mentioning. This neuromuscular principle says that when a muscle meets a resistance that it can't overcome, its opposing muscle will relax. This is used in physical therapy all the time and falls within the category of proprioceptive neuromuscular facilitation (or PNF) techniques. Using PNF, therapists take advantage of neuromuscular principles to get certain muscles to activate or deactivate, depending on the situation.

We can find the principle of opposing muscles anywhere in the body. We'll use our biceps and triceps brachii as an example of how the principle works. Biceps is a flexor and so bends the elbow. It is located on the front (or anterior) surface of the upper arm. Triceps brachii is on the other side of the upper arm, or posterior surface. It does the opposite action, extending or straightening the elbow. Bend your elbow and try to straighten it against resistance; try using the floor or whatever you happen to be sitting near at the moment. Push into the resistance by trying to straighten your elbow. If you touch your biceps with your other hand, it should feel very soft, like it is not engaging at all. If you put your hand on your triceps brachii, you should feel it engage.

Because your triceps brachii is meeting a resistance that it can't overcome, your body recognizes that it doesn't want to add to that resistance. In order to accomplish this task, it shuts off the signals to the biceps sent by the nervous system, in essence, asking it to relax more. Think about it, if the biceps were engaging, this would add to the resistance you were pushing against in trying to straighten the elbow.

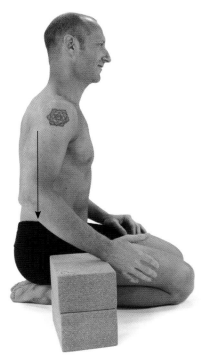

Figure 1.10: *Triceps contracts as it pushes into a point of resistance.*

Let's apply this to yoga. We have already discussed hamstrings and *Uttanasana*. The opposite group of muscles to the hamstrings at the hip and knee are the quadriceps (on the front of the thigh). When I do a forward bend, my quadriceps and other hip flexors try to pull me forward against the resistance of my hamstrings.

When this happens, if the hamstrings were activated or holding a contractile tension, the amount of resistance to the forward bend would increase. Increasing the resistance coaxes the nervous system into telling the hamstrings to relax or to stop engaging! This is the best time to stretch and lengthen tissue—when it is not being asked to contract. In this instance, therefore, we're using the resistance of the knee joint to shut off the hamstrings rather than trying to stretch the hamstrings during an eccentric contraction.

Like a physical therapist, we can consciously take advantage of this principle by actively engaging our quadriceps and other hip flexors while taking a forward bend. By doing so, our nervous system will reduce the stimulation to the hamstrings so that they relax more, allowing for a deeper forward bend. We will actually get deeper into the stretch this way rather than overusing the arms. Notice that I said *overuse*. I'm not saying we shouldn't use them at all. It is more effective, however, to use them only after we have engaged the entire front side of the body to draw us down and forward.

Gravity: The Forgotten Force

We have discussed the potential for muscles to contract and bring either end towards the other. We have also covered different types of contraction. However, we need to consider gravity. In a way, gravity's role in all of this is so obvious that it gets ignored. Think about it. If we lift a limb, it has weight because of gravity. If we release the muscles that we used to lift the limb, the limb falls back to our side. Why? Because of gravity. Simple, right? Yes. But things get complicated when we start considering different movements.

First, let's go back to our *Laghuvajrasana* example (see Figure 1.7). When I start to dip back and take my head towards the floor, I am using an eccentric contraction of the quadriceps to lower me down. My thigh muscles must work to resist gravity. In other words, the distance between the tibia and pelvis is getting longer as the knee bends and I move towards the floor. When I'm in the pose, I am maintaining an isometric contraction of these tissues: my muscles are working to resist the pull of gravity. When I come up, the muscle contracts and the distance between the ends of the muscles is shortened. We call this a concentric contraction. Again, gravity is the force against which the muscles are working.

Our first consideration of *Laghuvajrasana* provided an example of a muscle working in such a way that the commonly agreed upon origin was actually the one that moved relative to the insertion. Now we have layered the ideas of concentric, eccentric, and isometric contractions, plus the force of gravity, on top of that. Let's do the same for another pose to clarify the point.

A simple but effective example (and one that everyone is familiar with by now) is the standing forward bend, *Uttanasana*. When I bend forward to touch my toes, my muscles contract to resist gravity and the weight of my upper body. If these muscles did not contract, I would basically accelerate into the forward bend in a flopping motion because my muscles would not restrict my speed.

The anatomically named movement for the forward bend is flexion at the hip joint. Does this mean that the hip flexors are responsible for folding me forward? No. Gravity and the weight of my upper body are responsible for my forward motion. When I slowly fold, the muscles on the backside of my body, particularly the hamstrings, engage and lengthen against weight and gravity to lower me down with control. So, technically, the hip *extenders* (i.e. the hamstrings) are responsible for controlling my movement into the forward bend (flexion). Once I am in the posture, I can use the hip flexors to take me deeper, but the transition into the pose is actually controlled by what anatomists would consider the opposite muscles. To re-emphasize, this is because of gravity.

On the way back up from the forward bend, these same muscles (the hamstrings) contract and shorten. You might recall that the hamstrings attach from your sit bone (ischial tuberosity) to below your knee onto the tibia. Their main function at the hip joint is to extend it. When they do this in a forward-bending position, they work to stand you back up. This is an example of concentric contraction of the hamstrings. It is a contraction that lifts you against the force of gravity. It is also an example of the commonly considered origin being turned into an insertion.

Again, this action seems opposite to how we would normally learn the action of the hamstrings. Why? Normally we are taught to see the ischial tuberosity as the origin and the area below the knee as the insertion. Thus the femur is the bone that moves, not the pelvis. In the instance of the forward bend, the pelvis has rotated around the head of the femur (at the ball and socket joint). Therefore, when the hamstrings engage, the pelvis is pulled back up and around the head of the femur. As a result, the upper half of the body returns to standing.

This is cool stuff that you won't find in your average anatomy book, because we're working with a dynamic body in motion rather than a static body in anatomical position. You won't see it explained in this manner often, if ever. For those of us who practice yoga, this little concept is critically important. On our mats, we are rarely moving to or from anatomical position. We are sometimes upside down, sideways, or a combination of both, and our position can change which muscles we use to move.

WHEN THINGS GET STUCK

Chances are if you practice yoga, at some point or another you have hurt yourself. Maybe you pushed too far in a stretch. Maybe you woke up with a sore something. Maybe you injured yourself off your mat. No matter the reason, at one time or another we all have to deal with pain, discomfort, or injuries. Let's spend a little time exploring what these injuries are and the healing therapies we can take advantage of.

Although it's useful for us to understand what it is we're stretching and how long we should stretch it, realistically we are most likely to tune in and pay attention to our bodies when something is not functioning correctly. In the same way that the fascia, connective tissues, and muscular contractions allow for and create movement, so they taketh away. When irritated, injured, or just plain tight, these tissues can limit our movement. Because each cell, fascicle, and muscle belly is surrounded in fascia, the fascia itself can limit the ability of the muscle to lengthen or shorten.

It doesn't take an injury to thicken the fascia in a particular area of the body. High levels of use (or even over-use) can cause a restriction in movement or flexibility in that area as well.

RECONSTRUCTION – SCAR TISSUE

Muscles can also tighten or shorten in the healing process. Connective tissue itself is used to help fix and repair damaged tissues. For instance, when a bone breaks, connective tissue is laid down first to span the gap at the break point. Then bone cells are laid down in order to make the bone whole again. The same is true with fascia when we tear a "muscle."

Scar tissue is produced by fibroblasts, the same thing in our body that creates connective tissues. When a muscle is torn, it is connective tissue that needs to be repaired. If you take a piece of myofascia (muscle) past its ability to stretch, you can tear the connective tissue surrounding it. When this happens (and

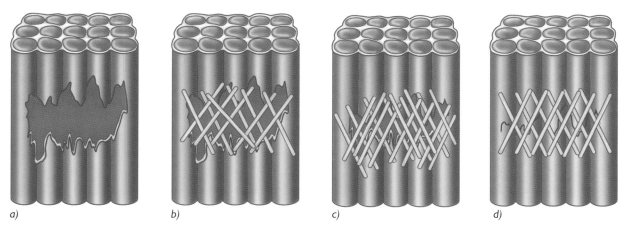

Figure 1.11: *Scar tissue: a) tear in the tissue, b) scar tissue lays down in random fashion, c) too much time and lack of movement cause tension to build around area of repair, d) scar tissue better aligned to the natural tension in the tissue.*

depending on the degree to which it happens), the body responds with inflammation, fluid, and swelling. Sometimes the area will even bruise.

On the connective tissue level, the fibers go in a particular direction, creating a "flow" of the fascia. When there is a tear, the responsive connective tissue (we call this "scar tissue") is laid down over the area that is torn. In order for it to make a strong connection so that the muscle itself can heal, the fibers are laid down in a cross-hatching type of pattern. In other words, the scar tissue goes against the flow of the torn fascia. While this makes for a more secure connection around the tear, it also creates some puckering around the site of injury.

The repaired area now has more tension around it because the surrounding tissues have been pulled toward the repair. This might account for why injuries seem to occur in the same place. Because of the added tension in the area, it becomes more likely that a subsequent injury will occur there.

The medical community has come to recognize this as well. Over the last 30 years, surgeons have slowly changed their approach to rehabilitation after surgery, which often causes huge amounts of trauma to tissue and the need for scar tissue to be laid down. In the past, people would lie in bed for a long time (4 to 6 weeks) after knee surgery. The idea was to let the person heal before putting weight on or rebuilding the tissues around the knee. With this approach, people built up a lot of scar tissue as they rested. Consequently, they would often lose range of motion (ROM) at that joint. Doctors have found that rehabilitating a patient sooner after the surgery creates thicker scar tissue. By "thicker" we mean scar tissue that is organized in the original flow of the connective tissue in that area. This leads to an overall quicker recovery time and better long-term mobility in the joint.

Students often ask me whether it is better to work through an injury or to rest and let it heal. This is a difficult question to answer, as there are countless varieties of injuries and scenarios. However, if someone has torn fascia, as we've described, I generally recommend movement. Obviously, there are injuries that you do not want to move around, like a broken bone, so I do not want to give an oversimplified answer to the question. I'd much rather you understand the individual, the injury, and enough anatomy that you can figure out what is most appropriate.

That being said, it's good to know that moving an area of "torn" tissues will quite often assist in the healing of the tissue. It can also have long-term benefits for strength and mobility. Yoga is a fantastic way to warm and then lengthen the tissues of the body.

THE NERVOUS SYSTEM

The nervous system is an extremely complex component of our physical body. Copious numbers of books have been written about it. My expertise is not in the physiology of the nervous system, but in its function. The nervous system itself brings up questions about mind and body that are integral to our understanding of yoga. Where and how are mind and body connected? Where does one begin and one end?

As we now know, all our parts are integrally connected and were formed from a single cell. In terms of formation, three layers of tissue come to be in a developing embryo—the endoderm, the mesoderm, and the ectoderm. Each of these layers is the beginning of different physical parts of a baby. The endoderm is responsible for creating our internal organs. The mesoderm creates the connective tissues, including bones, fascia, muscles, and all the other components already mentioned. The ectoderm creates the outermost layers of our body, our largest organ, the skin. But, that's not all. The ectoderm also creates our nervous system, intimately linking the outermost to the innermost parts of our body.

The nervous system embodies the connection of mind and body. Nerves reach from deep within the protected layers of the spine and skull to make their way throughout the body, getting into every nook and cranny. The nerves send information to the body and receive information via the brain/mind on all the activity going on in the system. Thus the mind and body are one, plain and simple. And now, enter yoga. What is yoga? Is it whatever we want it to be? Is it what Patanjali has told us it is?

Asana is the most popular way to interface into this great lineage of coming to know oneself. Even stripped down to its physical form, yoga has the power to change people physically, mentally, and emotionally. The reason for this seems to be the nervous system, which is ultimately what yoga is about.

The opening of Patanjali's *Yoga Sutras* states that yoga is the cessation of the fluctuations of the mind. The fluctuations referred to are housed within the nervous system. I sometimes have to argue with my Ashtanga friends that Ashtanga Vinyasa Yoga is a form of Hatha Yoga. Loosely translated, Hatha Yoga is a physical tool to control our wandering minds. It is the antidote to the modern malady we so often hear people complain of: "I just can't sit down, quiet my mind, and just be." Hatha Yoga allows us to use the body to help access and control our minds. How can this happen if not for the nervous system? Movement is a way for us to know ourselves. Practicing *asana* teaches us about ourselves through movement itself. The compression, stretching, and contraction of our tissues awaken the mind-body connection by stimulating the nervous system.

Sensory Receptors

There are different classifications of sensory receptors in the body. Any recent physiology book will outline all of them for you in detail. They are generally classified first by location (superficial, or closer to the skin of the body, or deeper and closer to the organs in the body). But there are also receptors that are specialized. We find these in our muscles, joint capsules, and tendons. Within these categories you will find that movement or change in shape, chemicals, temperature, and intense stimuli (such as pressure or pain) stimulate the receptors.

The type of receptor most pertinent to our discussion of movement and *asana* are called proprioceptors. These are found inside the body and more specifically in the joint capsules, muscles, and tendons. Within our joint capsules, receptors give us information about pressure, movement, and where things are in space. In muscles we have a specialized receptor called a muscle spindle. In tendons, it is called the golgi tendon receptor.

A muscle spindle is specialized tissue in the belly of the muscle that measures the length of a resting muscle. Based on that information, the spindle may cause a "stretch reflex" to occur. Note that this stretch reflex happens unconsciously. This type of receptor is not responsible for creating sensations such as heat, cold, or pain. An example of this is the classic reflex test that doctors give patients. Using a rubber hammer, doctors tap on the tendon below the kneecap with the leg draped over the end of a table. The rapid change in length of the resting muscle stimulates the muscle spindle in the quadriceps (the rectus femoris, particularly) and a stretch reflex is initiated, which causes a muscular contraction.

Golgi tendon organs are located in areas where muscle fibers become tendinous. Their role is the opposite of the muscle spindle. Instead of measuring the change in a muscle's length, they measure the amount of force produced on the tendinous area where they are located. If a muscle over-contracts and nears the limits of causing a tear (yes, tears can happen as a result of contraction, too), the golgi tendon reflex will occur, causing the muscle to relax in order to prevent injury.

All of the various types of sensory receptors feed information into the nervous system. This

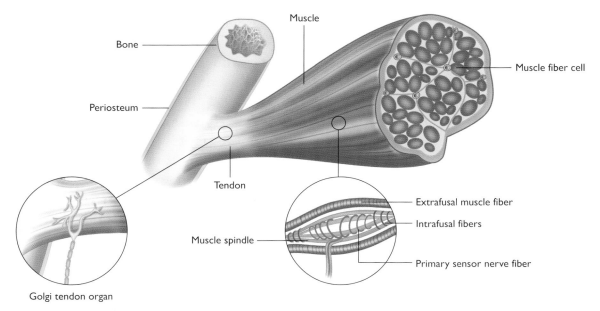

Figure 1.12: *Anatomy of the muscle spindle and Golgi tendon organ.*

information is used in different ways within the body. In all cases, there is a response to this information, for example a muscle contraction or release of certain hormones. Responses can be immediate or they can occur over time.

If we're sensitive enough and not moving too quickly, these proprioceptors may save us from injury while practicing *asana*. It is possible that lengthening tissues as we do in yoga postures can trigger the stretch reflex. If the timing and speed of movement are appropriate, this reflex might already have saved us from injury. The same is true of the golgi tendon organ. In strength-based *asanas*, straining can cause a sudden feeling of weakness. By asking the muscle to relax to avoid tearing, we feel weaker and come out of the pose.

When information is put into the body repeatedly, the nervous system creates certain "automatic" responses. For instance, a good friend of mine, in his younger years, ate a whole jar of sweet pickles. At some point his body got sick of all those sweet pickles being in his stomach and he vomited. Perhaps it was the over-stimulation of certain receptors in his stomach that caused this to happen. What interests me is that, even today, more than 20 years later, if you open a jar of sweet pickles and put it under his nose, he gets nauseous. The fact that his entire system "remembers" that event to such a powerful degree is both fascinating and enlightening. This could be correlated to physical and emotional reactions while in certain postures. It also plays into something we will talk more about, which are patterns of movement that become part of our *asana* practice.

This automatic response also happens on a physical level. Activities we do regularly cause an almost unconscious melding together of the nervous and muscular systems in the body. I call the results of these repeated activities "facilitated pathways." They are nervous system pathways that are repeatedly traversed for a similar action or movement of the body. This term can also be used to describe a feedback loop in musculoskeletal pain patterns. For our purposes, when an action is repeated, neuromuscular conditioning happens. What begins as a very conscious muscular action or perhaps a sequence of muscular events evolves into a more unconscious muscular event.

For example, learning to drive a car begins as a conscious activity. We take into consideration information about speed, direction, and what is happening beside and behind us. We may learn to drive on a manual transmission, which means we also need to coordinate clutch, gas, and shifting with braking. Driving is complicated. How then, is it possible that we can now drive while talking on a mobile phone, eating breakfast, putting on make-up, and maintaining control of the vehicle? The answer is facilitated pathways.

After doing these activities over and over again, the information that comes into the nervous system no longer needs to be processed with such awareness; it doesn't even need to reach the brain for processing. Being relayed to the spinal cord and back is enough.

We have created many facilitated pathways at different times in our lives by doing different activities. We consciously chose some. Others were less consciously developed. Some of these are physical, some are emotional, and some are energetic in nature. Either way, these groupings of facilitated pathways reveal themselves in the way we move; our patterns of movement illustrate our facilitated pathways. They're observable and, whether we like it or not, unconsciously habitual.

As well as being seen in movement, these patterns are even more observable on our mats when we stop moving and take a look at our posture. This is partly what continually brings our right shoulder down or our left shoulder up; it's partially what shifts our left hip higher or lower than the right. These are just a few possibilities. Think back to those converging histories. They all help to create the patterns we live with now, both on the physical and on the more subtle level.

Depending on the type of yoga we practice, we may be supporting our patterns, ingraining them even further. It is also possible to practice in a way that undoes or starts to balance out our patterns or even encourages positive and healing patterns. I wouldn't suggest there is *any* one practice or method that is beneficial to all; but it's important to take note that any practice that you do is in some way imposing another pattern onto your neuromuscular system.

In addition, the way we move into each posture, the technique if you will, creates a new facilitated pathway. Each and every time we do an Up Dog, our body learns to move in a particular way. When we enter other postures that ask our back to be in a similar position, similar muscles will naturally contract. We are creating new neuromuscular patterns each and every time we practice *asana*.

Is it possible to change or get rid of certain patterns? When patients in a hospital are put under anesthesia (the type that requires gas and respirators), the doctors and staff must be very careful when moving them around. Because the nervous system has been shut down to such a degree that there's no tone in the muscles, if the patient is moved too quickly or inappropriately, the bones can be dislocated. The patterns of movement and holding in the body are released. Those of you with tight hips

would have no problem doing a very nice *Eka Pada Sirsasana* (Leg-Behind-the-Head Pose) while under anesthesia (unless bone structure is the cause of your inability).

Just as our patterns disappear when the nervous system shuts down, when it comes back online, so do the tensional patterns. This has some interesting implications relating to our physical practice. For example, how much of the tension that we hold in our body is related to an over-stimulated nervous system? If we can undo nervous system activity on our own, can we remove held tensional patterns in our body? What can we do to continue to reduce this stimulation? The nervous system basically has two ends-the mind and body—that live on a continuum; they are not two separate parts or areas. Nervous system stimulation can happen through the physical body, but it can also happen via the mind. Our mind is directly related to brain function and thus the nervous system. The mind's ability to influence other parts of the body is also somewhere along that continuum.

We can use our mind to direct our body, that's obvious. But what happens to our body when we focus our mind on breathing, for example? This is a common way to begin meditation. We use our mind to focus on one thing. As we do this, the body responds. Our heart rate begins to change. Even the breath, our point of focus, changes.

If we sit long enough, even the perception of our physical form can change; the space that we sense our body occupying changes. Perhaps our limbs feel like they are a great distance away from us, or maybe they feel large, or maybe we don't feel them at all! Through the mind's attention and focus, we can change (or at the very least distort) our perception of the physical body. So what is it that brings us back from these meditative states? The edges of our physical body can blur as we sit in meditation. The moment we move, the boundaries are quickly reconstructed. In this way, movement itself informs our mind about whom and where we are.

In yoga *asana* we use physical movements to focus the mind. This differs from focusing on the body for its own sake. I'm referring to using the physical sensations of movement as a means to focus the mind. This is partly what yoga does to help us still the fluctuations that Patanjali refers to.

When we practice yoga, we explore layers of focus. As we start to layer on elements of movement, such as balancing our effort (contraction) and our release (relaxation), we train the neuromuscular system while enhancing our mind's capacity to focus. We take this further by layering on breath control, coordination, and the *bandhas* in our postures. How much do we learn about our mental patterns from practicing *asana* regularly? Does it not bring up issues of our own determination? Doesn't it reveal our negative or positive thought patterns? Can't it even help us overcome the negative ones? The impact that regular physical practice has on the mind is huge.

Physical *asanas* retrain and work on the peripheral nervous system. It trains the mind/ nervous system to be more focused and controlled. Working both the body and the mind systematically brings the nervous system under control.

The sophistication of the combined nervous and muscular system is astounding. Laying down new patterns in the body can be very challenging. In some cases moving out of old patterns can be challenging. Because our body is patterned to do something else, it can be resistant to change. This often happens when students receive an adjustment or correction from a teacher. Teachers often want us to change where our body is in space, or the way our muscles contract to get us there, or they want to hold us in a posture. Depending on how long we've been doing that pose in a particular way, our mind may object, saying something like "That doesn't feel right!" Or our nervous system and muscles might resist and not allow us to stay in the corrected position. This isn't surprising when we think about it— it's our normal pattern! We might even think our teacher is crazy to want us to move that way, but really we're just uncomfortable doing something outside of our 'norm.'

For beginners, creating certain new patterns is quite difficult. Lack of coordination, strength, or flexibility can be major hurdles. Luckily, the way the nervous system is designed means we don't always have to think about contracting specific muscles to do a particular action. We just need to have the desired goal in mind. Sometimes, however, the unconscious mind and a lack of strength override our intention to do something specific; for instance, lowering into *Chaturanga* with the elbows in.

From their very first Sun Salutation, beginners are confronted by *Chaturanga Dandasana*. Assuming the neophyte can actually lower down, they will almost always let their elbows move outwards or away from their body. No matter how many times I tell them, some of them simply cannot bring their elbows in while lowering into this posture.

As their teacher, I could continue to correct them or simply acknowledge that the triceps brachii are too weak to accomplish this on their own. The nervous system understands the goal, lowering down. In order to accomplish this task when the triceps brachii are too weak, it recruits other muscles to assist. Usually pectoralis major comes to the rescue. By moving the elbows out and away from the body, the pectoralis major is in a better position to help with the required action. Why turn to the "pecs?" They are larger, have more fibers, and with the shoulders abducted (the elbows out) have more leverage to work with.

As the triceps brachii get stronger, the student won't need to recruit the pectoralis muscle to help. Gradually, they will begin to keep the elbows in while they lower down. This is the start of creating a new pattern and breaking an old one. There are two ways of helping the triceps brachii in this scenario. One is to allow the elbows to stay away from the body. If you do so, then move your hands slightly wider as well. You can also invite the student to place their knees on the floor while lowering down, which will enable them to keep their elbows in.

Ultimately, our work as yoga teachers is to help create a pattern that serves the student and their progression through the posture. The progression through the posture then relates to a progressive understanding of the student's own body. This is the beginning of the interface of body and mind, as well as of physical *asana* and the larger idea of yoga.

Keep in mind that, if you are a teacher, you will relate to your student through your own nervous system. All of your observations of your students happen through your own nervous system. You deliver all of the corrections that retrain their patterns through your nervous system.

When teaching a group of students, it is natural (and necessary) to make observations about them—even simple things such as whether they are on time, whether they quietly lay down their mat or lay it down with noise. We are already using our senses of sight and hearing to get an idea of who these students are and how we will work with them. All of this is filtered through our own nervous system patterns and can be triggers of mental patterns that we hold about these things. If we are aware of this, then we might work with the different students differently. We might approach them differently or ask different things of them.

We will also observe their individual physicality. I often find myself paying attention to people as they move and walk around or into the space. Even more telling are the "preparations" that people make when they first sit on their mat before class has started. Are they rubbing their knees, their back, or their hips? Are they stretching certain areas of their body before they begin? All of these filter through my own nervous system, as I'm sure they do yours.

Then there are the observations we make while students actually perform the *asanas*. What patterns of tension or strength show up and, more importantly, are repeated throughout related *asanas?* These are telling clues about the patterns we want to work with on an individual basis.

At some point we decide to share what we have observed about our students in the form of adjustments or corrections. Now we must engage them through their own nervous system. If we use words, demonstrations, modifications, or actually put our hands on them, all of these ways of delivering information will be processed through the student's nervous system.

THE SKELETAL SYSTEM

The skeletal system is often understood by the layperson as some type of hard, dead, sort of "thing" that is nothing but the framework of our body. In fact, it is a complex, ever-changing system that deals with and reacts to stresses placed on it both anatomically and physiologically. Bones are alive. They have a blood supply. They have nerves running in and out of them. If they get bruised or hit hard, you feel it. If they break, you definitely feel it. The bone itself is constantly going through changes on a cellular level, as cells are created, broken down, and rearranged based on the stresses they have to manage.

Bone is yet another varied formation of connective tissue in the body. There is a thick layer of connective tissue surrounding the outer surface of bone called the periosteum. Inside the bone is the medullary cavity, which contains bone marrow. Along the inside of this cavity is another layer of connective tissue called the endosteum. Sandwiched between these layers of connective tissue are the crystallized minerals that make our bones hard. Primarily, these minerals are calcium and phosphorus. Within them are hollow areas that allow for nerves and blood supply to move through the bones.

The skeletal system has five basic functions: provides structure, produces red blood cells, stores minerals, offers protection, and enables movement. The skeleton is the internal framework of the body. It is relatively light for the amount of strength it provides; our bones are not particularly easy to break if they're healthy. Bones also provide attachment places for muscles and other tissues. The boney prominences you find throughout the body are created both by the genetic coding of the bones themselves, as well as by the tension placed on them by the muscles.

Have you ever wondered where your red blood cells come from? The technical name for the production of red blood cells is hematopoiesis. In adult life, most red blood cells are produced in the flat bones of the body, namely the pelvis and sternum. This function reveals how very alive and dynamic our bones are.

Protection is a simple yet vital function of bones. Our skull protects our brain with a hardened shell. Our rib cage protects the heart and lungs. Even our vertebrae have a ring of bone that is created to protect our spinal cord as it runs down the torso. Not only do the bones store minerals for the purpose of creating the bone itself, they also store minerals for use in the rest of the body when needed. The function of storing and releasing minerals is evidence of the constant change occurring in our bones.

Movement happens where two bones come together. We call this coming together a joint, or more technically, an articulation. And although we can make this general assumption about movement, there is a classification of joints (synarthrosis) that is considered to be immoveable. Some movement might be possible at this type of joint, but forces other than muscles must create it. For example, the bones that make up the skull are held together by a dense, ligamentous connection. We call these articulations sutures of the skull. These joints are considered immoveable, but it's possible that they can move relative to one another when impacted or by the subtle work of craniosacral therapists.

There are three types of bone cells: bone-building cells called osteoblasts, mature bone cells called osteocytes, and the cells that break down mature bone cells called osteoclasts. As bones are built, minerals are crystallized and built into the structure of the bone. If calcium or phosphorus is needed in the blood supply, then osteocytes may be broken down by osteoclasts to release these minerals into the blood supply.

A similar mechanism allows bones to recreate their structure based on the stresses placed on them. Stress placed on bones can actually cause them to change shape. I'm not suggesting that you can get a femur to end up with a 90-degree bend in the middle of it, but a bone under prolonged stress will react by shifting its shape. This affects how force runs through the bone.

At the ends of long bones especially (for example, the top of the femur), there is the amazing trabecula of the bones. This part of the bone transmits the force of the weight of the upper body from the pelvis into the shaft of the femur. The matrix of bones here is almost constantly adjusting based on how the bone cells are breaking down and rebuilding. It does this to manage and adapt to the changes in stress that have to pass through this area. Bones change. Some changes in bones are not always welcomed or positive changes. For instance, when a heel spur develops, it is often painful. Through tension or overuse, the outermost layer of connective tissue on the heel bone is pulled away and inflamed. The area becomes inflamed and tender. The development of bone spurs in different areas of the body is, in some way, indicative of the bones' ability to adapt and change. On a positive note, this ability to change also helps maintain or rebuild strength in the bones of people with osteoporosis.

So, the skeletal system reacts to stresses and stimuli placed on it. This stress is not a negative thing. It is just something outside of or greater than the norm. Bones change in size, mostly thickness, and density based on stimulus. For example, say I jumped up and down on one foot for a week without stopping. Not only would I be extremely tired, but the bones in that leg would have become denser and, in a sense, stronger, as a result of all that jumping. Just as miraculous is that if I never jumped up and down on that leg again, the density of the bones in that leg would return to roughly what it was before I started jumping.

On a cellular level, when I begin jumping, osteoblasts swing into action to create more osteocytes (bone cells) to help handle the stress being placed on the bones. If the stimulus is removed (if I stop jumping), the body will recognize that there are more bone cells than are required for normal daily activity. The body responds by having osteoclasts remove some of the osteocytes.

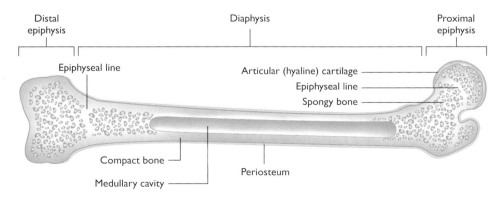

Figure 1.13: *Components of a long bone.*

Any repetitive action has an effect on the skeletal system, as well as other systems of the body. Conditions like osteoporosis, a breaking down of bone cells and therefore the density of the bone itself, can be improved by adding weight-bearing exercise to your days. This exercise stimulates osteoclasts into action to prevent further loss of bone cells and therefore density. Bones also have a blood and nervous supply that is part of all of this physiological function. In short, they are not dead and dry frameworks but rather living tissues in the body that react to stimuli.

MUSCLE STRETCHING AND LENGTHENING ... WHAT MAKES SENSE TO ME

We've covered a lot of ground within the muscular system. We have talked about muscle names, types of muscular contractions, how the nervous system integrates with the muscular system to create movement, and even how gravity impacts the muscles as they move our bodies. Further, because this is a yoga anatomy book, we have explored how anatomy in a moving body can be different than in a body that simply shifts in and out of anatomical position.

Our exploration of the muscular system would not be complete unless we addressed what happens when we stretch and lengthen our muscles by moving on the mat. There are many opinions about how one should stretch the tissues of the body. Which is the best way and why is highly debated. I let my anatomy knowledge, logic, and personal experience of stretching tissues in my own body guide me.

In yoga, we have simplified our understanding into words like stretching and lengthening.

This is not a bad way of describing what we are talking about. However, what does it literally mean?

What we are literally describing is increasing our range of motion (ROM). In our most simplistic way of thinking about this, we assume that ROM is based on muscle length, and therefore we "stretch" to increase it. In reality, we are talking about a complex combination of nervous system stimulation, connective tissue tension, and joint structures merging to create what we call our ROM. Therefore, we are re-training this complex combination how to be at a new ROM, not simply lengthening or stretching just the muscle.

From my experience, the best time to lengthen the tissues of the body is when they are relaxed. By relaxed, I mean when they're not being told by the nervous system to contract. In other words, you wouldn't actively try to engage and stretch a muscle at the same time. It just doesn't feel right. Of course, there is always a certain amount of tension in the myofascia. This is what we have already referred to as muscle tone.

Muscle tension changes as a result of two things: either the muscle is being stretched or it is receiving signals from the nervous system to contract. The second scenario is relatively obvious; most people haven't considered the first.

Tissues have elasticity in them, sort of like a rubber band. If you stretch a rubber band, the tension increases. If you flip your finger over a rubber band that was just mildly stretched out, the sound that you would hear would be more or less a low pitch. If you stretch the rubber band out further and flip your finger over it again, the pitch would get higher, showing the increase in tension.

The same thing happens with our myofascia when we lengthen it. As we fold into a seated forward bend, our hamstrings get longer, hence the tension in them increases. You might call it passive tension as opposed to the active tension created when you contract a muscle and change its tone. The passive tension in this scenario is unavoidable as you lengthen your tissues.

A common topic of conversation exists around the length of time one should hold a stretch for. Well, how long? I often ask this question in workshops just to hear the myriad of answers that are floated around. People usually respond with answers ranging from 5 to 60 seconds. Of course, the average length of time people think you should hold a stretch ends up being around 30 seconds.

If you do a Google search on how long to hold a stretch, you will see an even wider range of answers. Some even suggest holding stretches for 15 minutes or longer! Most seem to agree that approximately 30 seconds is the right amount of time—about 5 deep inhalations and exhalations.

Personally, I think this is oversimplified. We have already mentioned that there are four basic components that allow and restrict movement—connective tissue, muscle (we now know to lump the two together and call them myofascial tissue), the nervous system, and the skeletal system. On top of that, there is the amount to which you push yourself in a stretch. If you do not go into a stretch far enough, no change will happen. If you go too far, the reaction from the body can be the opposite of your intention. That is, your muscles may get tighter (or even injured) in response to being over-stretched.

In addition to the length of time a stretch is held and the number of repetitions we do,

other factors need to be considered. How warm your body is at the time of the stretch will impact its effectiveness. How often you stretch is a determining factor. Do you practice once a week, three days a week, or seven days a week? And we can't forget those converging histories and good old genetics. The bottom line? It's complicated. Ultimately you will find a frequency and depth that work for you.

TYING IT ALL TOGETHER

Before we move on to take a closer look at each of our body parts, I'd like to offer a tool for understanding the integrity of the whole. If we look at the potential for movement, posture, and integration of fascia and muscle, we should consider a principle developed by Kenneth Snelson and popularized by Buckminster Fuller in the 1940s and 1950s called "Tensegrity." The word *tensegrity* is made up of two words, *tension* and *integrity*. This concept posits that tension in a structure can maintain the integrity of the structure.

Let's use a suspension bridge as an example, maybe the Golden Gate Bridge in San Francisco. Imagine the long thick cables draping down from the large towers. Those towers are certainly important, but how long would it take for the road to collapse if we removed all of the cables? Not long at all. The tension provided by the cables is essential to maintaining the integrity of the larger structure. There are two components in this principle. First are the tensional members (the cables), which bind or hold the whole together. Second is the more rigid compression member (the towers and the road). In the tensegrity model, the wooden sticks are the compression members and the elastic bands are the tensional members. You will notice that the sticks aren't touching one another. The tension of the elastic bands keeps them in place.

If you change the tension in any of the bands, the tension around the entire model will change. This isn't the only effect. The change in tension would also make the compression members move in space. We could turn it around and move the compression members so that the tension all around the model would change. Thus the tensional and compression members are intimately connected. If one changes in any way, the entire structure must compensate for that change.

Let's make the leap from this model to our own body. We have both compression and tensional members in our body. Compression members are the bones and the tensional members are the connective tissues. In essence, our bones are suspended in connective tissue tension. When we practice *asana*, we change the dynamics between the tensional and compression members in our body. When our fascia gets stuck, in whatever way and to whatever degree, the entire body is affected. Potentially, the areas closest to the "stuck" spot will have to compensate more. The effects would decrease the further the areas were located from the source of the sticking. In addition, the compression members will adjust and move to compensate for the "stuck" area. If the restrictions in the tissue are released, the skeleton returns to its natural alignment.

Tensegrity begins to give us an idea of how the structures of our body interrelate. When we see postural patterns or distortions, it is the tensegrity of the body that has allowed the adaptation to occur while still maintaining the integrity of the structure.

Taking It Further

Each system of the body lives in and creates its own world. For instance, we listed the five functions of the skeletal system, which define the boundaries of the skeletal system's "world." This same simple analogy can be applied to the circulatory system or the muscular system, and even the nervous system. Each of the systems has their own set of activities and functions that they are responsible for. But this isn't the whole truth. Each of these worlds that they create lives in the universe of the body, so they must all co-exist harmoniously—not for world peace, but for the survival of the universe. What would happen if we removed any one of these systems from the universe of our body? Where would muscles attach if we removed the skeleton? How would muscles contract if we

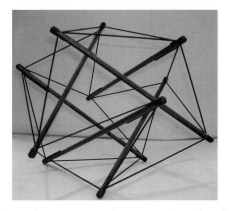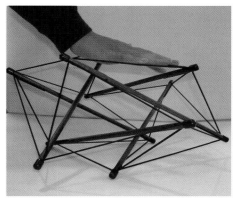

Figure 1.14: *Tensegrity structures, when stressed, tend to distribute rather than concentrate strain. The body does the same, with the result that local injuries soon become global strain patterns.*

didn't have a nervous system? How would we move if we didn't have a muscular system? You get the point. In this same way, we more deeply understand the importance of the skeletal system's function in movement, where it almost always plays second fiddle to the muscular system. In terms of generating movement, one doesn't do anything without the other.

FUNCTIONAL JOINTS

Let's use the same analogy of worlds and universes relative to systems in relation to the joints of the body. This will encourage an image that represents the path of interconnectedness over separation.

Each joint is a world of its own, with its own problems, specific functions, and structures that make it unique, relative to other joints. Each can be classified in one of six categories according to their function, shape, or both. Each joint is in its own world, but at the same time, it lives in a galaxy of joints that exist within the universe of the body.

Remember that the body has formed. The joint has also formed. It has formed in a particular shape, based on genetic coding as well as on stresses, stimuli, and input from other systems and factors of development. Structurally, the joint forms with cartilage in the right places. It also forms with the membranes (synovial membranes) that create the lubricant for the cartilage within the joint. Because that fluid must be contained, a sleeve that surrounds the ends of the two bones that have joined forms to keep the lubricant inside. The sleeve is flexible enough to allow the joint to move and function as it needs. The lubricant is squished around the cartilage through the movement of the joint itself. What brings movement to the joint? What stabilizes the joint? Well, as the joint is forming, the thick straps needed to secure those two bones together are forming as well. The sleeve is strong enough for some functions, but not all. Thicker straps of tissue form to allow for or restrict movement in different directions.

Something has to move the joint as well, otherwise the lubricant inside won't get moved around and the health of the joint will be compromised. So, longer straps are formed that anchor near the joint and influence that joint's movement. Some of these longer straps anchor themselves near two or more joints. The straps then connect the joints to one another; the function of one has an effect on the other. The straps sometimes act more like cables, not only with tension but also with information. The joint then gets used, based on its shape and the resultant function-like pulleys and levers being manipulated by the long cables and straps that surround and connect to it. In this way, function and movement are linked through a chain of joints. Tension created at one joint affects the function of that joint, which then impacts the joints closest to it. Although these joints do function individually, they also rely on and influence the other "worlds" that are part of their galaxy. It would be limiting to talk about the knee without considering the foot, ankle, and hip joints as well.

2
THE FOOT AND ANKLE

Consider for a moment that an entire branch of medicine has been created around the foot. This alone shows the demands placed on this structure. Not only does it sustain a large amount of our body weight, it also handles multiple, sometimes conflicting, functions. To these ends, the foot has a total of 26 bones and 32 joints. In total, the entire lower limb has 30 bones and 37 joints. There's a lot going on in the foot! Why are there so many bones and joints in such a small area?

The foot has to be stable, of course, as stability is at the heart of what the foot represents. It is our foundation, the platform upon which we walk

around. When standing, 100 percent of our body weight passes through the feet. It's not as if there is only one weight-bearing position. In fact, there are many—especially for those of us doing yoga. Think of the number of standing postures that place our feet at various angles, and then we ask them to hold our body weight. Sometimes we hold our weight on just one foot! This foundation, however sturdy, also has mobility built into it. The foot has to adapt to the changes and movements of the joints that are above it. Even as it functions in weight-bearing, the foot adapts and changes to absorb the weight. This is where those 26 bones and 32 joints come into play, giving the foot its adaptability.

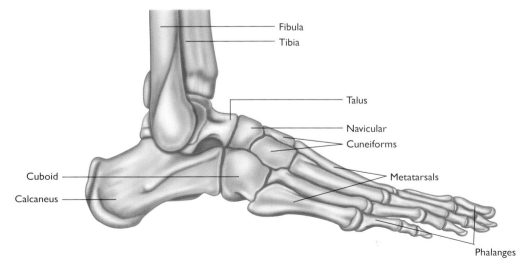

Figure 2.1: *Lateral view (from the outer side) of the foot and ankle.*

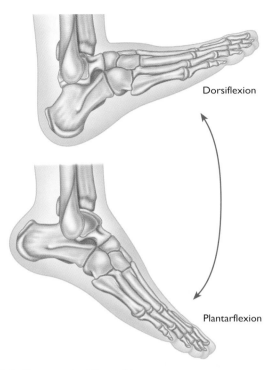

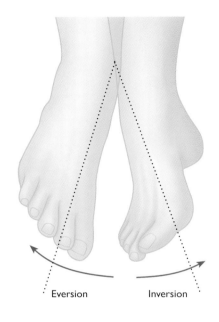

Figure 2.2: *Movements of the ankle.*

The foot is adaptable in two primary ways. First, it absorbs and distributes the body's weight. It literally changes shape to varying degrees depending on what we are doing. Second, it adapts to changes in the terrain beneath it; for example, when walking or running on uneven surfaces. The foot's mobility and adaptability is present in our yoga practice. Consider the numerous standing and sitting poses where one or both feet are compressed, twisted, or otherwise forced to adapt. None of this would be possible without the ankle joint that sits above the foot. The ankle is created by a bone that is part of the foot called the talus. The tibia (shin bone) sits right on top of it, with the smaller fibula off to the outside (lateral). The two bones create what is called a mortise, which basically looks like a monkey wrench.[2] The shape is important because it limits how much side-to-side movement occurs at this joint. This side-to-side motion is called inversion and eversion. The shape of the ankle joint allows for plenty of forward and backward movement, which we refer to as flexion (technically dorsiflexion) and extension (technically plantarflexion). These two movements are critical in walking.

By virtue of its position and what we ask it to do, especially in standing postures, the foot represents our connection to the ground, to the earth. As it keeps us rooted, we discover that it is not simply the foundation upon which the rest of the body is supported when doing standing postures. It must adapt and respond to our shifting body weight while we're holding these poses, too.

FOOT AND POSTURE

If we stand naturally, feet slightly apart, the forces of gravity pass through us in a straight line, whether we're straight or not. This magical line runs somewhere from the center of the earth out into infinity. If our bodies are in relatively good alignment, then that line flows through the body with few adjustments and compensations required by the tensional structures (tensegrity!).

The further our body moves away from this "perfect" alignment, however, the more the tissues of the body will have to respond to maintain an upright position in relation to gravity. Over long periods of time, the stresses and strains of misaligned bones and tissues can lead to chronic pain. Consider all of those "convergent histories" that have led us to where we are at the moment. Consider their role in our natural posture. Now consider the tensions that have to support our posture. This natural posture or basic alignment begins at the feet, since they are the structures that meet the earth. Everything else is, of course, stacked above the feet, and the line of gravity passes through it all.

To see how our body adjusts to the line of gravity and how our feet do not, consider the following: let's say we stand on an incline, readying ourselves to walk up a steep hill. As we stand facing the hill and its upward slope, our feet will stay flat on the ground and our body will shift position. Our feet would be parallel to the slope, while our body could not possibly stay perpendicular to the ground. Our body has adapted to that gravitational line.

For this adjustment to happen, some muscles will have to shorten (decrease the distance between the ends) while others will have to lengthen (increase the distance between the ends) in order for the bones to move around and maintain posture and balance. In this example, the main adaptation is around the ankle joint. Put simply, the calf muscles lengthen and the muscles at the front of the foreleg on the shin shorten.

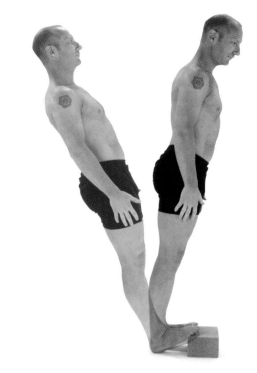

Figure 2.3: *The body adapts to the gravitational line.*

The feet are similar to the foundation of a house. The foundation of a house must be even, so that it basically aligns with gravity. If, however, the foundation settles in an uneven manner, the house itself will exhibit problems. If one side of the foundation settles a few inches more than the other, for example, stresses will be created in the structure. Instead of forces running through the center of the beams, straight down into the foundation, they may be running at slight angles. Doors and windows might not open and close properly as a result. These same principles exist in our body. What would happen if one of our arches fell? How would that impact the rest of the body? Just as the moveable parts of a house (the doors and windows) would be affected, so too would the moveable parts of our own "house" (the joints) incur change. If, for whatever reason, our right arch collapsed, there would be less support, the knee would fall in, and the hip joint on that side might actually tilt down and forward as a result. This, in turn, compresses the low back on that side, which could also set the sacrum off at an angle and become part of a scoliosis. The compensations for a fallen arch could go on and on.

EVOLUTION OF THE FOOT

To get some perspective on the foot, we'll go back in time to look at some evolutionary changes. We humans have made our way from walking on four legs to two. Chimpanzees are our closest relatives from the perspective of DNA coding. If we look at these primates, they come off of their front knuckles sometimes and use their legs and feet for bipedal walking. The difficulty of long-term bipedal walking for chimps is apparent when you observe their side-to-side sort of waddle. This reveals that the chimpanzee's pelvis and tissues surrounding it are not designed in an optimal position for walking this way.[3]

The human foot underwent three basic changes as we developed into an upright position. First, we lost the semi-opposable digit on our feet. Primates have the ability to grasp and hold onto different objects (often branches) with their back feet. In our feet, the semi-opposable digit has disappeared (at least in most of us). This has brought our big toe closer to the second toe and shifted the way our weight travels through our feet.

Second, the center or axis of the foot now runs directly through the second toe. Most people have a second toe that is slightly longer than the big toe (at least those who are more evolutionarily advanced. Ha! Notice my toe in the picture). This change has everything to do with how weight transfers through the foot during walking and how supination and pronation have developed with regards to our gait.

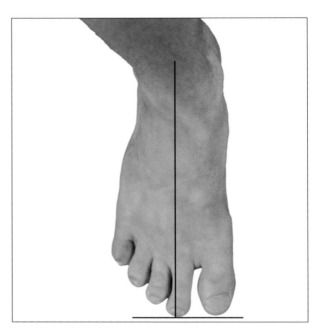

Figure 2.4: *Most people have a second toe slightly longer than the big toe.*

However, no change is more significant to the foot than the development of the arches. As a result of moving to an upright bipedal position, the feet adapted to handle the weight and stress of walking on these two relatively small areas all the time. The arches are perhaps the most significant part of the design that allows us to walk so quickly and adeptly. And we can do so for long periods of time. Primates, however, can only go so long on their own two feet. After a short time they have to put those knuckles back on the ground.[4]

ARCHES OF THE FOOT

Most people are familiar with the arch you see on the medial or inside of the foot, called the medial longitudinal (ML) arch or simply the medial arch. However, there are actually three arches of the foot. There is a second arch on the lateral or outside of the foot, called the lateral longitudinal arch (LL) and a third, called the transverse arch (TA), which runs across the distal end of the five metatarsals (base of the toes).

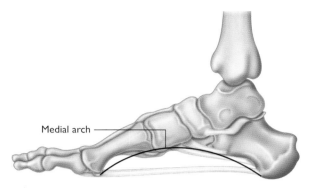

Figure 2.5: *The medial arch of the foot.*

Although the second and third arches mentioned are not as obvious or critical as the medial arch, together they create an important synergistic quality to the foot and its ability to support us where we connect to the earth. Let's look at them more closely to understand what maintains their shape and health.

If we were to play connect the dots to create these arches, we would look at three points: one at the heel (calcaneus), a second at the base of the big toe (the distal end or head of the first metatarsal), and a third at the base of the little toe (the distal end or head of the fifth metatarsal). This triangle outlines the three arches—medial, lateral, and transverse.

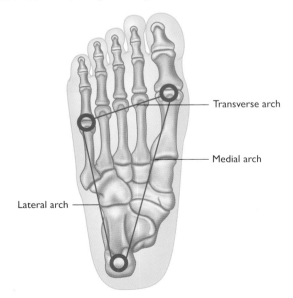

Figure 2.6: *Outline of the three arches of the foot.*

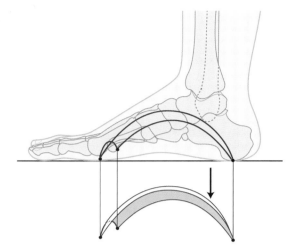

Figure 2.7: *The arch-like structure of the foot is three-dimensional.*

The arches do not function individually, nor are they static in the lines that we use to outline them. The medial and lateral arches are connected to one another as they both span the length of the foot together as a series of parallel arches. In other words, they form a continuous arch across the foot. In this same way, the transverse arch is actually a series of parallel arches running from the back of the foot across to the front (see Figure 2.7). This is a pretty sophisticated structure, and we shouldn't be surprised. For thousands of years, arches have been a very strong and powerful way of building structures. Envision the aqueducts in Segovia, Spain. This series of arches transported water through the city at the end of the first century. This aqueduct spans more than 3000 feet and is a living testament to the strength of arches.

In addition to the arches, there is another powerful and simple architectural shape found in the foot: a spot on the very top of the talus where the tibia meets the foot. Weight also passes through here, from the tibia through the talus and into the foot. So we now have an element of three-dimensionality with a three-sided pyramid.

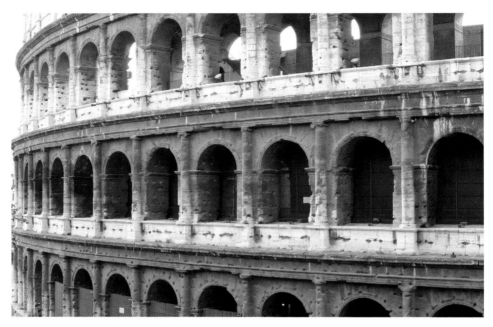

Figure 2.8: *Here is a testament to the strength of arches in the form of the Coliseum in Rome.*

When I think of a pyramid, I think of Egyptian pyramids, which have been standing since 3200 BC. I can't say I've ever heard of one of those four-sided pyramids falling over. So can we turn our foot into a similar shape? Of course we can. Just make the heel two points instead of one. Maybe you've heard a yoga teacher refer to the inner and outer heel? I don't want to stretch too far from what exists anatomically, but it's not difficult to imagine a four-sided pyramid. The point is, the strength and resiliency we find in pyramids also exists in the foot. Of course, our foot is much more dynamic, since it has to change shape as we use it. Practically all of our weight passes through either foot while walking, and if we're running, the equivalent of over three times our body weight may be passing through just one of our feet!

Every time you take a step or place your weight onto your foot, it spreads in three directions across the three basic lines we have discussed. It gets longer through the medial and lateral arch and wider across the transverse arch. As weight comes down through the tibia and into

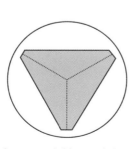

Figure 2.9: *The foot is arch-like, and the way it distributes weight is pyramid-like.*

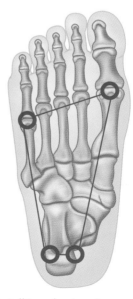

Figure 2.10: *By talking about an inner and outer heel, we now have a four-sided pyramid.*

the foot, about half the weight goes into the heel and the other half into the forefoot. The mobility and adaptability of the foot's 26 bones and 32 joints allow it to change shape and adapt to the surface beneath it.

Energetic Qualities of the Arches

Trees root into the earth, which is what our feet do in standing postures. They create a stable base or foundation for what has to happen above. The ideas of *mula bandha*, or root energy, and its opposing *uddiyana*, or upward flying energy, have been important concepts in my own yoga practice. The foot is a simple, microcosmic place to observe these two concepts.

If you look at a footprint, the dark area, the print itself, is where the foot touched the ground. It is the area that roots into the earth and has a downward *mula* quality to it. The arch, however, does not touch the ground. It is lifted upwards and has an *uddiyana* energy or quality to it. If the arch has fallen in a particular pose, we could say that the quality of the overall pose will suffer, because everything above the feet will also be affected. The balance of the foot and its arches provide clues into what's going on above it. After all, a pose is built upon its foundation, too, just as we are. Don't standing poses rely heavily on the feet? What quality is being exhibited in the feet, then? Is there a balance of down and up, *mula* and *uddiyana*?

If the foot has too much *mula bandha* quality (no arch) then there is an overpowering sinking feeling or look to the pose. When there is a balance between the *mula bandha* and the *uddiyana* of the foot, the pose can be balanced between sinking and lifting, suspended between these two energies. And not only does the energetic quality shift, but the physical body will also change with or without arches. The same problems that we mentioned earlier with issues in the feet will be seen in the poses. The lack of arches in a pose can mean that the tibia rotates, the knee faces inwards, and the hip joint changes, which could put the entire pelvis off.

An important component of standing poses is where we place our feet relative to one another. How far apart they are and how they align with one another effects the structure and thus the posture that lives above it.

Three Components

Three components create and maintain the arches in the foot. The bones, connective tissues, and musculature are responsible for the dynamic resiliency and the adaptability we find with each step. When there are problems in the foot, one must look to these components and their balance (or lack thereof) for remedy.

Bone

The bones are "genetically" designed so their natural shape creates the arches. The 26 bones fit together like a puzzle of interlocking pieces that play off one another through movement. There are times where this genetic code is not "perfect" and the resulting bone shape is created in a less than optimal way; in other words, people may be born without the genetic code for arches in their feet. There are often medical solutions provided for these people, from simple arches in shoes, to braces on the legs, or sometimes surgery.

That being said, the shape of the bones in the foot allows for or restricts movement in particular directions. The complex movements of supination and pronation are created through the interactions of several joints. Thus it is the bones *first* that create the structure or shape of the arches. The "interlocking" of these joints accounts for the strength we find in the back foot when we step forward while walking. This is sometimes called the toe-off position. During this part of walking, the foot is supinated. All of our weight is no longer just on our foot, but on our toes, or what we might call the ball of the foot. Without the bone shape and design, this strength would not exist to propel our bodies forward.

Connective Tissue – Component

The second component creating the arches of the feet is connective tissue. There are numerous small bands of ligaments that tie these 26 bones together. Both the top and bottom of the foot have small bands that create small straps knitting the bones (and therefore the joints) together. These ligaments create the resiliency, flexibility, and dynamic tension that allow for the spreading and adaptability of the foot. They are also part of the structure that makes the bones return to their "neutral" position. This is an excellent example of tensegrity in the body.

These small ligaments holding the 26 bones together are also a potential cause of having flat feet. If one has a genetic disposition to loose connective tissue, often termed hypermobility, these little straps aren't as tight as they should be. If the ligamentous bands are more flexible, than the bones more easily succumb to weight-bearing and we end up with flat feet.

The bottom (plantar surface) of the foot has some very important pieces of connective tissue. This makes sense, since this is the surface we're actually walking on. The force of our weight going through the longitudinal arches lengthens the foot with every step. These tissues add additional tension under the foot to resist the amount of spreading that happens between the heel and the base of the toes. These tissues and their tension, act like the string on a bow and arrow (the bow is the arch of the foot) and help maintain the distance between the ends of the foot. They also lift the arch by pulling the ends closer together. Heel spurs and plantar fasciitis are related to these tissues.

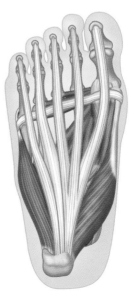

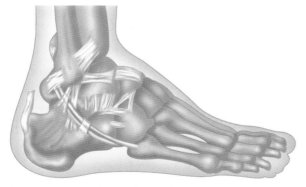

Figure 2.11: *Note the small strap like ligaments that hold the bones together and help maintain the shape of the foot.*

Figure 2.12: *The plantar fascia thickened connective tissue that crosses the ball of the foot.*

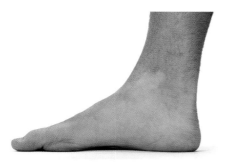 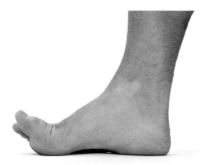

Figure 2.13: *Notice how lifting the toes changes the tension in the bottom of the foot and increases the arch.*

One of the simplest ways we engage our arches in yoga is to lift our toes. This action directly relates to the plantar fascia, which attaches from the heel, past the ball of the foot (metatarsophalangeal joint), and on to the ends of the toes (phalanges). With this arrangement, whenever the toes lift up (hyperextend), the tension in the plantar fascia is increased and the arches of the foot lift. As a result, the heel and the ball of the foot move closer to one another. You can see this quite easily on your own foot.

Muscles – The Third Component

Let's look at an overview of some of the muscles responsible for moving the foot and ankle, stabilizing it, and contributing to the arches. Please keep in mind that, although I'll refer to a particular muscle, we're really talking about a myofascial unit. The muscle is simply sophisticated connective tissue that has the ability to contract and relax. It's important to remember the muscles' ability to maintain a certain amount of tension. Maintaining tension is related to stabilizing various parts and pieces, not only in the foot but in all places in our bodies.

The foot is controlled by muscles that originate either from bones within the foot itself or from the foreleg, namely the tibia and fibula. We're not going to look at every muscle around this area, there are plenty of kinesiology books that already

do that. Let's just look at some of the larger main muscles that move the ankle and foot.

Within the foreleg there are three compartments: posterior, anterior, and lateral. The posterior compartment has a deep and a superficial layer. The design of this area of the body (along with the forearm and hand) is such that the bulk of the muscle is placed above (proximal to) the part that it moves. Think of how difficult it would be to move your foot around if you had large bulky muscles surrounding the joints. Instead, we have thin tendons that cross those joints to give it a larger range of motion.

The ankle does four movements: extension (plantarflexion), flexion (dorsiflexion), inversion (sometimes referred to as supination), and eversion (referred to as pronation). Remember that muscles pull on bones to move them, so pause for a moment to consider where on the foot you would pull to make it do those actions. Basically, the anterior compartment has attachments that go to the top of the foot and thus are primarily responsible for lifting the foot up (dorsiflexion). The posterior compartment has muscles that attach to the heel or just past the heel to the underside of the foot. They pull on the foot by lifting the heel or by pulling the foot down in extension (plantarflexion). The lateral compartment attaches from the outside of the fibula to the same side and under the foot to pull the foot

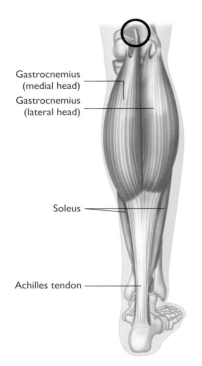

Gastrocnemius
(medial head)

Gastrocnemius
(lateral head)

Soleus

Achilles tendon

Figure 2.14: *Note that the gastrocnemius crosses the knee joint and attaches to the femur.*

into eversion. Supination or inversion is created by some of the muscles in both the anterior and posterior compartments attaching on the inside (medial) aspect of the foot.

Posterior Compartment

The strongest of these compartments is the posterior. Here we find two very powerful muscles—the gastrocnemius and the soleus (deep to the gastrocnemius). These two muscles attach to the heel bone (calcaneus) by way of the Achilles tendon. Most people are familiar with this thick and dense piece of connective tissue in the form of a tendon just above their heel. When these two muscles contract, they pull the heel up and the foot plantarflexes. Notice that when the foot is on the floor, the toes become a fulcrum around which the entire

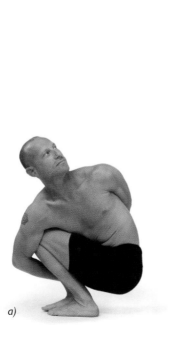

a)

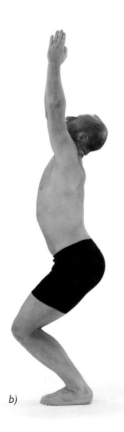

b)

Figure 2.15: *a) Pasasana, b) Utkatasana.*

weight of the body is lifted. The combination of actions at the ankle and toes is critical for walking and explains the power and size of the posterior compartment, which can easily lift twice our body weight.

There is, however, one key difference between the two muscles in the posterior compartment of the foot and that is the joints they cross and/or do not cross. Gasctrocnemius crosses both the knee joint and the ankle joint. This means that if the knee is flexed (a movement this muscle can contribute to), the gastrocnemius has less power to contract and extend the foot. The lengthening or stretching of these muscles is affected by the position of the knee. When the knee is straight, flexion (dorsiflexion) of the foot is restricted by both these muscles. When the knee is bent, dorsiflexion is only restricted by the soleus muscle and the general tension of the Achilles tendon.

When looking at a yoga pose like *Pasasana* or *Utkatasana*, you will see that the ankles are in a dorsiflexed position. This requires two things to happen: the posterior compartment needs to be long enough for the heels to be on the ground, and the muscles that create flexion (dorsiflexion) must be strong enough to keep the tibia in its position over the foot. This is an important concept. One side needs to be flexible enough and the opposite side needs to be strong enough to maintain the position.

Anterior Compartment

The anterior compartment is opposite of the posterior compartment. The muscles in the anterior compartment attach to various places on the top or dorsal surface of the foot. There is only one muscle from the anterior compartment that I'm going to mention. It is called tibialis anterior (you sometimes see

it named anterior tibialis). It is the strongest flexor (dorsiflexor) and inverter of the foot.

It is involved in "shin splints," a condition where the connective tissue layer around the bone known as the periosteum is pulled away from the bone itself and becomes inflamed. Overuse or strain of this muscle can lead to this condition.

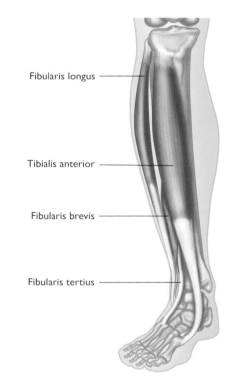

Fibularis longus

Tibialis anterior

Fibularis brevis

Fibularis tertius

Figure 2.16: *Anterior view of lower leg.*

The tibialis anterior has a proximal attachment on the outside (lateral) of the tibia, covering the upper two-thirds of the bone. It attaches distally on two bones, the medial cuneiform and the proximal end of the first metatarsal. Basically, it attaches to the peak of the arch. This attachment is shared with another muscle that we will look at in the lateral compartment called the fibularis longus.

The fibularis longus and tibialis anterior muscles comprise what is known as the "anatomical stirrup" of the foot; they are key

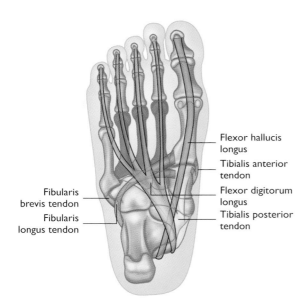

Figure 2.17: *The tibialis anterior and the fibularis longus tendons attach to the same bone to create what is called the anatomical stirrup.*

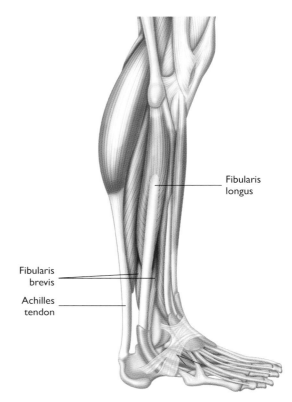

Figure 2.18: *Lateral view of lower leg.*

to balancing the body in our standing *asanas*. If you were to stand up and balance on one foot, you would note that your foot continually corrects itself in a side-to-side movement, not forward and back. The primary muscles working to manage the foot and ankle are the two that comprise the anatomical stirrup. This stirrup is crucial for maintaining a healthy and adaptable arch. They are also the foundation of our balancing postures.

Lateral Compartment

The lateral compartment is located on the outside of the foreleg and is made up of three muscles known as the fibulares. Fibularis longus is the largest and longest of the fibulares. It attaches onto the top and side (proximal and lateral) of the fibula. The two other fibulares are the fibularis brevis (meaning short) and fibularis tertius (meaning third).

The lateral compartment is responsible for eversion of the foot. We do not find our feet in an everted position very often, even

in our yoga practice, but it does happen. This movement and these tissues are critical in balancing the foot during walking and when doing balancing poses. I liken it to the abductors of the hip joint (which you haven't met yet in this book). Although we rarely find ourselves abducting our hip joints throughout the day, the abductors are crucial stabilizers. The muscles in the lateral compartment of the foot are similarly crucial to stabilizing the foot.

INTEGRATING ANATOMY INTO YOUR PRACTICE

So, how do we integrate this information into our practice? Slowly. More important than you reading this information is that you have an experience, a direct understanding of the material. Below are some ways to play with the concepts and ideas presented thus far.

Lift Your Toes

Stand with your shoes and socks off and simply lift your toes. You have probably done this at some point in a yoga class, but this time, look for the three points that outline the three arches: the base of the big toe, the base of the little toe, and the heel. Do you stand evenly on these points? Do you feel an obvious inner and outer side of your heel? Pay attention to how much weight you feel in your toes and in your heel. Do you stand predominantly on the inner or outer edges of the feet? You might even rock back and forth or side to side to get a sense of where weight passes through the feet comfortably.

Take a Look

Look in a mirror or have a friend, a partner, your students, or even your classmates stand in a row with their socks off and their pants pulled

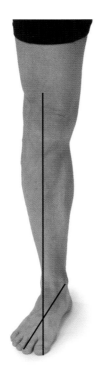

Figure 2.19: *Notice how my knee and foot are not pointing in the same direction.*

up over their knees. Can you see a relation between their feet, their arches (however high or low they may be or different on one side or the other), and their knees? How does one affect the other? Do the arches and feet affect your posture all the way up into the hip? Further?

Feel the Effect

Feel the difference between stretching your calf muscles with straight legs and with bent knees. With a straight leg, you will probably feel the stretch more superficially on the calf. If you sink into a squat, you might not feel much in the calf but your soleus muscle will restrict you from going lower and being stretched. You might only feel the sensation in your Achilles tendon.

Play with the Quality of the Pose

Go into Warrior 1. Now lift your toes and let them fall repeatedly while paying attention to what changes above them (maybe close your eyes). Does the entire structure seem to collapse and then lift again with the toes?

Play with the Arches

Look at the qualities that arches can bring to a pose. Use a simple *asana* like Warrior 1. Get into the pose and then let your arch collapse in the front foot. Watch the effect on the knee, and therefore the hip, in this leg. You probably find that your knee falls in a bit. While the knee is in, lift your toes up. Can you sense or see the knee trying to move laterally as a result? You may find that lifting your toes not only affects your arches but also repositions your knee and causes the hip joint to move.

PROBLEMS WITH THE FEET

Because they play such an important role in supporting our bodies, it's not surprising that problems in the feet get our attention in a dramatic way. Let's discuss four common foot problems: plantar fasciitis, flat feet, bunions, and ankle pain. There are many ways to help alleviate the discomfort of each.

Plantar Fasciitis

Plantar fasciitis typically creates intense pain in the bottom of the foot after a period of no use, often after sleeping. For instance, the first step out of bed after a night's sleep is usually intensely painful. The sensation has been likened to a sharp knife in the bottom of the foot. The pain is usually close to the deep part of the arch or near the front of the heel bone; it often subsides with movement, as the tissues on the sole of the foot warm and soften.

The intense pain of plantar fasciitis after a period of no use is a result of scar tissue, which the body has created overnight. Your body literally creates scar tissue while you sleep! Part of the condition itself is a fraying of the plantar fascia, which the body naturally tries to heal. This is why splints are given to keep the plantar fascia stretched overnight as the scar tissue lays

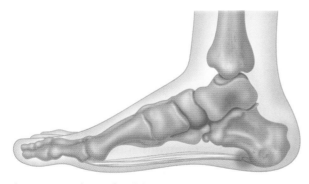

Figure 2.20: *Plantar fasciitis.*

down. This way the next morning it doesn't get torn again.

Why Does This Happen?

A number of factors play into the cause of plantar fasciitis. First and foremost, we need to look at what may be causing the tension in the plantar fascia in the first place. A very common component is tension in the calf muscles, which connect to the plantar fascia via connective tissue of the heel bone. This is why plantar fasciitis is quite common among runners, cyclists, and spinning enthusiasts. Additional factors, such as flat feet, misaligned feet, over-pronated or over-supinated feet, and obesity can create or exacerbate the problem.[5]

What to Do About It?

First, see a podiatrist if you think you have this condition. Also, there are a plethora of tools now available online to help you, including shoe inserts, splints, and guidelines on exercises. Because the calf muscles are generally involved in maintaining the tension that causes plantar fasciitis, stretching the gastrocnemius and soleus is often recommended.

If you already do yoga, focus on poses that rebalance the tension around the ankle. An excellent sequence of poses is *Surya Namaskara*. Use postures like Downward Facing Dog, *Utkatasana*, and forward bends to maintain length in the hamstrings, calves, and bottoms of the feet. Note: Heel spurs are often associated with plantar fasciitis; however, the latest research shows that the heel spur itself is not the cause of pain and is instead a by-product of connective tissue being pulled off the heel bone from the tension of a tight plantar fascia.

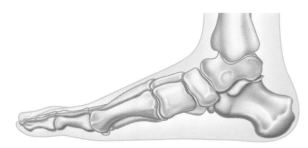

Figure 2.21: *Flat feet (pes planus).*

Flat Feet

The technical name for this condition is *pes planus*, which literally means "flat foot." The arch that is most obviously missing is the medial arch of the foot, but the other two arches are missing as well. This condition can be hereditary and passed through generations. It can be the result of the actual bone shape itself not being "ideal," or it can be that the ligaments holding the foot together are too loose to maintain their integrity of shape.[6] Either way, the foot loses its springiness in step. In other words, the foot doesn't flatten when weight is on it and then rebound back to the more arched shape, as it should. Several complications can arise out of flat feet.

Imagine the feet having to absorb the force of our body weight without having the shock absorption quality that healthy feet provide. The shock is essentially sent back into the body and up through the knees, hips, and spine. Flat feet have been connected to a number of problems located far away from the feet, including headaches.

When someone has arches but then loses them, it often occurs from trauma to the foot. If there is an imbalance of the tissues surrounding the foot and ankle that help to maintain the integrity of the arches, the result can be loss of the arch(es). In these cases, it is possible to rebuild the arches through physical therapy. In fact, many people experience significant gains in the health of their feet by practicing yoga.

I personally look to the fundamental movements found in Sun Salutations to maintain the health of the feet. There are different varieties of the movements, but any type that includes warrior postures takes the foot through a good range of motion. Forward bends stretch the calves as well as the hamstrings. *Chaturanga Dandasana* puts pressure on the toes, stretching the bottoms of the feet. Upward Facing Dog stretches the tops of the feet while strengthening the opposite muscles on the bottoms of the feet. Down Dog also stretches the calves, and if you lift your toes, you increase the tension in the bottoms of the feet and strengthen the fronts of the shins. If we mix a Warrior 1 into our Sun Salutation (with the back heel down), we invert the ankle and stretch and strengthen the inner and outer foot.

Although the warrior poses specifically benefit the feet, all of the standing *asanas* naturally call on the tissues surrounding the feet to work. These postures may be enough for students who are trying to rebuild an arch. Remember that people who were born with flat feet may not see the same results as those who have had arches and then lost them.

Bunions

Bunions are a condition where the joint capsule around the big toe is stretched and a callus grows over it. It manifests as a large protrusion coming off the inside of the big toe while the end of the toe itself points more outward.[7]

This condition is ten times more likely to happen to women, but men can have them as well. There is also a genetic component. People

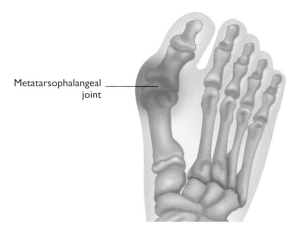

Metatarsophalangeal
joint

Figure 2.22: *Bunions.*

with loose joints and connective tissue are more inclined to develop bunions. The bigger culprit is what women put their feet in! Pointed, tight-toed, high-heeled shoes are a major cause of bunions. This is exponentially more likely if the women are genetically predisposed to the condition. There are many ways, some more invasive than others, to deal with bunions. As with most conditions, the sooner one intervenes and slows the progression, the better. As the bones start to misalign because of pressure on the big toe, uneven wearing down of the cartilage can occur, which can lead to swelling, inflammation, and arthritis—all of which create pain. There is no single solution.

Most people find that keeping the joints as mobile as possible helps. Instead of thinking what poses to do or avoid, think of consistently working with the feet. Do at least a little every day. As with most conditions, the stage of progression, whether one can stop contributing to the condition (by not wearing high heels or closed-toe shoes, for instance,) are all factors.

Ankle Pain

There is one yoga pose where ankle pain shows up more than any other—*Padmasana* (Lotus Posture). For some people, it occurs in Half- or Full-Lotus Pose. For others it only occurs in Full Lotus. Others still find pain when doing Half-Lotus postures such as *Marichyasana* B or D. Of course there are several reasons for this, but I'm going to address a few of the most common.

The first potential cause is tightness in the ankle. I'm not talking about tightness like you have in your hamstrings. I'm talking about compounded connective tissue tightness, or adhesions, if you prefer. When you feel a burning sensation or an ache over a large area on the outside of your ankle, there is a good chance you are dealing with adhesions.

Everyone has twisted their ankle at some point, some of us more than others. Gymnasts, runners, tennis players, football players, or any athlete who runs and changes direction quickly, are particularly prone to a twisted ankle, and some might have twisted the same ankle repeatedly. Is the ankle you twisted the one that hurts the most? Chances are it is. Every time you twisted that ankle, ligaments on the outside of the ankle were torn. The body's natural reaction to tearing is to lay down scar tissue. If you rested that ankle (as may have been appropriate at the time), it's possible that the scar tissue over-accumulated and created adhesions. This makes you more likely to re-twist your ankle because you have weakened the ligaments. Each twist results in more scar tissue building up on the old scar tissue.

Weakened ankles, in combination with two other contributing factors, foot placement, and hip tension, can create extreme pain on the outside of your ankle when in Half- or Full Lotus Pose. If this is the case, you likely have adhesions. Think about it this way, if your foot is "sickled" (inverted), you are compressing the inside and stretching the outside. The pain that you feel isn't a result of compression (or at least, it's unlikely). It is more likely to come from the tissues that are being stretched. As these tissues stretch, so does any scar tissue we might have from running around, and from growing up.

Where you place the foot when bringing it into Half-Lotus Pose is very important. Ideally, the outer edge of the foot lies inside the crease of your hip. There is a crucial limiting factor—how flexible your hip is. If your hip is not flexible enough, the foot won't land in the right place, and you'll end up with more pressure exerted on the outer side of the ankle. Trying to jam the foot up into the right place is the wrong thing to do. It is also not beneficial to avoid the real problem, which is a tight hip. The best way to alleviate ankle pain in Lotus[8] is to back up and work on opening the hip.

Note: The hip will be covered later in Chapter 4. You can read more about the specific placement of the foot in the posture section under Lotus and Lotus variations.

3
THE KNEE

Making our way up the body, the knee is the next major joint we come to. The femur and tibia, the two longest bones in the body, meet here to create one of the more complicated joints. Knee pain and dysfunction are almost as common as good old back pain. But what else should we expect from a joint that has to perform the type of demanding tasks that we ask of it?

In every workshop I have ever done, the knee is high on people's priority list. I can't say I blame them, since the ideal image of yoga in most of the world is someone sitting in Lotus. Therefore,

Padmasana becomes a measuring stick for a person's yoga practice. Of course, there is nothing less in line with a true yoga practice than a determined beginner trying to get into this pose and destroying their knee(s) in the process.

As my teacher John Scott points out, yoga has been plucked out of its cultural context and placed here in the West. In India, sitting on the floor has been a way of life for a long time. Although this is slowly disappearing with Western influence, you still regularly see women squatting to cook, or workers squatting to build things. And let's not forget the Eastern toilet: beautifully laid porcelain in the floor requiring that you squat to use the toilet! With all of this squatting and sitting in everyday life, Indian hips and knees stay more flexible than ours in the West. Therefore, it is practically assumed that Lotus can be done. Lotus variations are the norm in the culture in which yoga was created.

In the West you will find something completely different. Unfortunately, the transplantation of yoga into our culture often results in suffering knees. It doesn't mean that we can't do yoga or Lotus, of course. It just means that we may want to keep cultural differences in mind as we try to plant our own Lotus seeds. We have a different culture, and Lotus is not a natural part of it. It is important to understand all the

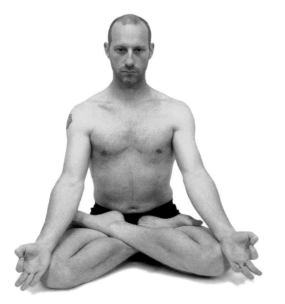

Figure 3.1: *The author sitting in Padmasana.*

components of the posture, work with them over time, and let your Lotus grow at its own pace.

THE BROADER VIEW

The knee is highly influenced by and connected to the joints above and below it, namely the foot and ankle joint below and the hip joint above. Often when injury occurs at the knee, there is some level of dysfunction (excess tension or weakness, or even a previous injury) in one or both of these surrounding joints.

The leg can be described as a kinematic chain. This means that the functions of the three main joints that comprise the leg are linked. Stand up for a moment with your book in hand and bend both knees at the same time; notice how the ankle and hip joints also move to accommodate the bend in the knees. Through its role as the central link in the kinematic chain of the leg, the knee is responsible for guiding and directing the movements of the leg in our daily activities, something as simple as walking or as complex as doing advanced *asana*.

The knee plays two somewhat contradictory roles: first it must be strong, because a great amount of our body weight passes through it. In addition to strength, it must also be flexible enough to deal with the adaptations of the ankle and foot, which change shape and position. It also must adapt to the hip and its role as we walk. When the balance between these joints and their roles (strength and flexibility) goes awry, the knee often receives the forces.

THE KNEE AND POSTURE

We started with the foundation of our standing posture, the feet. If there are dysfunctions at this level (for example, flat feet), the ankles, knees, and hips (the joints above it) will have to compensate. Now let's look at the second link in the chain, the knee.

A simple observation to make when studying the knees is to note the direction in which they face. You could look at the kneecaps as headlights and observe where they're "shining their light." Whether in *Tadasana,* Down Dog, or Triangle Pose, the knees tell a story. It may be a story about themselves, but it's more likely a story about the hip, ankle, foot, or a combination of them all. As we mentioned in the last chapter, problems below have an effect above. The knee is, therefore, the first joint to feel the effect of a fallen arch or pressure from an ankle that is stuck in Lotus.

Let me share with you my own foot/ankle and knee relationship. Remember my story of breaking my right femur playing soccer? I kicked the soccer ball at the same moment that my much larger neighbor was kicking it in the opposite direction. From my recollection, the soccer ball didn't move and I was vibrating like a cartoon character. The force of that mutual contact actually broke my femur. I wish I still had the x-ray to share with you here, but it has been lost over the years.

That event influenced that side of my body. My legs are slightly different lengths, which you may observe in an image of me in Headstand (see Figure 3.2). This could be a result of a stronger anterior tilt of the right side of my pelvis. My longer leg may be creating, or may be the result of, the slightly compressed arch in my right foot. This arch is visibly lower and more compressed looking. Who knows? My point is that there is an obvious relation between my foot, the arch, where my knee likes to point, and the tilt in that side of my pelvis; whether or not I can pinpoint the cause isn't important.

Of course this can change on a moment-to-moment basis. If you look closely, you may be able to see a twist below my knee, essentially

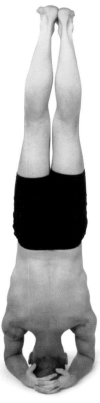

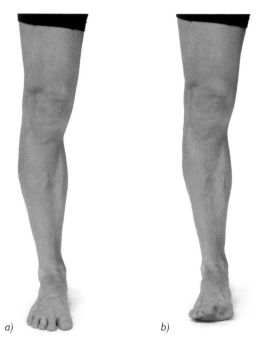

Figure 3.3: *Notice the effect on the knee when the arch is engaged; a) before lifting the toes, b) after lifting the toes.*

Figure 3.2: *Notice how my right foot is higher than the left.*

between the knee and the foot/ankle. If I add a bit of an arch to my foot, you can see how the direction of the knee changes (see Figure 3.3). Thus, due to the knee's relation to the joints above and below it, it often reflects what's going on (tension, weakness, injury, or other converging histories) in the joints surrounding it. This is a great example of the integrated nature of our bodies. Looking at the knee by itself does not give you the whole picture any more than feeling the trunk of an elephant gives you a clear idea of what an elephant looks like. To get the whole picture, we must also look at what is influencing it. This doesn't just mean the foot, ankle, and hip joints, but also the muscles that cross these joints and their influence.

BASIC ANATOMY OF THE KNEE

Three bones come together at the knee: the femur, tibia, and patella (kneecap). The technical

name for the "knee" is the femoro-tibial joint. It is the connection between the rounded ends of the femur and the relatively flat surface of the top of the tibia. Between and around these two bones are the meniscus, the cruciate ligaments, and the collateral ligaments that help support movement and stability around this joint.

The shapes and angles of the bones are part of the determining factor of the function of this joint. We do not often realize the shape of the femur until we take a close look at it.

If you look down the shaft of the femur from the top, there's a twist visible through the angle of the femoral head. The femur is also bowed forward in a slight arch (Figure 3.6). From its attachment to the pelvis, the femur angles in to meet the top of the tibia quite sharply (Figure 3.7). This angle evolved along with bipedalism (walking on two feet). It brings the feet in under the body and closer to the midline to facilitate walking.

Because of this angle, more weight is passed through the lateral side of the knee.[8] This is

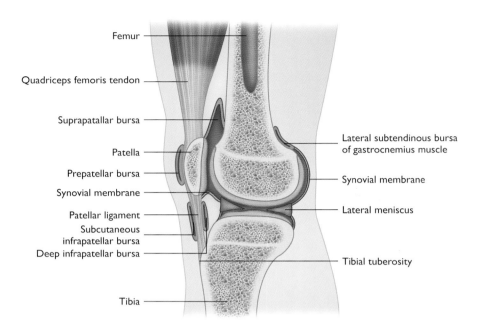

Figure 3.4: *The knee joint, mid-sagittal view.*

displayed by a larger knobby-shaped bottom of the femur on the outside (lateral condyle of the femur) and a slightly deeper depression in the top of the tibia on the outside. This seemingly small detail provides a glimpse into the evolutionary process. Chimps bear weight in the knees on the inside (medial), and their tibia is convex; their feet are spread more widely and the knees allow for more rotation than ours do.[9]

The tibia also has a twist in it that accommodates the twist in the femur and allows for proper placement of the foot. Needless to say, the femur and tibia come together in a fairly odd way. It's actually not a great fit, and it's surprising that more problems do not arise within this joint, given all the twists and forces acting on it. It is a particularly vulnerable joint.

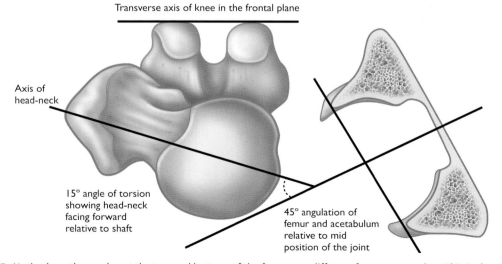

Figure 3.5: *Notice how the angles at the top and bottom of the femur are different from one another. This is the twist.*

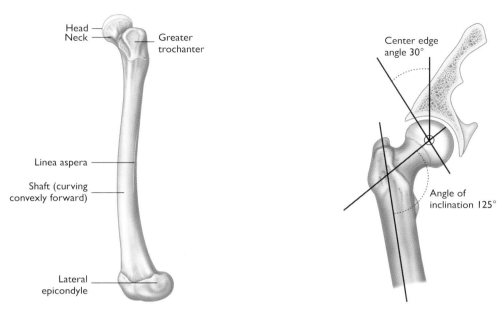

Figure 3.6: *The femur is bowed forward.*

Figure 3.7: *The angle of the neck and shaft are variable.*

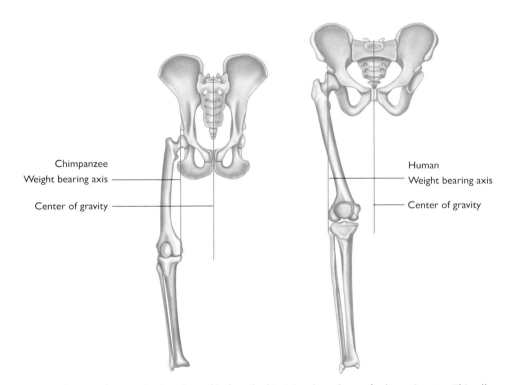

Figure 3.8: *Human legs are less vertically oriented below the hip joint than those of other primates. This allows our support to be closer to the center of gravity and leads to the adaptation of the enlarged medial condyle—a feature that is developed by walking rather than being inherited.*

The Patella

The patello-femoral joint is where the patella meets the femur. It is essential to the strength we have when we extend the knee. Without this little bone, it would be more difficult for the large quadriceps muscle group to move the tibia with the force and strength that it does. The patella becomes a point of additional leverage for the thick tendon of the quadriceps to lie over and around. It redirects force over the top of itself, thereby increasing the force of the quadriceps. By changing its angle, it also helps reduce friction as the thick tendon extends the knee joint. Consider how many times a day we bend and straighten the knees. Without this little bone, the tendon would rub on the bones as we move our knee joint. Eventually, were it not for the patella, the tendon would fray and tear from friction.

The underside of the patella has cartilage and thus easily and smoothly slides on the groove of the femur below. The shape of the underside of the patella is designed to fit into the shape of the space between the knobby ends (condyles) on the bottom (distal) end of the femur. The patella is held in place by the thick patellar ligament (sometimes called the patellar tendon). This ligament doesn't allow very much movement up or down the patella once it becomes taut; instead, as the knee bends in flexion, the femur slides under the patella. This helps to keep the movement as straight as possible.

Primarily, the patella aligns the movement at the knee. It keeps the flexion and extension as true to a straight line as possible. The patella is also designed for leverage, as discussed.

Injuries to the Patella

There is a condition, called patello-femoral syndrome (chondromalacia) that applies to the patella specifically. This condition can be a precursor to arthritis at the joint and is almost always associated with overuse. People with this syndrome usually have some type of trauma to the cartilage under the patella. Depending on how much cartilage you start off with (this is genetic), what seems like overuse to one person may be different to another. Regardless, if you have this condition, excessive amounts of activity will contribute to the wearing away of the cartilage on the underside of the patella.

Another factor contributing to patello-femoral syndrome is the alignment of the knee, as in what the knee does while we're moving it. If the tissues that control the patella (the quadriceps on the front of the thigh) are imbalanced, they add to the amount of pressure on the patella.

For instance, if the quadriceps muscle on the inside (vastus medialis) is too tight, relative to the muscle on the outside (the vastus lateralis), then the patella will naturally get pulled more medially. If this happens, there is more pressure on the medial part of the patella where it meets the surface of the femur. Tightness in the vastus lateralis would create the opposite effect. Either can lead to an uneven wearing of cartilage.

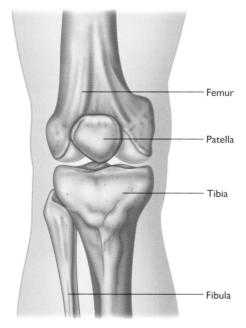

Femur

Patella

Tibia

Fibula

Figure 3.9: *Bones of the knee, right leg, anterior view.*

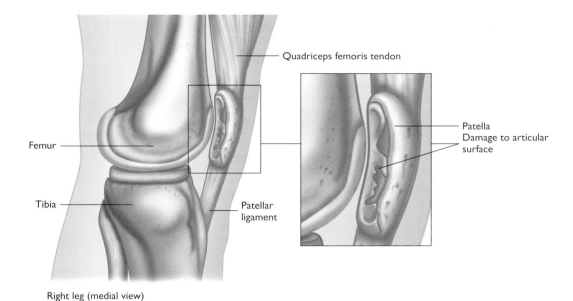

Right leg (medial view)

Figure 3.10: *Patello-femoral syndrome (chondromalacia).*

Symptoms of this syndrome include pain deep inside the knee and stiffness after long immobility or long sustained use. Of course there are many other reasons one might feel pain in the knee. If you have long, sustained periods of pain, talk to your doctor.

MOVEMENTS OF THE KNEE

The primary movements or actions of the knee are flexion (bending) and extension (straightening). But two other actions occur at that joint that are often misunderstood or perhaps not even known. The knee also rotates when it is bent. Technically, if you bend your knee 10 degrees or more, the tibia can rotate both internally and externally relative to the femur. If you sit on the floor with a straight leg and try to move your foot side to side, you will find your leg rotating from the hip joint. This changes when the knee bends.

If you bend your knee more than 10 degrees, you will find that your foot rotates from side to side fairly easily. Often this ability is met with

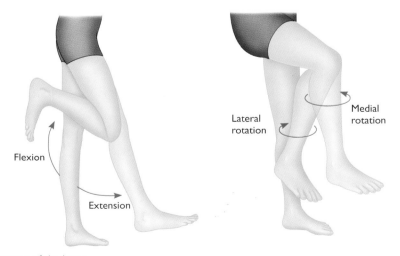

Figure 3.11: *Movements of the knee.*

some fear: "Don't twist your knee!" But we wouldn't walk the way we do, run the way we do, much less do complicated activities such as ski, play basketball, or play tennis if this wasn't how our knees naturally functioned. The joint is designed to adapt to the foot and the hip. That said, this rotation is responsible for many troubles in the knee joint.

Similar to the rest of our body parts, the knee is but one component of the whole leg. Flexion and extension at the knee are more pertinent to the strength role that the joint plays. These actions propel us forward as we run. These more or less straightforward movements do not put much strain on the ligaments and other structures within and around the knee. They're at the heart of our ability to walk and run and are fundamental to our mobility. It is the more complicated movements of rotation required while pivoting in basketball, skiing, or even yoga postures that make the knee as adaptable as it is to the actions of the foot, ankle, and hip.

LIGAMENTS

Ligaments allow for and restrict joint movements. The knee is no different. There are four main ligaments in and around the knee. When the ligaments around a joint are in a "slackened" position, they allow for movement. When the ligaments become more "taut," they restrict movement. In the knee, they are taut when the leg is in anatomical position (that is, extended or straight). Keeping in mind that ligaments play an important role in creating joint stability (by restricting movement), we shouldn't forget that they are part of a larger, integrated structure. The tension of the myofascia that surrounds the knee also supports the joint and allows for movement at the knee.

Two of the main ligaments of the knee are called the collateral ligaments. Both of these connect the femur (above) to the tibia (below). One is on the inside (medial) of the two bones and is thus called the medial collateral ligament or MCL for short. The other is on the outside

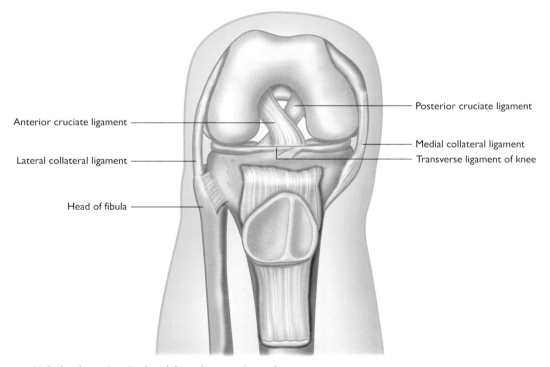

Anterior cruciate ligament

Lateral collateral ligament

Head of fibula

Posterior cruciate ligament

Medial collateral ligament

Transverse ligament of knee

Figure 3.12: *Right leg (anterior view) with knee bent at ninety degrees.*

(lateral) surface of the joint and is called the lateral collateral ligament, or LCL. The MCL attaches to the meniscus and blends into the joint capsule. The LCL is more independent in its attachments; that is, it is not part of the joint capsule the way the MCL is.

These two strap-like ligaments are primarily designed to prevent the tibia from moving sideways (medially and laterally) under the femur ends. They keep the knee from buckling inwards or outwards. If you remember the description of the angle of the femur as it meets the knee (the natural angle inwards of the femur), it becomes clear that the inside part of the knee tends to receive stress. Therefore, the MCL is thicker than the LCL because it has more work to do in resisting stress and maintaining stability as we move through life.

By virtue of their function to prevent side-to-side movements of the knee, the collateral ligaments naturally help maintain the alignment of straightforward and backward movements at the knee. They also aid in resisting external rotation of the flexed knee. Therefore, the MCL and, more likely, the LCL can be injured during both flexion and external rotation of the knee. This can occur in poses such as Lotus and *Eka Pada Sirsasana* (Leg-Behind-the-Head Pose).[10]

The Cruciates

The word cruciate literally means "crossing." When you look at these two ligaments from almost any perspective, they cross one another. Unlike the collateral ligaments on the outsides of the knee, the cruciates are on the inside of the knee. They hold the femur and tibia closely together and are named the anterior cruciate ligament (ACL) and the posterior cruciate ligament (PCL). If you look at Figure 3.13, you will see that the ACL attaches to the front part

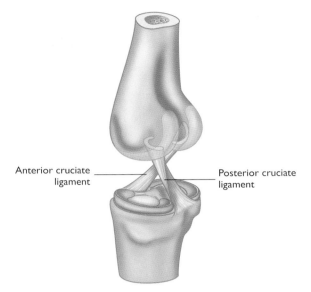

Anterior cruciate ligament — — Posterior cruciate ligament

Figure 3.13: *The cruciates with the bones separated.*

(anterior) of the tibia and then runs to the inner part of the big bump on the bottom of the femur (lateral femoral condyle). The PCL attaches to the back part (posterior) of the tibia and then attaches to the inner part of the bump on the inside of the femur (medial femoral condyle). Their attachments account for their names.

These strong ligaments are the primary stabilizers of the knee joint. As with the collateral ligaments, they are taut when the knee is extended. The ACL resists movement in primarily two actions. First, it keeps the tibia from sliding forwards under the femur. Anatomically speaking, this is referred to as an anterior displacement of the tibia under the femur. The ACL also prevents excessive medial (or inward) rotation of the flexed knee. As the tibia rotates medially, this ligament becomes more taut as it winds around the PCL. In lateral rotation, the ACL is lengthened and stretched over the PCL. There is a possibility that the ACL can tear when the knee is flexed and either internally or externally rotated.

Having said that, it is most common for the knee to be flexed and internally rotated when the ACL tears; it is common for this ligament to

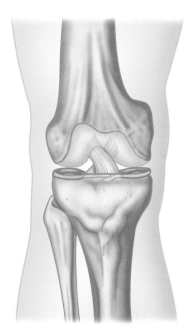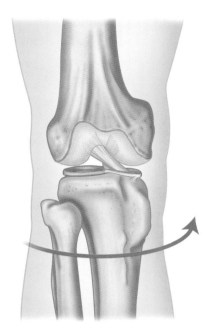

Figure 3.14: *Internal rotation of the lower leg showing the lengthening or resistance of the ACL.*

be torn while skiing. The skiing part itself isn't risky, however. It is when the skier is about to run into someone or something and stops rather quickly. For those of you who have skied before, you know to ski with the knees slightly bent. You have also trained yourself to slow down or stop by pointing the front of the skis towards each other. This is internal rotation of a flexed knee. If you do this suddenly and one ski happens to turn in more than you'd like and your body continues to go forward, the knee rotates internally *a lot*. You may pay the price by tearing your ACL.

The attachment site of the PCL lies opposite to the ACL. The PCL attaches to the back portion (posterior) of the tibia and attaches to the femur opposite the ACL. Its main purpose is to restrict the tibia from sliding backwards under the femur. When the knee is extended, it allows almost no room for give in the tibia and is the main force holding together hyperextended knees. In terms of rotation, it has minimal impact. This is probably why you don't hear about injuries to this ligament nearly as often as you hear about injuries to the ACL. In those cases where you do hear about PCL injury, it

often includes some type of hyperextension. For example, you can hurt your PCL when you miss a step and your knee buckles backwards.

Ligament Tears

Let's talk about what happens when ligaments in the knee become dysfunctional. A tear of a ligament isn't always what we think. Most people assume this means the ligament tears in half, like tearing a piece of paper in half. Don't get me wrong, this is possible, but it would require a very violent action or injury. Tears of tissue are categorized into grades or degrees. These grades apply to ligaments, tendons, and muscles. The type of tear referred to above would be classified as a Grade 3 tear. This is a complete tear of the ligament and would be associated with extreme pain, heat, and instant swelling.

Grade 1 tears are the most common. While they definitely cause pain, there is often no swelling or heat. Typically you just feel tenderness. The pain increases in certain movements, depending on which ligament is torn. Grade 2 tears step it up a notch in the pain department. You typically feel more significant pain and an increased amount of heat. Normally these tears involve swelling. Again, movements and positions will increase the pain and give some indication (if you know what you are looking for) of which grade of tear may have occurred.

We'll look at how the ligaments are created to better understand what happens when we tear one of them. When we go deeply into a ligament we find collagen molecules (proteins). These molecules interlink with neighboring molecules and create a functional coil-like shape, kind of like a spring. A ligament is a huge bundle of these coils—think of a Slinky(TM) or a metal spring. If you stretch a Slinky or a spring, it will return to its normal state after being lengthened. A healthy ligament works in the same way. There is some elasticity to it.

However, if you take the spring or Slinky and uncoil it too much, that is, if you overstretch it, what happens? When it springs back, there will be a gap between some of the coils, right? It never fully returns to its original shape or tension.

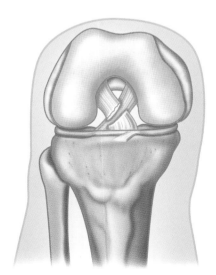

Figure 3.15: *Anterior cruciate ligament (ACL). Once the fibers are stretched beyond the point where they can return, we have a tear.*

This is what happens when we have a Grade 1 or Grade 2 tear of a ligament (or other tissues). The coils of protein have been pulled apart so far that they can no longer "re-coil" to their normal position. Consequently, some of the tension is lost in that piece of tissue. If this happens around the knee, stability between the bones may be lost. When you have an MRI and the doctor says that your ACL is 50% torn, what he or she is actually saying is that your ligament has lost 50% of its ability to stabilize your joint.

With the ACL in particular, this loss of stability is very important. The ACL keeps the top of the tibia against the bottom of the femur. When it is torn or overstretched, the knee may become wobbly and lose some of its inherent strength and stability. Depending on the severity of the tear, the person's health, and the patients' activity level, the muscles around the joint may have to compensate for this loss of stability.

If non-surgical strengthening exercises do not work for a torn ACL, surgery can be performed. The surgeon takes a piece of ligament (a ligament from another place in the body, or even a cadaver) and connects the ends of this "new" ligament to the places on the bone where the other ligament attaches. This will become your "new" ACL and will add stability to the knee. You should seek medical advice if you think you might have torn your ACL. Do not diagnose yourself.

MENISCUS

The menisci (plural) are two semi-circular pieces of additional cartilage sitting on the almost flat area of the tibia. There is one on either side, hence the terms medial (inside) and lateral meniscus (outside) of the knee. Menisci have two "horns," an anterior (front)

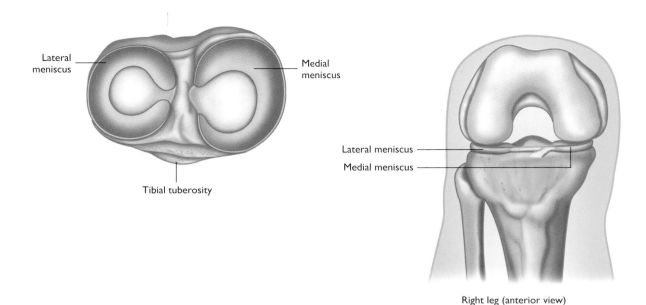

Right leg (anterior view)

Figure 3.16: *Meniscus from front between two bones.*

and posterior (back) horn. The horn is the rounded end facing the center of the tibia.

The menisci serve a few purposes. First, because of their shape, they create a deeper cup for the knobby ends of the femur to meet the relatively flat plateau of the tibia. This creates additional stability in the knee. Because they are flexible, they also play a shock absorber role in the knee joint. Finally, the meniscus also helps with the knee's functional movements, such as flexion, extension, and rotation.

Instead of being completely fixed in place, the menisci actually move and distort in shape depending on the movements of the knee joint. Every time the knee flexes, the meniscus must slide or be "squished" backwards on top of the tibia to help keep those knobby ends in place. The opposite happens in extension. The meniscus slides or squishes forward. Rotations of the knee also force the menisci to move and shift according to the direction of rotation.

So, we see that the seemingly simple movements of flexion and extension at the knee joint aren't really so simple. If the knee was exactly like a hinge, as it is often classified, when it bent, a large gap would be created between the bones at the front, similar to what you see on a door. If the femur simply rolled backwards and forwards on the top of the tibia, it would roll off the back or the front of the bone. Instead, the condyles (knobby ends) both glide and roll at the same time. There is, in essence, a controlled sliding at the knee joint during these movements.

As the knee flexes, the condyles basically roll up the ramp of the meniscus. Because it is a ramp and everything inside the joint is pretty slippery, the femur slides back down the ramp while the condyle is rolling up. In other words, the femur is forced to rotate in place on top of the tibia. Movements at the knee force the condyles and the meniscus to interact. The meniscus is forced to adapt. When they do not interact properly we run into trouble.

Meniscus Injuries

The menisci can tear from compression, movement, or a combination of the two. Compression happens when the condyles of the

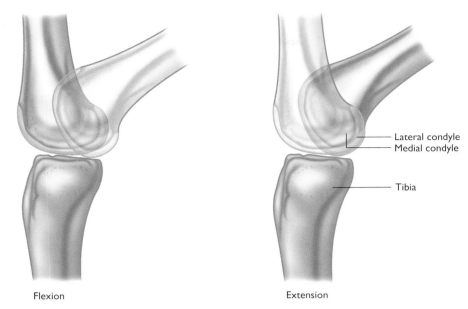

Flexion

Extension

Lateral condyle
Medial condyle

Tibia

Figure 3.17: *Flexion/extension of the femur on the tibia.*

femur pin the meniscus down against the top of the tibia. The pressure on this cartilaginous structure causes it to tear, split, or fray. Because this injury causes more than normal friction, some inflammation and pain often go with it. Depending on the situation, there may be an audible click or pop at the moment of injury. There are various types of tears that can occur to the meniscus. Many have interesting names such as a bucket handle tear, parrot beak, or radial tear. What's more interesting is that, of the two menisci, the medial meniscus is the one most commonly torn. It's not uncommon for such a tear to occur while going into *Padmasana* (Lotus Pose). More on this later.

There are some obvious differences between the medial and lateral meniscus. The medial meniscus is larger and more open at its center than the lateral meniscus. The lateral meniscus, on the other hand, seems ready to complete a circle. As it turns out, the lateral meniscus is

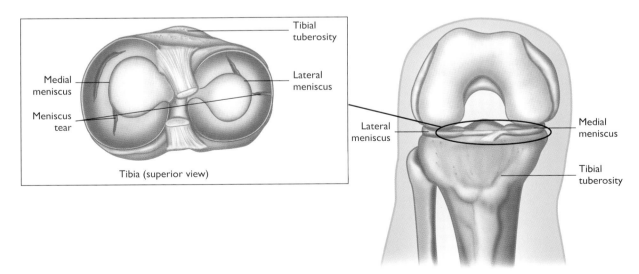

Tibial tuberosity

Medial meniscus

Meniscus tear

Lateral meniscus

Tibia (superior view)

Lateral meniscus

Medial meniscus

Tibial tuberosity

Knee in flexion (anterior view)

Figure 3.18: *Meniscus injuries.*

actually a bit more adaptable to the rotational movements of the knee. The medial meniscus is more fixed.[11] Because it doesn't adapt as much as the lateral one, the likelihood of it getting caught up and compressed by the femur ends is greater. This is partly why one of the most common places to have a torn meniscus is on the posterior portion of the medial meniscus.

The meniscus is designed to move with the bones. If it is compressed (for example, if the knee is completely flexed and then asked to rotate), the meniscus may be held down by the condyles and can stretch to the point of tearing. A similar thing can happen when the knee is moved very quickly. You often see this when people drop into a squat or stand from a squatting position quickly. None of this means that if you flex your knee and then rotate it or squat quickly that you will tear your meniscus. Other factors are involved.

One of the most common ways to tear the meniscus is to rotate a completely flexed knee. Does this sound familiar? It should. This is exactly what we do to move into Lotus. Now, don't go running in the streets screaming that Lotus is going to tear your meniscus! *If your body is ready*, it won't. But things get riskier if you try to do Lotus before your body is ready.

Can a Meniscus Heal?

A meniscus tear can happen anywhere. However, where it tears has a lot to do with whether it will heal itself or require intervention. If you look at Figure 3.19, you will see the meniscus divided into an outer, middle, and inner third. The outermost layer of the meniscus is made up of loose, fibrous connective tissue. This tissue maintains blood supply and circulation. For this reason, tears to the outer third often heal on their own if

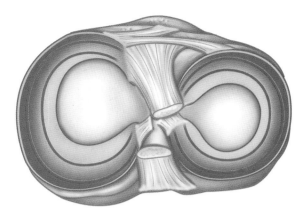

Figure 3.19: *The outer third of the meniscus maintains a blood supply and has the potential to heal.*

not too severe.[12] Unfortunately, the blood supply is limited by the time it gets to the more tightly packed connective tissues that make the cartilage in the middle and inner thirds. The inner third and most of the middle third are actually considered avascular (no blood supply). Consequently, it is almost impossible to get the elements required for healing to this area of the meniscus. Although nothing is impossible, it is unlikely for tears to the inner two-thirds to heal themselves.

Over time, small tears in the meniscus can get larger, be broken off, and float around in the knee. This is why common symptoms of a meniscus tear are pain, clicking sounds, or even locking of the knee. When left alone, a tear usually progresses; continued movement of the knee can create additional problems, such as uneven wearing of the cartilage surfaces on the bottom of the femur. Long term, this can contribute to arthritis in the joint.

MUSCLES AROUND THE KNEE

Let's talk about soft tissues (muscles/myofascia). The main muscles that cross the knee joint are the quadriceps, hamstrings, iliotibial band, and gastrocnemius (calf muscle). All of these muscles clearly demonstrate how well integrated

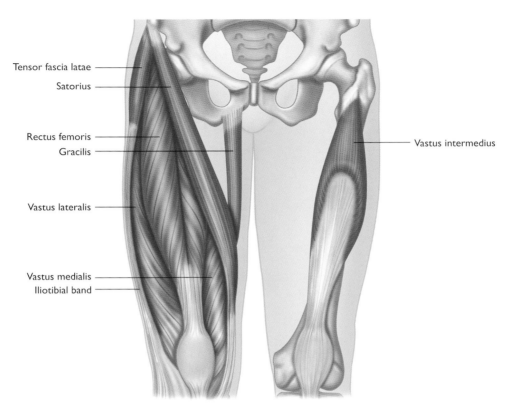

Tensor fascia latae

Satorius

Rectus femoris

Gracilis

Vastus lateralis

Vastus medialis

Iliotibial band

Vastus intermedius

Figure 3.20: *Muscles around the knee.*

the knee is with the hip and ankle. Most of the muscles here cross two major joints, either the knee and hip or the knee and ankle.

One of the largest groups of muscles in the body is the thigh muscle known as the quadriceps, which literally means four heads. The four heads are the vastus lateralis (on the outside), vastus medialis (on the inside), vastus intermedius (in the middle), and rectus femoris (on top). The first three cross only the knee joint (not the hip). Therefore, they extend (straighten) the knee. This simple action is essential for walking and running.

The rectus femoris crosses two joints, the knee (for extension) and the hip (to assist in flexion; i.e. lifting the leg forward and up from a standing position). These four muscles converge around and attach to the patella and then continue through a ligament (the patellar ligament/ tendon) to attach to the top of the tibia.

Although less obvious, the hamstrings in the back of the thigh also impact the knee. They create balance for the quadriceps. In other words, as the knee straightens, the hamstrings get longer. If the hamstrings shorten, the quadriceps get longer. Thus the hamstrings balance the forces impacting the knee joint.

Three muscles comprise the hamstring group. First is the biceps femoris (biceps means two heads and refers to a long and short head of this muscle). Semitendinosus and semimembranosus are the other two. I wouldn't worry too much about the names. It's more important to focus on what they do. All three of these muscles cross both the knee and the hip joints and perform the opposite actions of the quadriceps. They flex the knee and extend the hip joint. (If you take your leg backwards from a standing position at both the knee and the hip, you can feel the hamstrings working.)

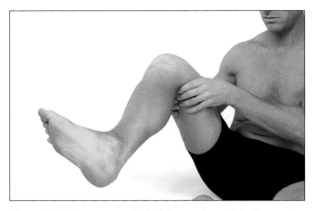
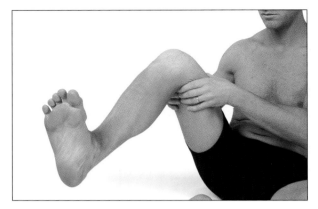

Figure 3.21: *You can easily feel the tendons of the hamstrings moving behind your knee.*

This group of muscles also rotates the tibia when the knee is flexed. You can easily feel this yourself. Place your hands on your hamstrings with your knee bent to about 90 degrees. Rotate the lower leg and you should feel the change in tension under your hands. Two tendons attach to the inside of the tibia and one to the outside of the tibia. Visualize the tendons as a cable or rope. As the tendons pull on the inside, the tibia rotates inward. As the outer "cable" is pulled, the tibia rotates outward.

THE ILIOTIBIAL BAND

The IT band or tract (ITB or ITT) is a piece of fascia on the outer part of the thigh. Its name describes its attachments. At the top it attaches to the ilium (bone of the pelvis) and below to the tibia in the foreleg. It attaches to the ilium via a muscle called the tensor fascia latae (TFL). If we look at the name of the muscle closely, it is the tensor of the lateral fascia which is exactly what the ITB is, the lateral fascia.

In addition to attaching at the ilium via the TFL, the ITB also attaches to the gluteus maximus and gluteus medius. The connective tissue runs down the outer part of the leg, over the lateral quadriceps (vastus lateralis), and attaches to the lateral part of the tibia as it crosses the knee joint.

The ITB is normally considered to be a stabilizer of the knee, especially during walking and running. With overuse, such as sometimes seen in runners, cyclists, and other sports enthusiasts, the ITB can adhere fascially to the lateral quadriceps beneath it. This can lead to a number of tensional isues that can affect hip and knee function. Avid runners and cyclists actually need an ITB that is taut to support the knee during those activities. If we recognize

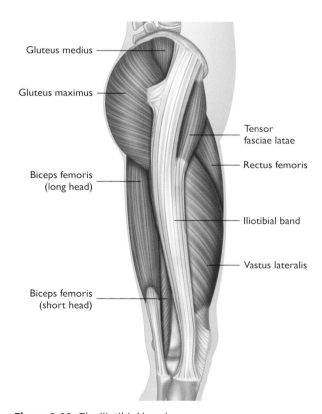

Figure 3.22: *The iliotibial band.*

that someone has an ITB that is too tight, simply stretching it out with yoga postures may lead to trouble in other activities. This doesn't mean that we want a super tight ITB either. It's about balance and what activities you want to do. A loose ITB can cause instability while running. A tight ITB can cause pain at the knee in postures like Lotus. Hips that are tight from either running or cycling are often the exact opposite of what we want them to be like in order to do Lotus Pose.

INTEGRATING ANATOMY INTO YOUR PRACTICE

We're all familiar with the advice to bend our knees when stooping down to pick up a heavy box. We do this to help distribute the weight from the lower back into the legs. This same concept can be used in our transition in and out of standing postures. Straight-legged standing postures themselves do not call for bending the knees, but in a standing forward bend, Triangle Pose, or any other straight-legged standing pose for that matter, bending the knees distributes the weight in the legs.

Play with entering and exiting a number of standing poses with the legs straight and then with the knees bent. Compare the difference. Bending the knees to transition between postures can be extremely helpful to students with SI, lower back, or knee problems. Once in the final pose, however, you should at the very least be trying to straighten the knees.

Your knees may be indicative of what is happening at the joints and structures that surround them. Take a look at your knees in a simple Downward Facing Dog and see where they point. Bend them slightly, and see if they point straight forward, inwards, or outwards.

Better yet, lift your toes and see if this has any effect on your knees. Is there a connection between the feet and the knees?

Try this one. Step into a simple Triangle Pose, and before your reach out to move into the posture, notice where your knee tends to point. Chances are it points inwards. If you bend the knee slightly, you'll notice that it unlocks the hip and brings the knee to point straight forward over the foot.

Pain in Your Knee During Lotus?

At a workshop, when I ask who has knee pain, approximately 80 percent of those who complain about knee pain in a Lotus type of posture (where the leg is flexed and rotated) say they experience pain on the inside (medial) of the knee. Approximately 10 to 15 percent complain about pain on the outside (lateral) of the knee. The rest usually complain about pain through the centerline of their knee or around the kneecap. All three areas express stress in the knee in different ways.

Pain on the inside of the knee is the most common knee pain associated with the leg being in Half- or Full-Lotus Pose. Using statistics from my own personal observations, I've come up with a working hypothesis: the most common cause of pain on the medial knee is compression of the medial meniscus. Please note that I am not suggesting that all pain on the inside of the knee is coming from the medial meniscus. Nor am I saying that pain on the inside of your knee during Half- or Full Lotus means you have already torn your meniscus. You may simply be irritating it. There are other structures in this area that can get inflamed or irritated and cause pain on the inside of the knee. For instance, the MCL and various muscles crossing the inside of the knee, and even the joint capsule itself, can get compressed and irritated.

One reason I first suspect medial meniscus compression is that I've heard stories of many people who complain about pain on the inside of their knees who eventually experience a "pop" in Lotus position. Swelling in the back of the knee and sometimes a regular clicking sound follows the pop. It is also possible that the knee will lock intermittently after the original pop occurs. All of these are classic signs and symptoms of a meniscus tear. The best way to confirm if the meniscus has torn is to go to the doctor and have an MRI scan taken.

The other reason I tend to (at least initially) suspect medial meniscus compression, is that Lotus requires the two movements which, when combined, put the most amount of pressure on the medial meniscus: flexion of the knee and internal (medial) rotation of the tibia. Both the femur and tibia have to rotate externally. If the tibia doesn't have enough outward rotation, there could still be enough in the hip to make up for it, or vice versa. If, however, both the tibia and the femur lack the ability to rotate externally, you end up with more internal rotation, which can put pressure onto the medial meniscus. When you combine this with a flexed knee, as in Lotus, you end up with even more pressure on the medial meniscus. If the hips are tight, it is common to feel pressure in the knees.

There are two ways of dealing with this. The first is an immediate response: the moment you feel the sensation of pain, place one hand on your thigh near your knee and the other on your calf muscle.

Try externally rotating both of them, as if you are creating space between the ends of the two bones rotationally. You could also prop the

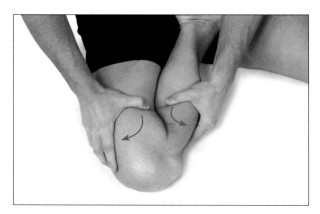

Figure 3.23: *Externally rotating the upper and lower leg usually alleviates pressure on the inside of the knee.*

knee higher with a block or a bolster to see if that alleviates the pressure or pain.

The long-term solution is to lengthen the tissues in the hip that are restricting external rotation of that joint. [See Chapter 4, pages 106–107 for specific stretches to lengthen the muscles around the hips].

What if you have pain on the outside or in the centerline of your knee around the patella? If you have pain on the outside of the knee, you're in a club of your own! When I meet people who have pain here, I often find (although there are exceptions) that rotation internally of both the tibia and the femur actually decreases their pain. (Note: this is the opposite of what to do if pain is on the inside.)

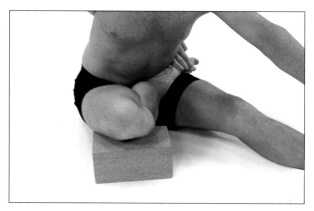

Figure 3.24: *Elevating the knee often works regardless of where the pressure is.*

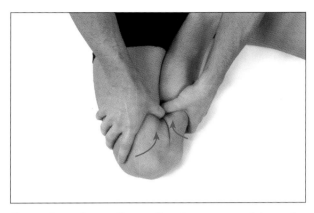

Figure 3.25: *Internally rotating the upper and lower leg usually helps with pressure on the outside of the knee.*

Upon further questioning, many of these people currently are or used to be runners or cyclists. My working hypothesis is that a tight ITB is the culprit. Again, I am sure there are exceptions, but this is a good place to start. A tight ITB seems to place rotational force on the knee. I assume the force is rotational in nature because when I help rotate the femur and tibia internally, their pain is reduced or goes away. Another option is to once again elevate the knee and support it with a block or bolster. This almost always alleviates pain anywhere in the knee in postures like Lotus or Half-Lotus. However, a long-term solution will still require that tension at the hip joint be released and that the muscles that create excess tension in the ITB be addressed. Remember, you want to balance the strength and flexibility of these tissues, especially for runners and cyclists.

If the pain is through the midline of the knee, I tend to focus on the quadriceps first. This group of muscles literally wraps around the patella to get to its final destination on the tibia. Therefore, they are intimately associated with the functioning of the knee, particularly extension. When the quadriceps are dysfunctional, students either lack flexibility or lack strength. Either of these situations can cause trouble in the knee. I realize this is unspecific, but in order to determine the

cause and treatment of the problem, an actual assessment of the individual is required. Having said this, there are several other issues that can show up on the midline of the knee and around the patella, including arthritis and a build-up of scar tissue under the patella itself.

Pain through the center of the knee usually shows up in *Virasana* (Hero's Pose). Just about anyone with tight quadriceps will feel a generalized pressure or pain through the centerline of his or her knee in this posture. If this is the case, elevate the pelvis so that the knee is not as deeply flexed.

Locked or Hyperextended Knees

I often get asked about "locked" knees and what that means. First off, it could mean a number of things. But I believe most people are referring to hyperextending the knees. Keep in mind that a hyperextended knee is usually that way genetically. In other words, the shape of the bones lends itself to this position. In a hyperextended knee the natural position of the bones requires less muscular effort. But in this position, the tensegrity or supporting tension surrounding the joint is also gone. Without this support, the adaptability of the knee is weakened. The joint loses its critically important ability to respond to changes and demands from above and below. Additionally, bone compression and tension are being loaded onto the PCL and hamstrings, which must resist the bones moving into hyperextension.

It is this adaptability, or lack thereof, that I focus on when looking at the knees. I avoid using the word "locked" because it is a loaded word, and people have preconceived ideas about what it means. Instead, I look at the knee's ability to adapt and change through movement. If the person moves "robotically" through the legs, I'll have them soften their knees a bit to help reintroduce the tensegrity of the knee by forcing the muscles to engage. This also helps to realign the femur and tibia relative to one another. If they're being soft in their knees statically (keeping them bent when they should be more straight), I'll often have them straighten their knees more and engage the quadriceps, as this is a stronger position for the knee.

Even if you don't have hyperextended knees, it's easy to see how a slight bend in the knees can help realign the tibia and femur. Let's use Triangle Pose as an example. When you set up to do *Trikonasana,* you will often find that the extended leg you are about to fold over is internally rotated. To see this just look at the knee and note what direction it is pointing. Most people's knee will be pointing inward. However, if you put a slight bend in the knee, you will find it then points straight ahead, aligning the two bones and the knee with the direction of movement.

4
THE HIP JOINT

For all of its strength, the hip joint is an extremely moveable joint. The potential range of motion is quite large and diverse considering its location, the amount of weight it supports and the force it generates. The hip joint is at the heart of the propulsion system of our bodies. Huge amounts of force are generated at this joint to move us forward when walking and running.

The hip joint itself is the meeting of the ball (known as the head) at the top of the thigh bone (femur) with either side of the pelvis.

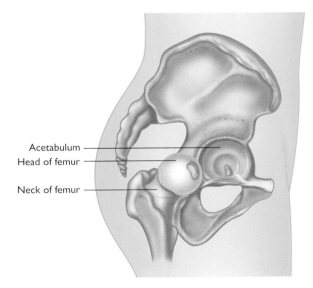

Acetabulum ———
Head of femur ———
Neck of femur ———

Figure 4.1: *The hip joint.*

More specifically, the ball meets the pelvis in the large depression called the acetabulum, which is derived from a Latin word meaning "vinegar cup." The deep depression or socket on the pelvis and the nicely shaped ball on the end of the femur contribute greatly to the strength of this joint.

The hip joint is also designed to support the upper body, including the spine, while standing and while on the move. If you look closely at the socket, you will notice that the top portion is like an overhang, but the bottom is open. It looks as if the pelvis has two shelves that stick out and rest on the top of the femur for support.

On the surface of the acetabulum is a kind of meniscus, or additional piece of cartilage, called the labrum, which is Latin for "lip." This added piece of cartilage deepens the acetabulum and results in a more stable connection between the two bones. It functions much like the meniscus in the knee. The labrum can be damaged and torn, although this isn't particularly common, unless you're a dancer or gymnast. A labrum tear is often associated with pain and clicking in the hip joint, similar to what you find in a knee with a damaged meniscus.

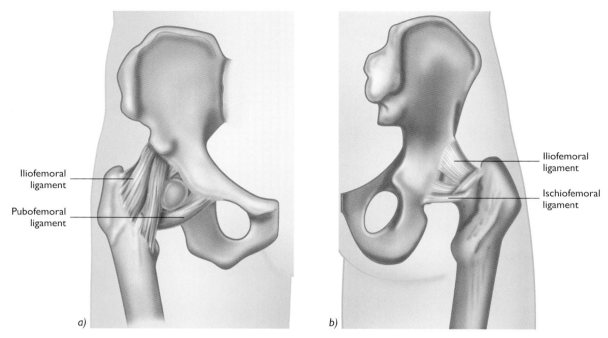

Figure 4.2: *The ligaments of the hip joint, a) right leg, anterior view, b) right leg, posterior view.*

LIGAMENTS OF THE HIP JOINT

The ligaments around the hip joint are particularly strong and dense. They lie on top of and are integrated with the joint capsule itself. There are two in the front (iliofemoral and pubofemoral ligaments) and one in the back (ischiofemoral ligament). As in many places in the body, there is debate as to how much each ligament restricts movement in a particular direction. For our purposes, know that every movement is checked or restricted by at least one portion of these three ligaments and that together with the joint capsule they provide incredible stability at the hip. This joint is so stable that dislocation at the hip is quite uncommon. There is only a little hip joint distraction (creating space between joint surfaces by pulling the femur away from the pelvis) even under extreme forces. After all, the ligaments and joint capsule support approximately two-thirds of your body weight when you are standing![13]

MOVEMENTS OF THE HIP JOINT

The possible range of movement in the hip is tremendous. It moves forward and backward, which we call flexion and extension. It moves sideways, which we call abduction and adduction. It also rotates both internally and externally (medial and lateral rotation). But just because a joint has the *potential* to move in all these directions doesn't mean that it does. So what restricts the joint so much?

We face the same restriction in the hip as we do in every other joint in the body. In addition to taking a look at our converging histories to see what is holding us back, we must also look at the structure of the joint (the bones themselves) and the tissues that surround and support it. As always, the very elements that create the joint can also restrict our ability to move it to its fullest potential.

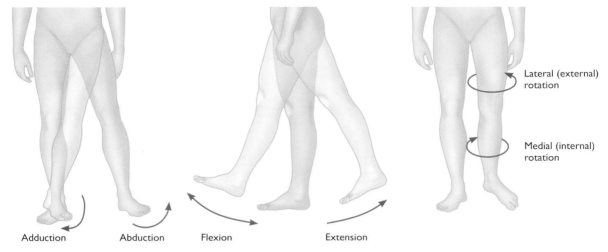

Adduction   Abduction   Flexion   Extension   Lateral (external) rotation   Medial (internal) rotation

Figure 4.3: *Movement of the hip joint.*

BONE SHAPES AND ANGLES

Bone shapes and angles, that is, the structure of the joint itself, can sometimes limit our ability to get into a yoga pose. The hips are one of two places in the body where we see the most variation in bone shape and its effect on movement. (The shoulder is the other.) Because the hip is one of our most mobile joints, it is an easy place to observe our restrictions relative to other people.

There is no doubt that people are built differently. Their bones have different shaped ends, lengths, and proportions. While it is true that some people will never do a pose the way it is seen in yoga books because they have a different bone structure or shape, this is less common than you would suspect. We need to look closely to determine whether our limitations are a result of bone-on-bone compression or another reason.

In some joints, limitations due to bone structure are pretty obvious. In the elbow, for instance, it is easy to see the end range of motion when bone bumps into bone. (Please note, "bumping bones" is not painful.) In other joints, it is less obvious if the end range of motion is due to bone-on-bone compression. I find that making this determination is most challenging in the hip. In my mind, the only way to know for sure if you have hit bone on bone in a forward bend would be to have an X-ray taken while in the pose.

Most people (80–90% of the population), even with all of our slight differences, tend to have a "normal range of motion." In essence, if you apply a bell curve to a particular joint, most people will fall in the center of it. Then you will have 5% to 10% on one end of the curve, with less range of motion due to bone shape, and another 5% to 10% on the other end, who have more range of motion due to bone shape. If you take the 10% with less than normal range of motion and compare them to the 10% at the other end of the spectrum, the vast difference between them doesn't accurately reflect the remaining 80% of people. So not everyone will look the same in a particular *asana*, and trying to get them to would be fruitless, not to mention being completely out of line with what yoga is about.

These anatomical variations do not make a huge impact on range of motion unless you are at the extreme ends; we definitely see a great deal of

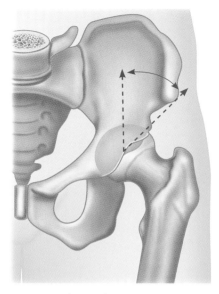

Figure 4.4: *Center edge angle.*

The angle of acetabular anteversion measures how much the socket points forward instead of straight out to the side. The average for men is 18.5 degrees and for women is 21.5 degrees. Increases in this angle are normally associated with decreased joint stability. As yogis, however, an increased acetabular anteversion could create a larger range of motion in the hip.[15]

The angle of inclination of the femur is the angle created by the shaft of the femur and the angle of the neck of the femur. In early infancy, this is about 150 degrees. It decreases to an average of 125 degrees by adulthood and then to 120 degrees for the average elderly person. Again, this angle definitely varies among people and between sexes; women tend to have a smaller angle than men due to their wider pelvis.[16]

variation in the angles that come together at the hip. There are two angles of the acetabulum itself, the angle of the neck of the femur in two directions, and the length of the neck of the femur. The first angle of the acetabulum measures whether it is facing more laterally or pointed downwards more. This is technically called the center edge angle. Given the differences between the male and female pelvis, it is somewhat surprising that men and women have fairly similar angles here. The average for both is about 38 degrees. The ranges in both sexes vary from 22 to 42 degrees.[14]

Now let's look at the angle of torsion of the femur. If we lay a femur on a table and kneel at the edge of it so that our eyes are in line with it, we would normally find that the head of the femur was sitting up at an angle. This is the angle of torsion. Again this angle changes as we age. The change is dramatic when we're very young and slows as we grow older. The angle of torsion is about 40 degrees in a newborn and decreases

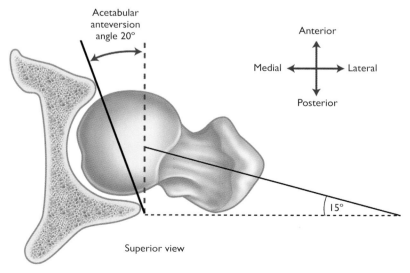

Figure 4.5: *Acetabular anteversion.*

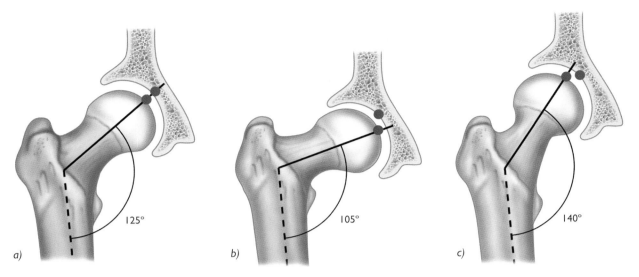

Figure 4.6: *Angle of inclination; a) normal, b) coxa vara, c) coxa valga.*

approximately 1.5 degrees per year until growth ends in a child. In adults, the average angle is between 10 and 15 degrees, but can vary from 7 to 30 degrees. That's a large variation![17]

The last measurement that we need to pay attention to in the femur is the length of the neck. Although I can't find any specific measurements on an average neck, there are definitely differences in length. You can argue that different lengths of the neck force the greater trochanter to hit the pelvis sooner or later in movements of abduction and adduction. However, some individuals have a notch on the neck of their femur called an iliac impression, which allows for more flexion.[18] In addition,

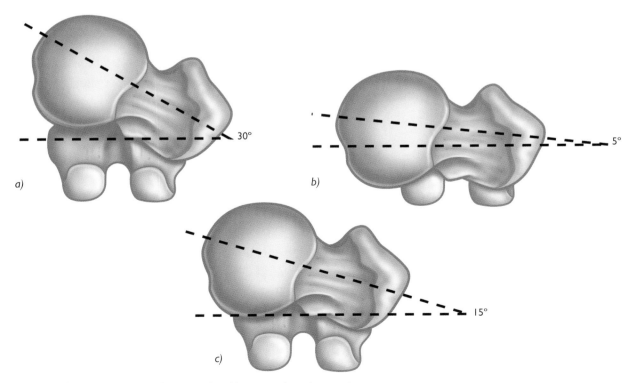

Figure 4.7: *Angle of torsion; a) antetorsion, b) retrotorsion, c) normal.*

there are two "types" of hip configuration. These types are extremes of the variations we have been discussing and represent the result of functional adaptation. They are known as Type 1 and Type 2. In a Type 1 configuration, you find a fuller femoral head. In other words, the head is almost a full sphere. This creates a larger angle of inclination and a larger angle of torsion. In "Type 1s" you also tend to find that the shafts of the femur are slender and the pelvis is generally smaller. In this type, you typically find a greater range of motion and speed of movement.

You see the opposite angles and sizes in "Type 2s." The head of the femur is more like a half-moon and the angle of inclination and torsion are both smaller. The shaft of the femur is thicker and the pelvis is larger and broader. The range of motion is decreased, but the joint is stronger. This configuration is considered more powerful.[19]

If we were to look at a row of femurs and see all of the variations present in these two types and everything in between, we would find ourselves right where we began this discussion. We should be asking, "How old is this person?" "Are they male or female?" "What activities did they do as children?" "What culture are they from?" and so on. We should go back to their converging histories.

It is tempting to take all these questions to the next level and ask which femur and hip configuration is a boon to the yoga practitioner and which is detrimental. But the reality is that, without an X-ray, we will never know for certain the details of our hip. We will never be able to say for certain that our bone structure is holding us back. There is no easy answer. We are more than bones. We're complex and integrated creations, and all of our facets play a role. To really learn about how we're made, we have to research through experience. We have to practice.

MUSCLES OF THE HIP JOINT

The hip joint is a multi-axial joint. This means that it can move around more than one axis. Not only can it flex, extend, abduct, and rotate, but with its ball and socket configuration, it can also move on any axis between these basic movements. With a joint that has the possibility to move at so many different angles, you must have muscles that can pull the femur in all of these directions, too. The tissues around the hip joint do just that-they attach to and cross the hip joint at all of the angles necessary to move it effectively. It goes without saying that any of these muscles, if tight, can also limit the hip's range of motion.

There is more than one way to describe the muscles and group them. We can label them based on location (anterior, posterior, lateral, or medial), and we can classify them by function (abductors, adductors, flexors, extensors, or medial or lateral rotators). We could even discuss them by muscle group (gluteals, adductors, quadriceps, or hamstrings). Because things get complicated and we don't want to miss any of the tissues around this joint, we will use a combination of labels, and I'll mention the overlaps as they occur.

The Quadriceps

Most people are familiar with the quadriceps muscles, located on the front of the thigh. The name *quadriceps* comes from the four distinct parts or muscles that are grouped together. "Quad" means four and "ceps" refers to divisions or heads. In sum, the name tells us this is a four-headed muscle group. All four parts of the quadriceps group share the same distal attachment on the big bump (tibial tuberosity) located just below the kneecap (patella) on a straight knee. The same is not true for the other end of each of these muscles.

To keep things simple, we'll start with the quadriceps that only attach onto the femur (there are three). Their function is dedicated to extending the knee. These three muscles are named by their location. They are vastus medialis (inside), vastus lateralis (outside), and vastus intermedius (between). The word *vastus*, by the way, means vast.

The fourth of the quadriceps, rectus (straight) femoris (femur), does not attach onto the femur. Instead, its proximal attachment is on the front of the pelvis on a little bump called the AIIS (anterior inferior iliac spine). This is a significant difference. Because it attaches onto the pelvis, it crosses the hip joint. It has the ability to create movement at the hip, as well as at the knee. Due to its attachment on the pelvis, the rectus femoris is also capable of moving the pelvis into an anterior tilt. This muscle is a two-joint muscle. It crosses the knee and the hip. Keep in mind that, in two-joint muscles, the position of one joint affects the amount of tension through the muscle and thus impacts the other joint's ability to move. For the same reason a muscle can move two bones relative to one another, they can also restrict movement at the joint.

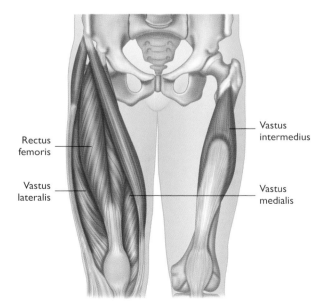

Rectus femoris

Vastus lateralis

Vastus intermedius

Vastus medialis

Figure 4.8: *The quadriceps.*

The quadriceps can restrict several movements that we see in yoga postures. They can restrict our ability to do Hero's Pose by not letting us flex the knees completely. In some backbending postures, the quadriceps can restrict our ability to posteriorly tilt the pelvis.

The Hamstrings

Where does the word hamstring come from? Apparently these same muscles (really their tendinous end near the knee joint) were used to hang pigs in the market years ago. There was also a medieval method of "hamstringing" your opponent in battle. You would do this by severing these unprotected tendons just above and behind the knee in battle. You rarely see this group of muscles referred to by any other name, but their Latin name is the ischiotibialis group. The name makes perfect sense considering the muscles attach from the ischium to the tibia.

Like the quadriceps, the hamstrings are two-joint muscles. Because they affect two joints, the positioning of one joint will affect the tension at the other end of the muscle and therefore the joint that it crosses.

There are three hamstring muscles in the group: the semimembranosus, semitendinosus, and biceps femoris. The biceps femoris has two parts to it (hence the word *biceps*, meaning two heads). These muscles attach at the top (or proximal end) directly to the sit bone (the ischial tuberosity). On the opposite (or distal end), the three muscles cross the knee joint, two going to the inside and one to the outside of the knee. The semimembranosus and semitendinosus attach on the inside. The biceps femoris attaches on the outside of the knee at the very top of the fibula.

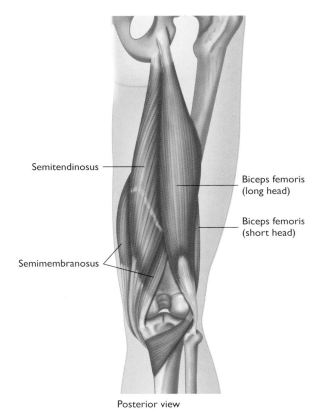

Semitendinosus

Biceps femoris (long head)

Biceps femoris (short head)

Semimembranosus

Posterior view

Figure 4.9: *The hamstrings.*

The hamstrings are best known for two main functions. They extend the hip joint by pulling the leg backward. They also flex or bend the knee. Two lesser-known functions of the hamstrings are internal and external rotation of the knee when the knee is bent at 10 degrees or more. The hamstrings also assist in rotating the hip joint internally and externally.

Of course, the type of posture most often restricted by the hamstrings is the forward bend. If we look at a forward bend more closely, we see the concept of the two-joint muscle in play. Bending the knees in forward bends shows how changing the tension at one joint (the knee) allows greater freedom at the second joint (the hip). These same muscles also restrict our ability to move our pelvis in an anterior tilt, as we can sometimes see in a Downward Facing Dog, where the pelvis is in a posterior tilt and the lower back is rounded.

Palpate Your Hamstrings

It is easy to feel the hamstrings behind the knee. You can palpate the tendons of these muscles just before they cross the knee joint. If you'd like to feel this for yourself, sit on the floor and bend your knee about 90 degrees. Place your fingers (spread them apart a bit) on the back of your thigh so that both index fingers are just touching your calf on both sides. Now, gently pull your heel into the floor and you should feel the hamstring tendons tighten against your fingers. They are surprisingly hard, almost like bone.

The most obvious tendon toward the middle and inside of the knee is that of the semitend-inosus muscle. If you slip off it towards your inner thigh, you will land on another obvious tendon,

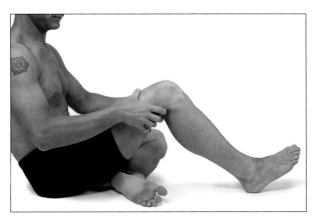

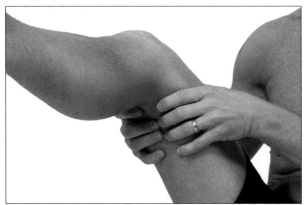

Figure 4.10: *The tendons are obvious when you pull your heel into the floor.*

this one belonging to the semimembranosus muscle. Lastly, on the other side of the knee is the biceps femoris tendon, which you can pretty easily feel as it attaches onto the head of the fibula. Now that you are clear on where these tendons are, and your fingers are still on them, rotate your lower leg internally and externally to feel the tendons move.

The Adductors

The adductor group of muscles is located in the front and inside of the thigh. The primary action of this group is, as the name suggests, adduction. In conjunction with adducting, they are also flexors. Although it is debatable, the adductors are also generally considered to be medial rotators of the hip joint. As a group, they help lift your leg in front of you (flexion), bring it towards the midline (adduction), and rotate it inwards (medial rotation). Thus the adductors collectively restrict the leg from moving backwards, moving outwards, and rotating externally.

The adductor group attaches at a relatively small area at the top of the pubic bones on either side of their two branches. At the bottom end of the muscles, they attach to a ridge running down the back of the femur known as the linea aspera. The following muscles are part of the adductor group: adductor longus, adductor brevis, adductor magnus, pectineus, and gracilis. Because these muscles attach to the pubic bone, they also have an effect on the positioning of the pelvis. That is, they can pull down on the front of the pelvis and contribute to an anterior tilt. This can happen on one or both sides.

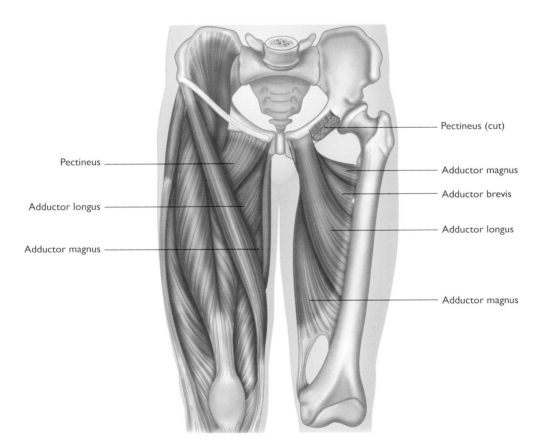

Pectineus

Adductor longus

Adductor magnus

Pectineus (cut)

Adductor magnus

Adductor brevis

Adductor longus

Adductor magnus

Figure 4.11: *The adductors.*

The most common yoga pose in which people are limited by their adductors is *Baddha Konasana*, or Cobbler's Pose (see opposite). This posture requires two actions that are the opposite of what these muscles do. In *Baddha Konasana*, we abduct (opposite) and externally rotate (also opposite) the femur. We experience the limiting effects of the adductors as tension in the "groin." We can also easily see or feel the tendinous attachment of these muscles popping up when we are in the pose.

These muscles restrict movement in other postures as well. One that comes to mind is *Virabhadrasana* II (Warrior II). At first glance you may not see the connection between Warrior II and the adductors, but if you take a closer look at the pose and imagine the pelvis under the skin in the front leg, you will see that the hip joint is both abducted and externally rotated relative to the pelvis. Yogis often look at how much tilt is in the pelvis in Warrior II. The tighter the adductors, the more likely it is that the pelvis will tilt anteriorly (making the butt stick out). The more open and flexible the adductors are, the easier it is to keep the pelvis in a neutral position.

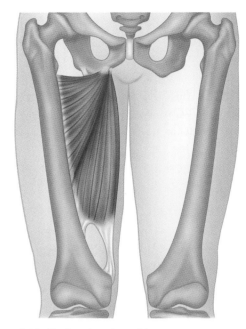

Figure 4.13: *Notice that the adductor magnus attaches to the same place (sit bone) as the hamstrings.*

The adductor magnus has an attachment on the lower of the two branches of the pubic bones and is closely related to the hamstrings. Technically, this point of attachment is called the inferior ramus. If you look closely, you will see that the inferior ramus becomes the sit bone. The attachment of the adductor magnus is far enough back that you often find the most posterior parts of this muscle function right along with the hamstrings in extending the hip. For this reason, it is sometimes referred to as the fourth hamstring.

The Gluteals

The gluteal muscles (glutes) work opposite the adductor muscles on the front and inside of the hips. There are three glutes on the lateral side and back of the pelvis. Most people are familiar with the largest of them, the gluteus maximus. There are two others that are smaller and partially covered by the gluteus maximus. The smallest and deepest of the group is the gluteus minimus. The third is the gluteus medius, and as its name suggests, is in the

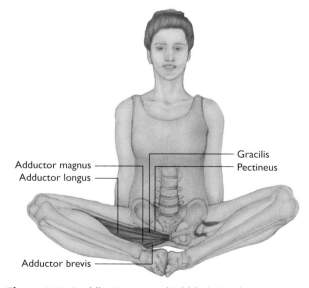

Adductor magnus —
Adductor longus —
Gracilis
Pectineus
Adductor brevis —

Figure 4.12: *Baddha Konasana (Cobbler's Pose).*

middle of the other two glutes, both in terms of size and depth.

As a group, the gluteals internally rotate, externally rotate, and abduct the hip. They also flex and extend the leg at the hip. That's right— the same muscle can have different sections that do opposite actions.

First, let's look at the gluteus minimus and medius together. They are quite similar to the deltoids of the shoulder. If you look at these muscles from the side, you will see that a portion of their fibers attaches more forward on the pelvis while other fibers attach further back. Where they attach on the femur reveals whether they pull the leg forward or back. Those fibers of the glutes that are closer to the front of the pelvis attach to the front of the greater trochanter. They have the ability to pull the femur forward and internally rotate it. The fibers further back on the pelvis attach towards the back of the greater trochanter. They pull it back and externally rotate it.

The glutes are collectively responsible for abduction from anatomical position. Now, while we don't often find ourselves doing that

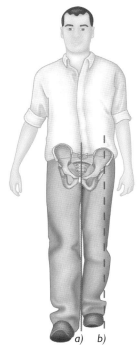

Figure 4.15: *The line of gravity (a) shifts toward the leg that is bearing weight (b) while walking. The gluteals prevent us from falling over by stabilizing the hip joint.*

particular action, we do contract these muscles regularly. Every time we take a step forward, we have to stabilize the pelvis and torso relative to the leg. As we walk, our center of gravity shifts from both legs to one leg. As a result, the bulk of our weight pulls us off the standing leg towards the other side of the body. This pull on our body happens primarily at the hip joint. The glutes on our standing leg contract and stabilize the hip. Through their stabilization, they prevent adduction at the hip. If they didn't contract, we would fall over or we would walk more like primates, throwing our weight from side to side when upright. You could say that preventing adduction is equal to creating abduction even when there is no actual movement occurring.

Large amounts of walking, running, cycling, and other activities that rely heavily on this repeated motion can create tight hips. There are always exceptions, but when you ask the average runner who comes into a class to sit down on the floor (much less try to do a Half-Lotus or

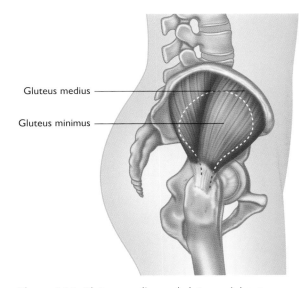

Gluteus medius

Gluteus minimus

Figure 4.14: *Gluteus medius and gluteus minimus.*

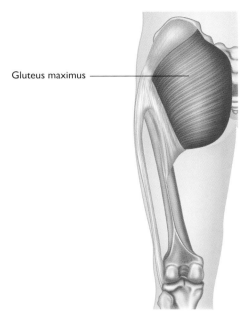

Figure 4.16: *Gluteus maximus.*

Baddha Konasana), you will quickly observe overall tension in their hip joint. In any of these postures, a runner's knee will commonly stick up at about a 45-degree angle.

So why do the abductors of the hip play such an important role in our ability to cross the legs in a Half-Lotus position, for example? Well, as I mentioned earlier in this section, the same muscle fibers that are so involved in walking and running also flex/extend and internally/externally rotate the hip. If the muscle is tight due to one of these repeated movements (as in the examples above), it naturally influences the joint's ability to do other movements. Thus tight hips from running and other activities can make it difficult to rotate the hip as well.

As its name suggests, the gluteus maximus is a large muscle. It extends and externally (laterally) rotates the hip. However, it doesn't assist in these actions until the demands are high enough. For instance, in regular walking, the gluteus maximus does not contract. But in running, it would contract to help extend the hip. You can see this phenomenon in yoga postures that require effort in this area, such as backbending and Warrior 1. Although not everyone needs to, most people will naturally tighten the buttocks to help extend the hip joint when pushing up into a backbend. In Warrior 1, the gluteus maximus resists flexion at the hip joint of the front leg, supporting the body weight and essentially keeping our hip from dropping too low.

The Deep Six Lateral Rotators

The deep six lateral rotators are a group of muscles under the gluteus maximus. They are

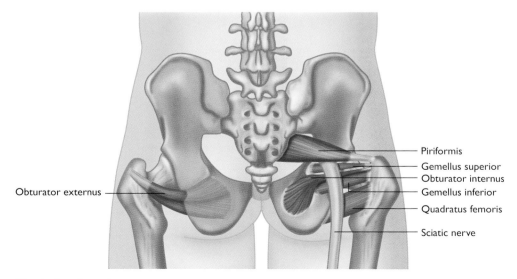

Figure 4.17: *The six deep lateral rotators.*

at the same depth as the gluteus minimus and the deepest part of the gluteus medius. In fact, when you look at an image of these muscles, you will notice that the minimus and medius are part of a fan of tissues that are on the back and side of the hip joint.[20] Most of these muscles are not well known, so here is the list from their orientation top to bottom: piriformis, gemellus superior, obturator internus, gemellus inferior, obturator externus, and quadratus femoris. The deep six lateral rotators attach in various places on the pelvis and then head off to attach to the back part of the greater trochanter.

The first muscle in the list, the piriformis, is the most well known. It has gotten a lot of attention in the yoga world and for good reason: the piriformis can create significant problems because of its relationship with the sciatic nerve. However, because of its popularity, any pain or problem in the buttocks is often associated with the piriformis. While this muscle may sometimes be the culprit, it can be easy to obscure the effects of the other deep six rotators on this area of the body or dismiss the possibility that something else is creating the problem.

The piriformis lies directly on top of the sciatic nerve as it comes out of the greater sciatic notch on the back of the pelvis. The sciatic nerve normally runs under the piriformis muscle before heading down the back of the leg, under the hamstrings, splitting just above the knee to feed the lower leg. However, there are variations; and in a very small percentage of the population, the sciatic nerve runs over or through the piriformis.

If the piriformis muscle is tight, it can compress the sciatic nerve and create any number of sensations, including pain, tingling, and numbness. Essentially, this is one of the causes of sciatica (although technically referred to as piriformis syndrome). The

other main cause of sciatica is compression of the nerves as they exit the vertebrae in the spine. Because the piriformis attaches from the sacrum (on the inside of the pelvis) to the large bump (the greater trochanter) near the top of the femur, it crosses (and therefore affects) two joints, the hip joint and the sacroiliac (SI) joint. Let's tackle the SI joint first.

Because the piriformis attaches inside the sacrum and then travels forward (anteriorly) to attach to the top of the greater trochanter on the femur, its tension pulls or holds the sacrum forward. A similar movement at the SI joint would be called counter-nutation. Normally the piriformis helps maintain the position of the sacrum relative to the pelvis. You could think of it as a stabilizer of the SI joint, as opposed to a mover. Whenever the SI joint finds its way out of place or is causing pain, it's a good idea to look at what's going on with the piriformis.

From the anatomical position, the piriformis is said to perform two actions: lateral (external) rotation of the hip and abduction of the hip. Therefore, the opposite actions of internal

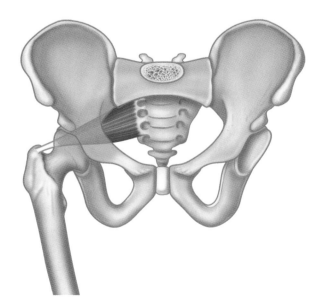

Figure 4.18: *The piriformis attaches to the anterior surface of the sacrum.*

rotation and adduction stretch the piriformis (along with the other deep six lateral rotators) in this position. Interestingly, this isn't true when the hip joint is in a flexed position. (Normally if we do the opposite of a muscle's primary action, we will stretch that muscle. However, if we're not in anatomical position, that could change.)

When the hip is flexed, the orientation of these muscles changes and the deep six lateral rotators actually require lateral (or external) rotation to stretch. Think of Pigeon Pose. In the front leg, the hip joint is flexed and laterally rotated, so you will feel the stretch or pressure in the buttocks. Stretching these tissues actually helps increase the amount of lateral rotation at the hip joint when the leg is in a flexed position. The deep six do not exist in a vacuum; other muscles, such as the adductors and any other internal rotators, also need to be flexible enough to allow these actions to happen.

The Psoas

Chances are you have heard of the psoas, but do you know where on the body to locate it? The typical response to this question is a lot of pointing. I normally see a room full of people pointing to various places on their body. Most people point at their stomach. Others go to their back. Some get a blank look on their face because they've never heard of it or because they're ashamed that they *have* heard of it (possibly even used it in a sentence) but aren't sure where it is. If there is one muscle every human being should be aware of, it's the psoas. It is the single most important postural and structural muscle in the body and has a powerful effect on how you move. The psoas lies deep in the body, at the very core of who we are physically. In fact, its

functions are related to posture, movement, balance, breath, and energy. Its connections span across the pelvis and connect the upper half of the body to the lower half. It crosses no fewer than nine joints on the journey from its proximal to distal attachments. If we intend to move in a way that is both strong and soft, both floaty and grounded, we must bring our attention to the psoas.

Psoas literally means "muscle of loin" (Greek). Three muscles are associated with what we refer to as the psoas: the psoas major, psoas minor, and iliacus. The psoas major refers to the larger of the two psoas muscles, and the psoas minor refers to the smaller of them. The psoas minor is present in perhaps half the human population and is fairly insignificant for our discussion.[21]

The third muscle is the iliacus. Iliacus refers to the ilium or pelvic bone. The iliacus and psoas major are often combined and called the iliopsoas muscle. We group them together for two reasons: first, their distal ends merge together into one common tendon and attach to the same place; second, because they share the same attachment and create the same action (flexion and external rotation) when they contract and shorten. For the most part, when you hear the word psoas thrown around in a yoga context, people are generally talking about the psoas major, even though functionally the iliacus is involved.

Attachments

(We will not discuss psoas minor here.) The psoas major's proximal (closest to the head) attachment is on the bodies of the vertebrae (the bones of the spinal column). Finger-like projections extend from the psoas major and

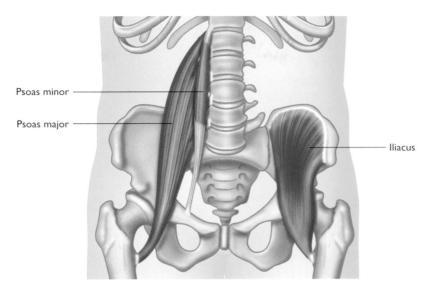

Figure 4.19: *The iliopsoas group.*

attach onto the lateral part (the outside) of the bodies of the vertebrae from T12 through L4 or L5. The muscle then sweeps down the sides of the spine (tapering its way there), drapes over the front of the pubic bone (off center), and then heads back to attach to the lesser trochanter of the femur (its distal attachment).

The proximal attachment of the iliacus muscle is on the inside of the pelvic bowl

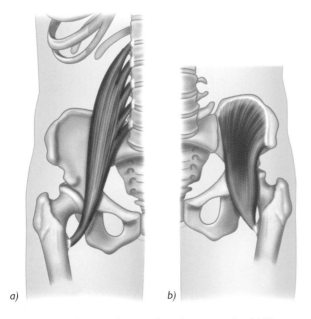

a)   *b)*

Figure 4.20: *The attachments for; a) psoas major, b) iliacus.*

(the ilium). It is worthwhile to note that the attachment site of a muscle isn't always a small spot on a bone, which is a fairly common perception. Instead, some muscles have very broad attachments where the muscle tissue itself covers the tendons that connect them to the bone. This is exactly how this flat, broad muscle is. From its proximal attachment, the fibers of the iliacus head both medially and distally and slowly weave together with the fibers of the psoas major to attach in the very same spot on the femur (the lesser trochanter). Because they both share the same attachment site, they both have the same actions at the hip joint. The psoas major crosses several joints: T12–L1, L1–L2, L2–L3, L3–L4, L4–L5, L5 – sacrum, sacrum and ilium (SI joint), pubic symphysis, and hip joint. That's a total of nine joints crossed and thus potentially affected by the psoas muscle.

Actions

The iliopsoas is a powerful hip flexor. Raising the leg to grab your toe in *Utthita Hasta Padangusthasana* and a pose like *Navasana* both engage the psoas. People often think the quadriceps and abdominals are doing the work here. In fact both are engaged but the quadriceps are working primarily to keep the knee straight while the abdominals stabilize the pelvis so that the psoas can flex the hip(s).

Lateral rotation and abduction of the hip are also associated with the iliopsoas muscle. However, these are secondary functions, and the position of both the torso and the leg matter in using the psoas for these actions. For instance, a pose like *Navasana* requires strong hip flexors to keep the legs raised. When we activate the iliopsoas, the legs typically want to rotate externally. Thus we must consciously internally rotate the legs against the force of the external rotators. Why? The iliopsoas is also a powerful external rotator that is actively used for flexion; if we don't use other muscles that create internal rotation, the strength of the psoas will dominate.

If the upper part of the attachment (say T12–L2) is tight or contracts, then the psoas would pull the upper lumbar/lower thoracic region of the spine down and forwards, creating less space between the lower ribs and the pelvis (spinal flexion). If the lower portion of the muscle with its associated attachment sites (say L2–L5) are tight or contract, it pulls the lumbar region down and forwards, creating an anterior tilt in the pelvis and a stronger lordotic curve. You could say this is spinal extension.

Perhaps more significant and more difficult to see is the psoas' potential to affect the SI joint. We have already talked about the piriformis muscle and its not-so-obvious effect on the SI joint. Well the psoas is the other side of this equation. If you are looking at the pelvis from the side, the piriformis would pull the sacrum and coccyx forward towards the pubic bone, creating a force of counter-nutation on the SI

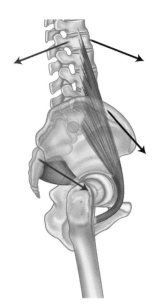

Figure 4.21: *The SI joint acts like an axis and the psoas and piriformis help maintain the balance of the spine around it.*

joint. The psoas creates the opposite action. Because it wraps over the pubic bone as it comes down from the spine and then heads back to attach onto the femur, the tension it places on the SI joint via those vertebrae, moves the coccyx backwards, or away from the pubic bone. This causes the top of the sacrum to move forward (nutation). This becomes clear if you look at the SI joint as an axis of rotation, with the piriformis and psoas on either side of the wheel of the sacrum. These two muscles help maintain balance around the SI joint.[22]

The iliopsoas crosses and sits on either side of our center of gravity. This spot is around the top of the sacrum (it changes slightly from one individual to another based on sex, height, weight, and other anatomical considerations). The bisecting line of the center of gravity is basically through the center of the spine. So, we have a gravitational line ideally running through the spine and dropping through the center of the sacrum and coccyx that crosses a horizontal line that essentially divides us into two equal halves.

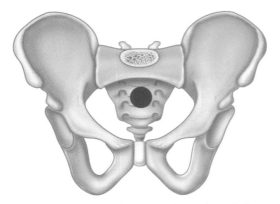

Figure 4.22: *Our center of gravity is located just in front and near the top of our sacrum.*

Because the psoas lies on both sides of this intersection and continues above and below it, it is a strong determinant of where and how this area moves. If you want to move your center of gravity forward or backward, you'd better believe that hip flexion or extension is involved. Even a sideways movement will involve a bit of flexion and stabilization from the psoas muscle around the center of gravity.

This means that the iliopsoas is the functional core of our movement. When practicing, we are either stabilizing or moving into and out of our postures. In order to maintain stability in a pose, the muscles closest to the center of gravity are the primary stabilizers. If we are moving, these same muscles are used to make the movement more efficient.

Evolving this idea, postures always combine movement, technique, flexibility, focus, and integration. Even though certain poses require us to use muscles in our arms or legs, these are attached to a torso that needs to be stabilized. Sometimes this happens while the entire body is in motion. The iliopsoas does not function by itself.

Intentionally focusing on creating movements from this area of your body can be a major step forward in efficiency of movement. By this area of your body I mean the location of the center of gravity as well as those muscles that are closest to it and help stabilize, control, or create movement. These include the psoas on either side, the pelvic floor muscles beneath, and the abdominals in front.

Other Elements

A multitude of other elements are associated with our "core." We have already mentioned the gravitational point that is surrounded by the iliopsoas. Now let's discuss the more subtle qualities of energy. The beginning of the psoas at T12 and its distal attachment on the femur is an energetically critical area. Here you will find the lower three chakras as well as *mula bandha* and *uddiyana bandha*.

The anatomical area of the pelvic floor and the base of the spine both represent the roots of our energetics. The first (root) chakra, or *muladhara*, is located at the base of the spine and is associated with survival, self-preservation, stability, groundedness, and trust. The element associated with it is Earth. *Mula bandha* is associated with preventing the escape of energy through the bottom of the pelvis. *Uddiyana bandha* brings the element of lightness, an upward flying from the roots that have been established. Watching an advanced yogi moving through a dynamic sequence of poses with lightness of limb illustrates correct application of *mula bandha* and *uddiyana bandha*. We must access energy, not just physical strength, to move in this way.

Every time I give a lecture on the psoas in workshops, I ask my students to do a few Sun Salutations with specific instruction to move from and in this place. Most people feel more lightness in their movements, especially in jumping forward and back. They also mention a feeling of focus and calm. It definitely seems a worthy place of putting one's focus. In terms of accessing the *bandhas*, we often look to the physical body for guidance. *Mula bandha* is normally associated with contracting the pelvic floor. Can you guess what muscle would most likely be associated with *uddiyana bandha*? The psoas. This is not to say that you need to contract your psoas to access *uddiyana*, but if there was a physical manifestation of it in the body, the psoas is a strong candidate for its functional representation.

Finding Your Psoas

Let's try to find and access the psoas muscle. First we'll attempt to connect to it with our fingers. (**WARNING!** Do not do this exercise if you are pregnant or have problems of any kind in your abdominal area, including, but not limited to, colitis, constipation, kidney disorders, etc.) The simplest way to find both the iliacus and the psoas major is on the floor. Sit with your legs out and let them relax and roll outwards slightly with a little bend in the knee. Fold a bit at the hips and relax your abdomen. Take both of your hands and find your hip points (the anterior superior iliac spine [ASIS]). Curl your fingers towards the inside of the pelvic bowl so that your fingertips stay as close to the bone on the inside of your pelvis as possible. Sink in maybe an inch, and press gently outwards onto the bone from the inside of the bowl.

Once your fingers are in place, lift one leg. Put it down and then try to lift the other leg. You should feel the tissues under the fingers quite obviously contracting. This is the iliacus. Finding the psoas major may be slightly more challenging. Let your fingers move away from the pelvis itself and towards the spine while

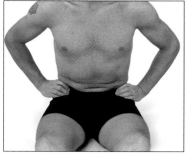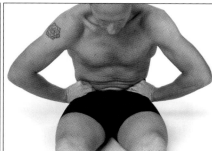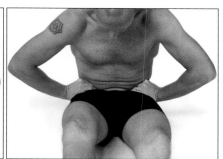

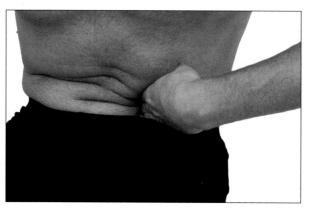

Figure 4.23: *Finding your psoas.*

maintaining the original depth you had when palpating the iliacus. If you lift a leg while doing this, you should feel a line running parallel to the spine pushing up into your fingers. Move your fingers over it from the hip point to the spine. You should be flipping over it if that leg is slightly lifted. This is the psoas.

INTEGRATING ANATOMY INTO YOUR PRACTICE

Exploring the Quadriceps in Warrior 1

The quadriceps are powerful stabilizers of the knee joint and we can feel them at work in the warrior poses. Most people feel the quadriceps working hard in the front leg to prevent the knee from bending (flexing). The position of the leg in Warrior 1 is an example of isometric contraction. No movement is really happening; instead, the prevention of an undesired movement (too much flexion/ bending of the knee) is taking place. The quadriceps don't exist in a vacuum; there are always other muscles helping them. In Warrior 1, the gluteals and hamstrings (hip extenders) also work to prevent further flexion at the hip joint. In other words, these muscles keep the hips from sinking further towards the floor. The quads are in a position of less leverage crossing the knee and thus feel the effects more greatly than the other muscles working to maintain the posture. If you were to stay in any warrior pose for more than about 10 minutes, not only would your quadriceps start to fatigue, so would your glutes and hamstrings.

Exploring Two-Joint Muscles in Virasana, Supta Virasana, and *Uttanasana*

As discussed, both the quadriceps and the hamstrings are two-joint muscles, which means the position of the joint at one end of the muscle will impact the mobility of the joint at the other end of the muscle. This is particularly true when looking at how to lengthen either of these two muscle groups.

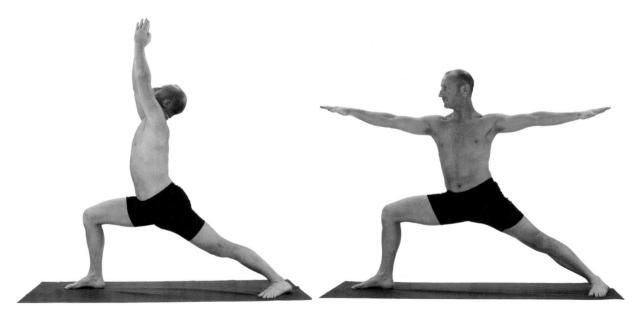

Figure 4.24: *Warrior pose.*

Quadriceps Example

Because the quadriceps extend the knee, if I sit in *Virasana*, the portion that attaches over the front of the knee is maximally lengthened because the knee is completely flexed. If I lay back into *Supta Virasana*, I now start to extend the hip joint. This means that the portion of the quadriceps muscle that attaches across the hip joint and onto the pelvis is also getting stretched. Because I have already lengthened the knee-end of the quadriceps in *Virasana*, as I move into *Supta Virasana* the stretch intensifies because I lengthen both ends of the quadriceps. By taking advantage of the fact that the muscle crosses two joints, I get maximal pressure on the quadriceps in *Supta Virasana*.

Bhekasana is another pose that lengthens the tissue at both ends as it crosses the two joints.

The hamstrings function in a similar way. If you stretch one end first, it is a little more difficult to lengthen the other end. A simple standing forward bend (*Uttanasana*) illustrates this point quite well, especially if your hamstrings are tight. Have you noticed that when the knees are straight, it is harder to fold forward completely at the waist? What happens if you bend the knees? You can usually get your abdomen closer to the thighs, which is full flexion of the hip joints.

What if you bend the knees, place the abdomen on the thighs, and then try to straighten your

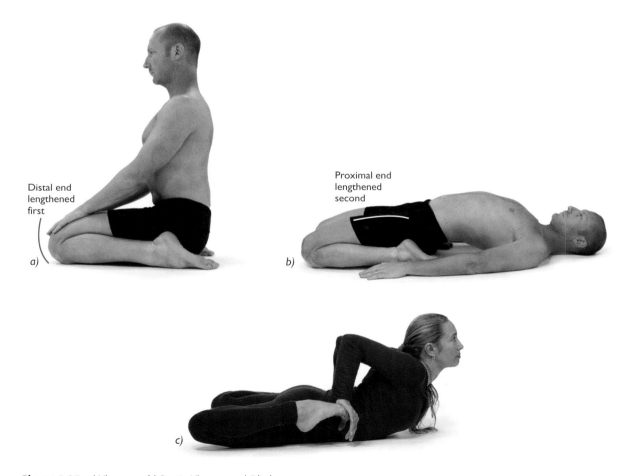

Distal end lengthened first

Proximal end lengthened second

Figure 4.25: *a) Virasana, b) Supta Virasana, c) Bhekasana.*

knees? If you do this slowly, you may feel the tension coming into the area just behind your knees first until the pressure is distributed more evenly throughout the whole of the hamstrings.

That said, forward bending with the knees bent tends to put more pressure on the sit bone end of the muscle group (the ischial tuberosity end) because there is less tension on the muscles as they attach to the knee. In other words, the stretch comes into the upper end more quickly. This can be alleviated very simply. Just try to straighten the knees in *Uttanasana*, even if they remain slightly bent. The action of *trying* to straighten them in this situation increases the tension on the backs of the knees and evens out the pressure between the two ends.

Exploring Torn Hamstring and Sit Bone Pain in *Asanas*

Pain at the sitting bone is a fairly common complaint among yoga practitioners. Sometimes it develops over time, and sometimes it happens after a minor tear to the hamstrings. Sometimes sit bone pain has nothing to do with the hamstrings at all.

I was teaching a workshop when I met a student who had recently "pulled a hamstring." When I saw her again almost a year later, she was still suffering with the same injury. Her major symptom was pain at the sit bone (the ischial tuberosity) when folding forward. It also hurt when sitting for long periods, especially in the car. At times the pain radiated down the back of her leg.

People are often taught to deal with a torn hamstring and sit bone pain by bending their knees in forward bends. The idea is that by bending the knees, you reduce the tension in the hamstrings. It sounds good in theory and might be recommended in some situations, but it's not what I typically advise students when there has been some level of tear.

Because the hamstrings are two-joint muscles, changing the position at one of the two joints (the hip or the knee) changes the end of the muscles that will receive more force from the actual stretch. When you bend your knees in a forward bend, you add more force to the end of the hamstrings that connect to the sit bones. Assuming that you have actually torn your hamstrings (usually a minor tear) close to the sit bones, it would not be wise to put more pressure on these same tissues. So what should we do? I will preface the following example by saying that it may not work in every situation for every individual; however, it has proven to work for a number of my students suffering from this particular irritation.

When I re-entered my student's story, she had been softening her knees in forward-bending postures for almost a year. Her lack of improvement indicated that it wasn't the right advice for her. She had mentioned pain when sitting in the car for long periods of time; in this position, the part of the hamstrings that receives the most pressure is the bottom (distal) end, closest to the knee. I took a moment to gently squeeze that area of her hamstrings (the opposite end of where she felt discomfort in forward bends) and could see in her face that those tissues were particularly tender. With this important information, I figured this technique would likely work for her. It's very simple: keep the knees straight! I told this student it would be worth trying for two or three weeks to see what happens. When you bend forward, either when standing or in seated postures, keep the leg extremely straight and do not go as deeply into the forward bend as you normally would. By keeping the knee straight and the quadriceps engaged, you equalize the stretch in the hamstrings between both ends. In the situation mentioned above, a year of bent-knee forward bends had created hamstrings where their distal end (closest to the knee) had become too tight. Tension in this end leads to consistent tension in the hamstrings as a whole, particularly near the sit bones.

After just four days of practicing in this way, the student's pain had reduced and no longer bothered her when driving. She could also fold deeper in her forward bends with less fear and less pain overall. This is a telling example of the kind of success we can have by looking beyond the body and considering our students' converging histories, by considering what has and has not worked so far, and by being willing to try something new.

Adductors: Are Your Adductors Limiting You in Forward Folds?

Because of its location, part of the adductor magnus is lengthened in a forward bend, and it is possible to have a minor adductor magnus tear that creates sit bone pain. This pain usually manifests in a wide-legged forward bend. In this position the adductors are already lengthened due to the abduction required to take the feet apart. A portion of the adductor magnus attaches onto the ischial tuberosity (sit bone) in a place that makes the posterior portion of the muscle function similarly to the hamstrings, as an extender of the hip joint. Keep in mind that a muscle may perform more than one action. Adductor magnus isn't only an adductor, it also extends and helps to internally rotate the hip. Thus when you add flexion at the hip joint, you further lengthen the adductor magnus.

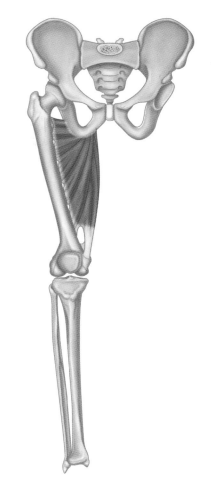

Figure 4.26: *The red area shows the attachment of adductor magnus.*

If you have sit bone pain in a wide-legged forward bend but not when your feet are together, you have most likely torn the fibers of the adductor magnus. If the opposite is true, that is, you feel pain when your feet are together in a forward bend but not when the legs are wide, then you are probably feeling the hamstrings, as we discussed above.

If you keep the knees straight in a forward bend, as suggested for the hamstrings, you will not have the same impact on the adductor magnus because it is not a two-joint muscle. If it does not cross the knee, then bending or straightening the knee will not directly impact the pressure on the sit bone. Nevertheless, you still want to gently stretch the adductor tissues in a variety of ways to avoid letting scar tissue build up. The wide-legged forward bends and other poses that stretch the adductors should help.

Exploring the Piriformis and Deep Six Lateral Rotators in *Asanas*: Double Pigeon or Fire Log Pose

The simplest way I've found to focus on these powerful tissues in my practice is a posture I often give for Lotus preparation. I've heard a couple of names for it, usually Double Pigeon or Firelog. It doesn't really matter what you call it, just how you use the stretch. I also find that the more closely you can approximate a particular pose, the more naturally you can put pressure on the tissues that need to open.

In my workshops I set this up as an experiment to determine what muscles affect Lotus. The experiment has shown over and over again that the deep six rotators and the gluteus minimus and medius are the key culprits restricting access to Lotus Pose. Over the years, in fact, a number of people have managed to get themselves into Lotus on their own for the first time in workshops just by doing this experiment. Depending on where you are in the evolution of the pose, this may be all you need to finally access this holy grail of *asanas*. Those who are miles away from the pose should adopt this position daily. And if you have no problem getting into Lotus, you will still benefit from understanding where your personal restrictions come from. You might even notice a sense of ease and comfort while in Lotus after taking this experiment.

Let's set it up. The first part is to put your legs into a Full Lotus, which means you need to sit on the floor. If you find this difficult, try Half-Lotus on one side and then the other. While in Lotus or Half-Lotus, note the positioning of your top foot, the angle in which your knee is pointing away from the body and the height of your knee from the floor. In addition, absorb the sensations in your buttocks, knees, ankles, feet, and where the shins lie over one another. Feel the general tension of the pose. Now, don't stay here too long or you will be tempted to argue that being in *this* position is what loosened your Lotus.

Now, stack your legs one on top of the other, and put the right leg and shin on top of the left; call that the first side. Make sure not to tuck your feet in too close to your pubic bone. You want your shins to be parallel to the front edge of your mat. There is a tendency for people to put their shins in the correct position and then scoot their butt forward … don't do that! It is also possible that your right knee is floating a little bit off of the left foot. If it is elevated just a few inches, don't worry. If it is more than a few inches, roll up a towel or put a block under the knee. If you are extremely tight, use the variations shown here.

Most often, pressure felt in the knee arrives when the joint is fully flexed. What I like about this prep is that we keep the knee close to 90 degrees, thereby minimizing this pressure. But there are exceptions. Those who already have knee issues might still feel a pinching on the inside or outside of the knee. If this is the case, put something under the knee to lift it a little higher. If that doesn't resolve the sensation in the knee when you move to the next step, instead of folding straight forward, fold at an angle away from the knee that has pain.

Now that you are set up, fold forward over both legs, trying to get your chest to touch your shin (it's ok if it doesn't) and reaching your hands for the floor in front of you. Ninety-eight percent of all people will feel this in the buttock

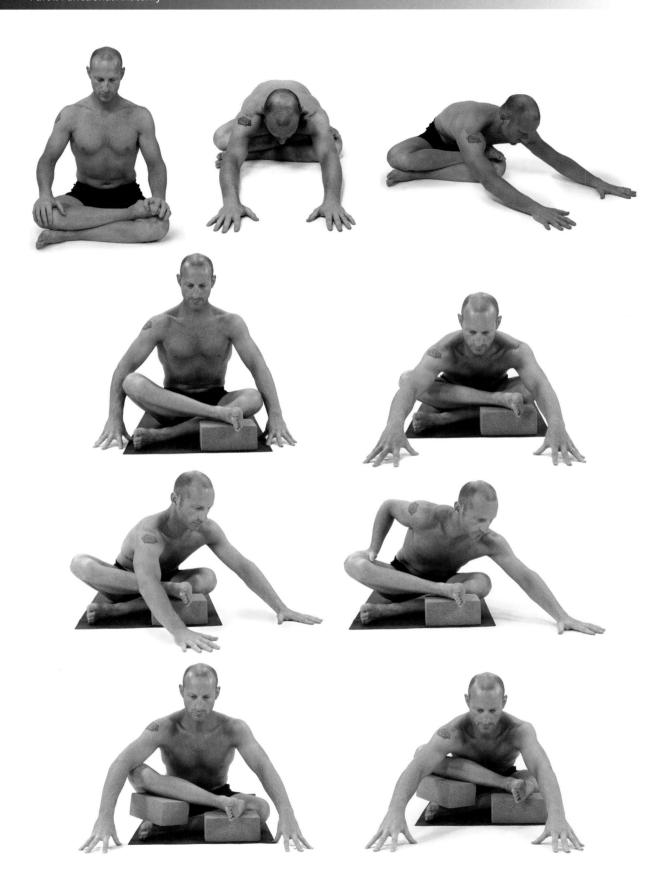

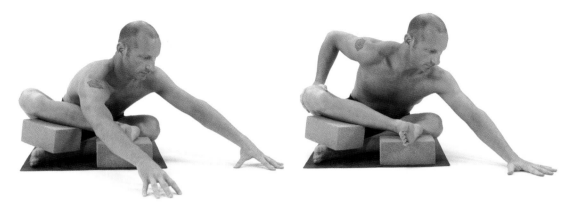

Figure 4.27: *Double Pigeon and Firelog Pose. If you need it you can also use a block, under foot and/or knee to avoid pressure or pain in the knee.*

of the top leg. In this case, if you have done as instructed and put your right foot on top of your left knee, you are feeling it in the right buttock. A small percentage will feel it in the opposite or both sides of their buttocks (which means the person has really tight internal and/or external rotators). Still a few more will feel nothing in the buttocks and only feel something in the hip crease or groin area. This is usually a sharp, pointed sensation. These people may need to stretch the hip flexors first, primarily the psoas. It's also possible that you feel restriction in your adductors.

You should stay in this position for approximately 30 seconds. After 30 seconds, return to an upright position and rotate your torso to the left so that you are facing the right foot as it sits on top of the left knee. Folding again, try to bring the center of your chest to the foot with your hands reaching for the floor. This should increase the amount of pressure in the buttocks and to the deep six muscles we have been talking about. Stay another 30 seconds here. You can take this one step further if you place your right hand on the right thigh about halfway down to your knee or a little beyond, and press your thigh down, externally rotating it with your hand while you continue to reach with your body and the other arm towards the

right foot. Again, stay here for about 30 seconds. Switch sides and repeat on the left.

We have now tested our Lotus to see how much tension is in the hips overall. We then felt the stretch primarily in one place, the buttock. This stretch put pressure on the deep six rotators and the gluteals. Now let's do Lotus again to see what it feels like. So, take the Lotus or Half-Lotus you originally did and again absorb the sensation of the leg in this position. Hopefully it feels more comfortable the second time around.

Exploring the Psoas and *Bandhas* While Jumping Back and Up

One movement ties together the concepts of center of movement, center of gravity, *bandha*, and the psoas. The movement is jumping back from *Uttanasana* into High Plank (or *Chaturanga*) and the returning to *Uttanasana* from Down Dog. These movements are commonly found in Sun Salutations. They are also a place where you can observe someone "floating" back using their *bandhas*.

At its most functional level, the movement back from *Uttanasana* to High Plank is extension of the hips. The returning jump forward is flexion

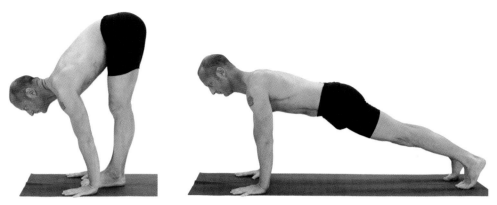

Figure 4.28: *The psoas eccentrically contracts to control the movement at the hip joint as we jump back from the look up position to high plank.*

of the hips. What is moving through the air is the center of gravity. Control of the pelvis, or more specifically, the center of gravity at the sacrum, is what is necessary. What muscle is closest to this area and has the ability to control the hip joint? You got it. The psoas.

The jump back to High Plank requires the practitioner to resist gravity at the hip joint, especially upon landing. The hip flexors engage in an eccentric contraction to prevent extension from happening too quickly or too strongly. We slowly lengthen with tension to prevent the pelvis from sagging and falling as the feet hit the floor.

Going the other way, once we jump from Down Dog into the air, it is the pelvis (center of gravity) that must lift and be balanced in the air. The center of gravity is located at the center of the pelvic bowl, thus intimately tying these two together. Once this happens with support from the arms, the legs must swing in against the resistance of the hamstrings and other hip extenders. This is harder to do in the air because there is less leverage. The action is concentric contraction of the hip flexors. And what is the strongest hip flexor? The psoas. Thus without a doubt, the physical aspect of the float that you see in yoga practitioners is related to the psoas.

Exploring the Psoas in *Asanas*

Everyone always asks, "How do I strengthen my psoas?" Or "How do I stretch my psoas?"

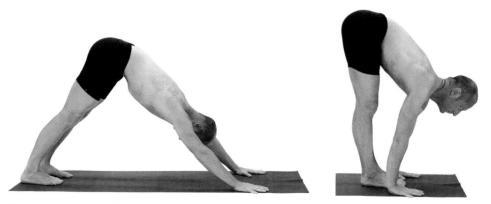

Figure 4.29: *The psoas concentrically contracts to bring the legs forward as we jump forward from downward dog to the look up position.*

First, you shouldn't focus on strengthening this muscle as you would, for example, the quadriceps. This is probably the single most important postural and structural muscle in the body. Changing the tension of it (and thus the tension of all the joints it affects) in a short amount of time is not a good idea. I have had clients over the years who over-zealously tried to strengthen their psoas, and it seemed to lead back to trouble. Alternatively, I suggest that you create a good working relationship with the psoas. *Relationship* means something much different from treating the muscle as if it has something wrong with it. So, how do you do this? It begins with a clear mental intention. Use the simple example of a Sun Salutation to begin.

To answer the second question, "How do I stretch my psoas?" most people need to lengthen this muscle, especially during or before building strength. The muscle is a hip flexor, which means that any strong extension of the hip joint should stretch the psoas. Lunges are a great one. You could also use Warrior 1 with the heel up, or take advantage of the back leg in a Pigeon Pose to stretch the hip flexors, including the psoas.

5
THE PELVIS

In Latin, pelvis means "basin" or "large bowl." The pelvis is not completely fused together until puberty, which is about how long it takes for the fusing to complete. In puberty the bones that comprise each side of the pelvis become completely fused together. This is why we talk about three bones, even though the pelvis looks like it is made of just one.

Your pelvis is at the very center of your body's design; it is at the center of all movement and is key to how we manage gravity. The hip flexors attach both onto and across the pelvis (rectus

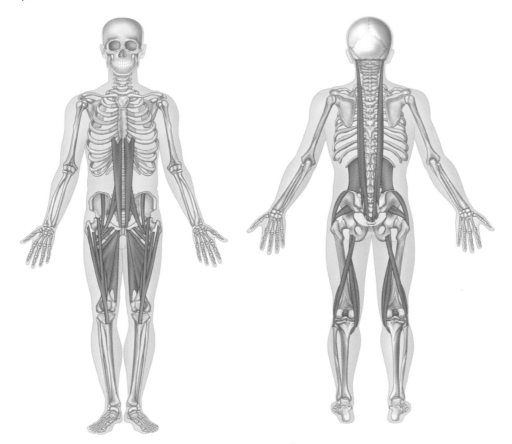

Figure 5.1: *The pelvis is the central hub of attachment for many muscles.*

femoris attaches on the pelvis at the AIIS, and the psoas major goes across it to attach onto the spine) and are responsible for our most important movements—walking. At the back of the bowl, the wedged sacrum is considered the body's center of gravity. The legs dangle from this bowl-shaped structure. The sacrum is literally wedged between the two sides of the pelvis, creating a steady and stable foundation for the spine, which grows upwards from the pelvis like a tree. The spine supports the rib cage as well as the arms, indirectly, which hang off the rib cage.

Many muscles connect from the pelvis and extend both upwards and downwards. The erectors of the spine head up the back of the torso and the hamstrings head down the backs of the legs. The abdominals, quadriceps, and adductors are all located on the front of the body and head off from the pelvis in different directions. Deep inside, part of the iliopsoas attaches to the inside of the pelvis.

In addition to its anatomic centrality, yoga philosophy also emphasizes the importance of the pelvis. The *bandhas*, chakras, and main energetic *nadis* are clustered within this region of the body. This makes it a critically important place to understand and explore from a yogic perspective.

LANDMARKS AND SKELETON

You often hear the word "hips" used to describe the pelvis. Although anatomically correct, the reference is too general for our purposes. As we explored previously, the hip is the joint created by the femur and the pelvis. Used more colloquially, the word "hips" can include the entire pelvis and the muscles and bones of the upper thighs. Sometimes each side of the pelvis is referred to as the hip bone. For our purposes, we will limit our study of the pelvis to the pelvic bones and tissues themselves. The three fused bones of each side of the pelvis are the ilium, ischium, and pubic bone. Other ways of referring to the ilium are the ilia, ilio, and iliac. Other words for the ischium are the ischia, ischio, and ischial. Finally, other words you might hear for pubic could be pubo and pubis. The ilium is the large flat area that I often refer to as the section of the pelvis shaped like an "elephant ear." The pubic bone is located in the front and is associated with the "pubic" region of the body. The ischium is the "rear end" and

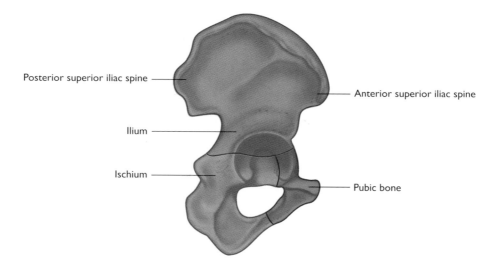

Posterior superior iliac spine

Anterior superior iliac spine

Ilium

Ischium

Pubic bone

Figure 5.2: *The bones of the pelvis.*

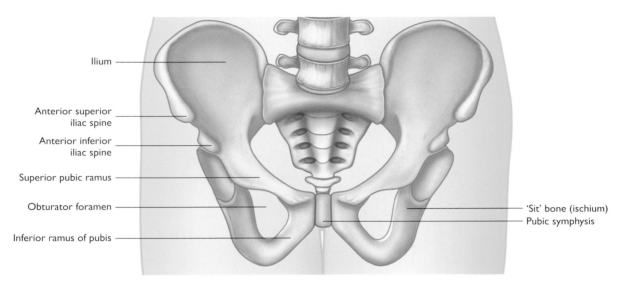

Ilium

Anterior superior
iliac spine

Anterior inferior
iliac spine

Superior pubic ramus

Obturator foramen

Inferior ramus of pubis

'Sit' bone (ischium)
Pubic symphysis

Figure 5.3: *Landmarks of the pelvis.*

back of the pelvis, what we often refer to in yoga as the "sit bones."

These three bones merge together at the center of the deep depression on the pelvis called the acetabulum. This is where the large ball on the end of the femur fits into the pelvis. The two sides of the pelvis are connected in the front by a disc-like piece of cartilage called the pubic symphysis and in the back by the sacrum. The sacrum meets the ilium at the sacroiliac joint.

There are several boney landmarks on the pelvis. I'll describe the most common, including how they got their name, which should help you to remember them. Let's start with a couple that are often referred to in yoga. The "hip points" are the two prominent bumps on the front (one on each side) of the pelvis that are officially known as the ASIS of the pelvis.

There is an iliac spine both on the front and the back of the pelvis. The ASIS is a ridge that runs up the front of either side of the ilium. The ASIS sits at the top of the anterior iliac spine, hence the word superior in its name. The bump below (inferior to) it is called the anterior inferior iliac spine (AIIS). This is the

location for one of the quadriceps attachments. The ASIS has a counterpart on the back of the pelvis known as the posterior superior iliac spine (PSIS). This is the bump on the top of the posterior iliac spine. We most commonly relate this bump to our SI joint. The area between the anterior and posterior iliac spines is commonly called the crest of the ilium. This is the section of bone that you can easily feel on yourself on either side of the body as the top of the pelvis.

In the front of the pelvis we find the pubic bones. They are connected in the middle via the pubic symphysis. This is technically classified as an amphiarthrotic joint and is considered semi-moveable. Fibrocartilage connects the two bones. This piece of cartilage is similar to the discs you find in the spine, except that there is no fluid nucleus. The cartilage is round and held in place by the bones and a wrapping of connective tissue. The pubic bones have two branches (ramii), one above and one below called the superior ramus and inferior ramus, respectively.

On the back and bottom (posterior and inferior) of the pelvis we have the ischium on both sides of the pelvis. The most visible part of the ischium is the ischial tuberosity. In yoga we refer to these as the sit bones. The ischial tuberosities are important attachment sites of the hamstrings. On the lateral side of the pelvis, as we already mentioned, is the deep socket that the head of the femur fits into. This socket creates the actual hip joint and is called the acetabulum, which means "vinegar cup."

PELVIC DIFFERENCES BETWEEN MEN AND WOMEN

There are some differences between the male and female pelvis that are worth mentioning. The shape of the pelvic bowl, the shape of the pelvic inlet (the hole where the pelvic floor muscles reside), and the angle at which the pelvis normally sits all differ between men and women. The female pelvis tends to be slightly wider, and the socket where the thigh bone attaches, the acetabulum, faces slightly more forward than in men. The shape of the pelvic inlet is normally more rounded in women to allow them to give birth.

When we look at the pelvis from the side, we see the two bumps sticking out that we looked at earlier. The ASIS is in front and PSIS in back.

If we draw a line between these two points and measure the angle, in most men the line sits at 0 degrees. In most women, the line tilts down, because the ASIS is lower than the PSIS. The average angle for women is 15 degrees. There are variations among men and women. This is simply a rule of thumb. Factors such as genetics and tensional patterns can create larger or smaller angles between the ASIS and PSIS.

MOVEMENTS OF THE PELVIS

The pelvis sits on top of the heads of the femurs. If the pelvis moves, there is a corresponding movement at the hip joint. Because the pelvis is connected to the sacrum and sits under the spine, movements of the pelvis also lead to movements in the sacrum or spine. When the pelvis moves, it does so at the hip joint and lumbar spine simultaneously.

Movements associated with the pelvis are anterior and posterior tilt, hip hiking, and pelvic rotation. In an anterior tilt, the pubic bone moves down. You can see this best when looking at someone from the side. When the pelvis tilts anteriorly, the pubic bone drops and the lumbar curve is accentuated. This is a

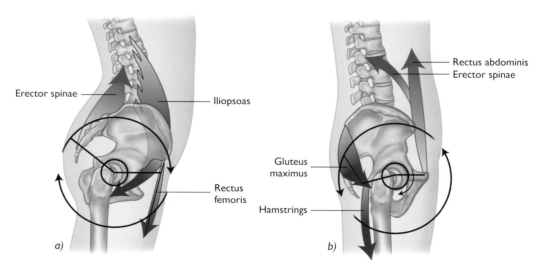

Figure 5.4: *Pelvic tilt; a) direction of anterior tilt, b) direction of posterior tilt.*

good example of the interrelationship between pelvic and spinal movements. A posterior tilt of the pelvis is obviously the opposite movement. Looking again from the side, the pubic bone lifts and the lumbar curve in the lower back flattens.

Having read more than my fair share of anatomy books, you might be interested to know that it is rare to see muscles described as anterior or posterior "tilters" of the pelvis. This is mainly because the pelvis is so often seen as the origin rather than as a more neutral attachment for muscles. In order to create pelvic movement, the muscles that move the legs, spine, and torso flip their origins and insertions as typically defined by anatomists. You might recall that we spoke about this in the muscular system section. I often describe the pelvis as a pulley wheel to clarify this point in workshops. A pulley wheel moves around one axis and can spin in either direction, depending on where the force is coming from. With a pulley, the rope that wraps around it loops around the pulley and heads off in the same direction that it came from. This way, when you pull on one of the two ropes, the pulley rotates. The pelvis is not literally a pulley, but it does rotate. In the case of the pelvis, the "wheel" will either be pulled on from above or from below. Using the pulley metaphor, the ropes end up both above and below and therefore in the front and back of the pelvis. If you take a moment to visualize this pulley wheel, you will see that pulling on it from the front and below will cause the same rotation as pulling on it from the back and above.

Translating this idea onto the pelvis, some muscles that attach to the front of the pelvis extend downwards. These are the adductors, quadriceps, and psoas. They pull the pubic bone down into an anterior tilt. They work in conjunction with the muscles that attach to the back of the pelvis and head upwards. These are

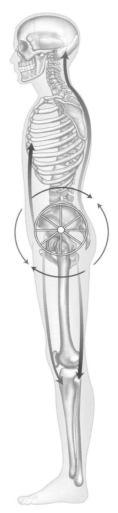

Figure 5.5: *Notice how the front below and back above the pelvis work together to rotate the pelvis down and forward. The opposite is also true, back below, and front above work together to rotate the pelvis back.*

the erector spinae group (the thick muscles on either side of the spine) and the quadratus lumborum (often known as the QL). They take the pelvis into an anterior tilt; you can see them at work in *Utkatasana*.

There are muscles in the front and above the pubic bone that lift the pelvis to create a posterior tilt. These muscles are the abdominals, all of which attach directly or indirectly to the pubic bone. They work in conjunction with the hamstrings. The hamstrings attach to the ischial tuberosities and pull the sit bones down, creating a posterior tilt.

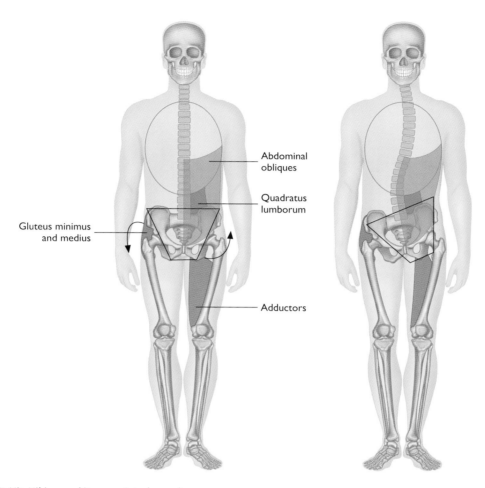

Figure 5.6: *Hip Hiking and its associated muscles.*

Gluteus minimus
and medius

Abdominal
obliques

Quadratus
lumborum

Adductors

"Hip hiking" or lateral pelvic tilt is another movement of the pelvis. When we hike our hip, we lift one hip up towards the rib cage. Although we don't often use this movement in yoga *per se*, it is not uncommon to find that our ribs relative to the pelvis have shortened in certain postures, for example, in Triangle Pose. Although not described as a "hip hike" that is in fact what has taken place. This reveals the interrelationship of the pelvis and spine. In a lateral pelvic tilt, the spine naturally bends to the side (lateral flexion). Pelvic rotation is another pelvic movement that occurs to some degree when we walk. When standing, this movement is normally seen when one side of the pelvis rotates forward around one of the two femurs.

To visualize this movement in *asanas*, we can look at Revolved Triangle. While doing the right side of this pose, not only does the right hip tend to move closer to the ribs, but the left side of the pelvis also tends to drop down. Because the *asana* asks that the pelvis be parallel to the floor, we could say that the pelvis has rotated forward on the left side, or forward towards the floor.

CENTER OF THE BODY

The pelvis is the crossroads of the upper and lower halves of the body. The legs hang from below it and the spine is supported above it. All the muscles that move the thigh bone

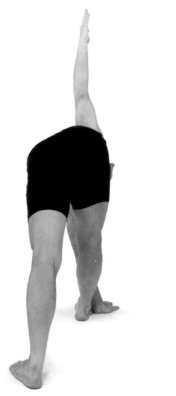

Figure 5.7: *Revolved triangle with the left hip dropping is an example of pelvic rotation.*

(femur) attach to or cross the pelvis. Many of the muscles that move the spine, such as the abdominals, attach to the pelvis. Even the thick and powerful erector muscles (the muscles on either side of the spine), attach to the sacrum.

I think of the pelvis as a secondary or elevated foundation for the body when standing, with the primary foundation being the feet. The feet indirectly support the pelvis. Think of the pelvis as a bowl. Below the bowl are two sticks (the legs) supporting it. If one of those sticks moves forward, it is going to shift the position of the bowl, causing it to tilt one way or another. Any movement that affects the position of the pelvis will affect everything above the pelvis as well.

SACROILIAC JOINT

As a result of the change in sacral positioning, the SI joint is essentially the single place

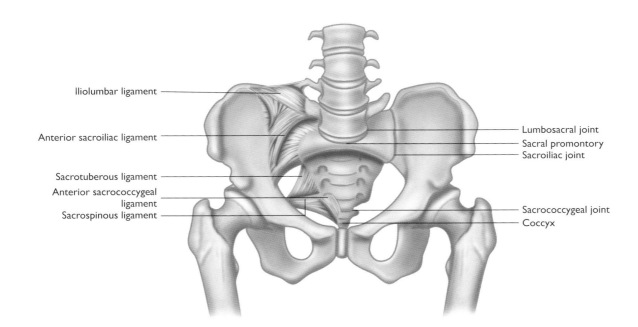

Figure 5.8: *Ligaments around the pelvis and the sacroiliac joint.*

where we have become "upright." To maintain this upright position, dense ligaments are required to hold this joint firmly in place. If they were magically removed for a moment, it is at the SI joint that we would fall forward. Different ligaments in the front (sacroiliac and sacrospinous) and on the back (sacrotuberous) secure the sacrum to the ilium.

At the heart of the joint is the contact between the sacrum and ilium. The surface of the sacrum has a sort of boomerang shape to it that matches up with a similar surface on the ilium. The joint surfaces do have hyaline cartilage and are bathed in synovial fluid, implying that some movement is possible. However, this joint is classified as being a plane or sliding joint. These joints often don't move a great distance.

Movements of the SI Joint

Between these thick, dense ligaments and the actual shape of the joint surfaces, the average person has, at most, a few millimeters of movement at the SI joint.[23] Despite this, there is a lot of talk in the yoga world about SI joint movement. I think it's fair to say that people who are naturally flexible will probably have more than average range of motion at this joint as well. A small portion of people might have an exceptional amount of movement and some might have none at all (some SI joints can

fuse). But overall, the average person has only a few millimeters of available movement at the SI joint.

Within the world of anatomy, the great debate about how movement at the SI joint is created, the type of movement that it is, and the degree of movement continues. Personally, I think the debate continues only because of variations among individuals and the fact that the joint itself changes through the span of our lifetime. If you looked at the movements of my SI joint when I was ten years old, compared to now at age 40, you would see differences, even though I am the same person (or am I?!).

In any case, movement at the SI joint is known as nutation and counter-nutation. Both refer to the tipping of the sacrum forward and backward between the two sides of the pelvis. When the top of the sacrum moves forward and down (anterior and inferior) with the pelvis stable, we call this nutation. Counter-nutation is the opposite movement. In other words, the top of the sacrum moves back and down. To clarify, we are talking about the sacrum rotating within the confines of the two sides of the pelvis. This movement does not involve pelvic tilting. Both nutation and counter-nutation can happen at the same time as pelvic tilting, but the occurrence of one does not imply occurrence of the other. This can get confusing. Keep in mind that the movement

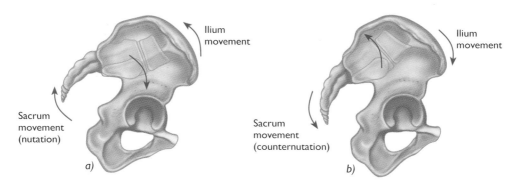

Figure 5.9: *Sacrum forward relative to pelvis is nutation. Sacrum back relative to fixed pelvis is counter-nutation.*

is at the SI joint itself. If the sacrum stays in place and the pelvis rotates forward at the SI joint, this is counter-nutation of the SI joint. Similarly, if the pelvis stays fixed and the top of the sacrum rotates back and down, this is also counter-nutation.

I've never seen a muscle labeled as a nutator or counter-nutator. Movements of the SI joint are passive. This doesn't mean that certain muscles do not have an effect on the joint. In fact, as we will discuss, the psoas and the piriformis do affect where the sacrum sits between the two sides of the pelvis. So what do I mean by passive? I mean that forces generated outside of the SI joint put pressure on this joint. What are these external forces? The first one is weight, which is related to gravity. The second is the build-up of forces generated through movement. It is not only pelvic movements that impact the SI joint. The interrelated movements of body parts that connect to the hip joints and the lumbar vertebrae also affect the SI joint. In other words, when we get to the end range of motion either in the spine or the hip, pressure is placed on the SI joint.

Let's take this concept of passive movement a step further. Imagine a pelvis with a spine sticking up from it, no arms, no legs, but include a rib cage and skull. Now look at it from the side so that you can see the curves of the spine in the lumbar and thoracic regions. Now put the pelvis and spine on the floor so that the spine is upright and perpendicular to the floor. Let's say that the floor magically grabs the ischium and the pelvis cannot move. The two sides of the pelvis are completely stuck and immobile. There is a natural line of gravity that passes through the spine and sacrum. If nothing else were holding the spine up, when it lined up with the force of gravity, it would fall neither forward nor back. It would be in balance.

Playing with the idea of passiveness at this joint, if the majority of the spine were to move in front of the gravitational line, what movement or force would be placed on the SI joint? If it helps, let's say all the ligaments surrounding the SI joint are also gone. Would the spine fall to the floor in front of the pelvis? Would this falling not eventually happen at the SI joint? Yes. Although this scenario isn't "real," it demonstrates how force is created at this more or less immobile joint. At some point, as the weight of the spine goes forward, it forces the vertebrae to get shorter in the front as the movement makes its way down towards the SI joint. As each vertebra goes further forward, it takes more weight with it. The last joint of the spine is the SI joint. If all the vertebrae of the spine have gone forward above it, then it seems evident that this one would move forward as well. In a way, the SI joint is the last and largest facet joint in the spine.

Personally, I don't feel any movement in my SI joint, although I have students who definitely do. As it turns out, they are on the hypermobile side. They are naturally very flexible and find that they need to work on strengthening and stabilizing within their practice. When they do feel this joint move, it is almost always in a deep back-bending type of pose. Being Ashtanga practitioners, they are all too familiar with the depth of postures such as *Kapotasana* as done in Ashtanga's second series.

In the depth of this pose if they feel the joint move, it's as though it is moving in a way that takes them further into the backbend. In other words, the top of the sacrum moves with the spine behind the line of the pelvis in counter-nutation. This is not to say that I tell my students to try and move from this place. Personally I do not think this is a very good idea. It can lead to further instability and potential problems down the road. More on forward folds and backbending relative to this joint in the Integrating Anatomy into Your Practice section.

PELVIC FLOOR MUSCLES

Although there will be some overlap between this section and the *mula bandha* section below, it seems worthwhile to clearly define what these muscles are and where they are located. The pelvic floor muscles act as a diaphragm, and this pelvic floor diaphragm is in exactly the opposite position as the respiratory diaphragm above. The two diaphragms effectively create the top and bottom of our abdominal cavity and, in a sense, regulate the amount of pressure within it. The perineal muscles include the transverse perinei, bulbospongiosus, and ischiocavernosus, but for the purposes of this book, there is no need to go into details of their attachments.

A term often used in yoga classes is the perineum. The perineal muscles are the most superficial of pelvic floor muscles; they are thin and indistinguishable, unless you are highly trained. They do contribute support to the pelvic floor, but they are not the muscles we really use to help stabilize this region.

What we're really using when we talk about the pelvic floor in yoga is the levator ani group. The term "PC muscles" (pubococcygeal muscles) is also thrown around a bit and, well, it's a bit more palatable then talking about the "elevators of your anus," which is what levator ani literally means. Technically speaking, the PC muscles are part of the levator ani group. Other muscles in this group are the iliococcygeus, puborectalis, and pubococcygeus.

Because we're studying a dynamic body, we're going to look at the function of the pelvic floor muscles as a group. The PC muscles, which we now know to technically be part of the levator ani group, are the real support system of the internal organs. Stop and think about the name of the group—levator ani, or lifting the anus. What happens when you do this? When is this used in your yoga practice? To answer the first question, when you engage these muscles, the contraction is not limited to the muscles of the pelvic floor. There is also a corresponding contraction in the lower abdomen. Try it. Tighten your pelvic floor muscles. You should also feel a coordinated contraction just above your pubic bone in the lower abdomen.

The SI joint is also at play here. This brings us back to the word *pubococcygeus*, which means

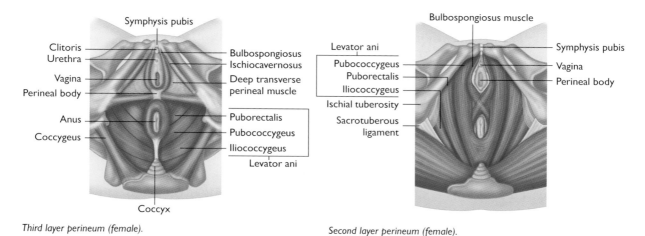

Third layer perineum (female).

Second layer perineum (female).

Figure 5.10: *The pelvic floor muscles.*

that the muscle spans from the pubic bone to the coccyx. There are sacral attachments as well. Therefore, tension in this muscle has an effect on the coccyx and sacrum, which articulates with the pelvis. If contracting a muscle could make the sacrum counter-nutate, this would be the one that would do it, though I've never seen this listed as one of its actions.

I am going to make a qualitative leap here. Tone in the PC muscles translates into stability for the sacroiliac joint and the spine. If we factor in the change in tension in the lower abdomen, then we also have increased stability from the front, as the abdominal muscles also stabilize the spine. Thus you could say that when the PC muscles engage, they help lift or tighten the anus, which has stabilizing repercussions into the spine.

INTEGRATING ANATOMY INTO YOUR PRACTICE

The Pelvis and the Feet

As we've said, the pelvis is an elevated foundation or second foundation, especially in standing poses. In these *asanas*, the first foundation is our feet. Where we position the feet will impact where and how we position our pelvis. Different factors can play into this, most significantly the general tension or openness in the front, back, and sides of the hip joints. The more open and flexible the tissues surrounding the hip joints are, the more adaptable the position of the pelvis relative to the feet.

If we look at how we set up our stance for a standing pose such as Triangle or Revolved Triangle, we can easily see the effect and relationship between the lowest foundation (the feet) and the elevated foundation (the pelvis). If I set my feet up so that the heels line up with one another, my pelvis is in a particular position. If I line the heel of the front foot up with the arch of the back foot, my pelvis is in another position. If I take it even further and line my front heel with the toes of the back foot, my pelvis is in yet another position. Depending on the individual and the tension in their hips, the foot placement may have more or less of an effect on the pelvis. Also, in each of these scenarios, you can see how the body parts above the pelvis compensate for the positioning of the pelvis.

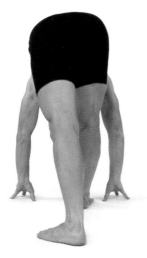 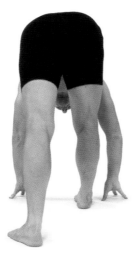 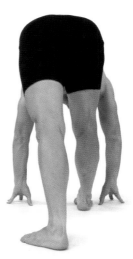

Figure 5.11: *Changing the position of the feet can have an effect on the pelvis and spine above.*

If the pelvis is not straight or square relative to the feet, then the spine must compensate. Where the spine goes, so goes the head, and slowly everything must rearrange itself using muscles and tension in ways that aren't necessary. Even in a simple forward bend, the position of the pelvis determines whether the spine will be straight or curved. This applies to both standing and seated forms of this posture. If the pelvis can't rotate freely over the heads of the femurs (usually because of tight hamstrings), then the spine is more likely to become part of the forward bend.

Pelvic Tilting

We often see the relationship between the spine and pelvis when we talk about pelvic tilting. We can see the effect of tight hamstrings and a posteriorly tilted pelvis in seated forward bends. In Down Dog, when the lower back is rounded, the pelvis is also in a posterior tilt. Often, but not always, if the student bends their knees, taking some tension out of the hamstrings, the pelvis settles into a more neutral position. It could also be said that bending the knees and removing the tension from the hamstrings allows the pelvis to tilt more anteriorly.

Keep in mind that what we are often looking for, are the muscles that are not allowing a particular movement to happen. For example, if we're working to create more anterior tilt in a posture such as Down Dog or a seated forward bend, we need to determine what muscles are not allowing this tilt to happen. In this case, it is the muscles that create a posterior tilt, namely the abdominals and the hamstrings. When I observe a student in Down Dog with a rounded back as we're describing, I almost always find their abdominal muscles and hamstrings to be tight.

We can take this example in the opposite direction and look at a pose where we might want to add a posterior tilt to the pelvis. As always, it is helpful to search not only for the muscles that create this movement, but also for those that restrict or prevent the pelvis from moving in that direction. Let's say we're in *Supta Virasana* (Reclined Hero Pose) and our back is significantly arched. To remove that arch, we need the pubic bone to move closer to the ribs. To do this, the abdominals and the hamstrings need to contract while the "anterior tilters" release. These "tilters" include the psoas, the adductors, the quadriceps, and their corresponding muscles in the low back.

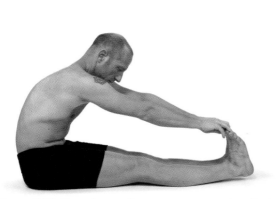
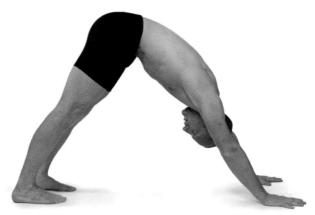

Figure 5.12: *These two patterns are common when the hamstrings are tight and cause a posterior tilt of the pelvis.*

Movement at the SI Joint in *Asanas*

SI Joint and Forward Bends

In a forward bend, at some point, as I move at my hip joints, my pelvis stops moving because the hamstrings are only so flexible. At some point, their tension won't allow my pelvis to rotate around the heads of the femurs anymore. The tension comes into my hamstrings because of the weight of my upper body combined with gravity bringing my torso towards my legs. This movement begins at the hip joint, but moves on to the spine. When that happens, my spine is well in front of my pelvis, my arms might even be acting to create leverage if they grab hold of my feet, and my lower spine may round a bit in flexion. In other words, the force of the hamstrings prevents movement of the sit bones and, thus, the rest of the pelvis. In fact, their tension actually pulls the pelvis in the opposite direction from where it wants to go naturally.

We see this with students all the time who have tight hamstrings. Their pelvis is posteriorly tilted (even though they are encouraging an anterior tilt). This forces the low back to round. If the pelvis is rotating backward (posteriorly) and the spine is in front of the pelvis and connected to the sacrum, then isn't this the same as my more simplified scenario from the section titled Movements of the SI Joint? The weight of the upper body pulls the spine and sacrum forward while the hamstrings (at the very least) hold the pelvis in place. This puts a force of nutation into the SI joint.

It makes sense to me that the exact opposite would apply if we put most of the spine behind a fixed pelvis. Because of the weight of the upper body and the forces of gravity running through the spine, counter-nutation will occur at the SI joint.

SI Joint and Backbends

In Wheel Pose, the pelvis is in the air, lifted by the force of the hands and feet pressing into the floor. The hip flexors are being stretched in the same way the hamstrings were in the forward bend. Their natural force pulls the pelvis in the direction of an anterior tilt as their tension increases. When this happens, while the spine is heading in the opposite direction (into a backbend), counter-nutation occurs at the SI joint. This statement may elicit some controversy. It is commonly asserted that when the lumbar spine moves into extension, the sacrum naturally moves into nutation; I agree. But in a backbend, the pelvis is not in neutral, nor is the lumbar spine just in extension. It is a step further and we have to remember that we are looking at the relationship of the sacrum to the pelvis, not just the sacrum or just the pelvis.

How do you prevent counter-nutation? Well, you get your pelvis to move in the same direction as the sacrum. The sacrum itself is moving back because of the natural force that takes your pelvis into an anterior tilt. If you can posteriorly tilt your pelvis, or reduce the amount of anterior tilt it creates from the beginning, you will reduce the amount of pressure at the SI joint. I know we are often told to tuck our tailbone, but I personally think that most people respond to this suggestion by squeezing their buttocks. When they do this, they actually end up adding extension to the hip joint and increasing the pressure of the hip flexors. This in turn can create more pressure at the SI joint. It is not the wrong intention; it is just an inability to execute a sophisticated movement.

Tightening your pelvic floor muscles puts tension on the coccyx, pulling it towards the pubic bone. Assuming for a moment that these very thin muscles have the strength to move your SI joint, the movement created by them would be counter-nutation. These muscles by themselves likely don't have enough strength to overpower the dense ligaments that surround the SI joint. If, however, you add the force of the spine and/or hip joint moving to the end of its range of motion and putting pressure on the SI joint, then squeezing these muscles might add to the amount of movement.

There are challenges to studying this joint. First, there are varied shapes of the SI joint and angles at which the sacrum meets the pelvis. Second, the SI joint sits at an oblique angle, which makes it difficult to observe during movement with present equipment that can see under the surface of the skin. Third, the amount of movement we are trying to observe is tiny.

It is conceivable that the way we test for movement at the SI joint is impacting the discussion. None of the testing for nutation or counter-nutation is done in extreme forward or backward bends. Rather, most testing is geared towards looking at SI joint pain and dysfunction. These tests usually work with the normal range of motion of the joint when moving from a sitting to a standing position. It may be that the normal sacro-spinal rhythm of movement is taken outside of the norm when we end up in Wheel Pose. After all, the spine is below the pelvis and the pelvis is being pushed up into the air by the legs and arms.

I remain perplexed at the amount of energy put into analyzing the joint that moves the least in backbends. SI joint movement is certainly important (when addressing SI joint dysfunctions, for example), just not in terms of increasing range of motion in backbends.

SI Joint Dysfunction

More people are familiar with the SI joint because of its dysfunction rather than its function. When people have pain at this joint, they want to know more about it. There are several factors that can play into SI joint dysfunction including gender, whether you have had a child, flexibility in the spine and hips, as well as what type of movements you do.

Structural factors can also contribute to SI joint dysfunction. If one side of the pelvis is tilted lower or higher than the other, force or pressure will impact the SI joint on either side. This can cause or be related to scoliosis in the spine. As the sacrum gets nudged off to the side and tilted, the spine corrects for this with a counter curve to the one created by the crooked sacrum.

I mentioned gender as a defining factor for the pelvis. Women are much more likely to have SI joint dysfunction than men, especially women who have been pregnant. During pregnancy, hormones are released that soften the ligaments around the pelvis for childbirth. When this happens, the SI joint, which is held together by thick ligaments, moves more than it normally does. This movement is good for childbirth, but if the ligaments are overstretched, they may not return to their "normal" amount of tension after birth. When this happens, the increased ROM that was desirable during pregnancy remains, placing these women at a higher risk of irritated SI joints.

SI joint dysfunction can cause pain in a variety of areas, not just at the location of the SI joint itself. Pain is known to radiate down the front and back of the leg, as well as up into the lower back. As with all conditions, good assessment is the key to resolution.

The movement most likely to irritate the SI joint is twisting. Forward bending and backbending are not far behind. The SI joint sits in the middle of a small kinematic chain. Its function and dysfunction are partly the result of the two joints that surround it—the hip joint and the lumbar joint.* This section of the spine moves forward and back (flexes and extends) easily, but is not very good at rotation.

When we twist, our lumbar spine rotates to its maximum. In many yoga postures, you find that the hip is also fixed in place, such as in a *Marichyasana C (III)* or *Ardha Matsyendrasana*. In twists like these, the hip is essentially pinned into place in a way that pulls the pelvis in the opposite direction of the twist. This is very effective for transmitting the force of the twist into the vertebrae of the thoracic area that are meant to twist, but if the SI joint is compromised for some reason (loose ligaments, for example), then the twist may irritate that joint.

If you have intermittent problems or pain at the SI joint, there are things you can do to alleviate the irritation. When working with postures that put pressure on this joint, let the hip joints (if they will) do more of the work. For instance, if you are doing a seated twist, allow more of the twist to happen at your hip joint; do not over-twist through the lumbar spine, which naturally puts more pressure into the SI joint.

The Anatomy of Energetics: Breath and *Bandha*

The *bandhas* are perhaps the most difficult aspect to grasp in the practice of Ashtanga Vinyasa Yoga. Personally, I think I know what they are. But then I look back at my little life as an Ashtangi, amazingly at 13 years now, and realize that I thought I knew what they were ten years ago. Even in the last six years my understanding of them has changed. I am assuming my understanding will continue to evolve and that yours will, too.

As an anatomy teacher, I try to bridge the gap between the subtle, esoteric aspects of the energetic system and Western terminology. In the area of *bandhas*, I am careful not to make it into a physical, anatomical "thing." Instead, I acknowledge that *bandhas* are both energetic and physical—as is our entire body. We are not just energy, not just emotions, not just spiritual, not just thoughts, not just physical. We are all of these at once.

Mula Bandha

To discuss *mula bandha*, or the root lock, we talk about the pelvic floor. Some people refer to the perineum and others talk about the PC muscles (pubococcygeal muscles). As mentioned earlier, this web of tissue at the base of our torso "container" is actually a diaphragm, or a ring of tissue. The opening at the base of our bowl-shaped pelvis is more or less circular and filled with thin layers of muscles and fascia, creating a "trampoline" of layered tissues. Technically, the perineum lies under the pubococcygeal muscles with a layer of fascia between.

Contraction of these muscles is often associated with *mula bandha*. There is great debate about whether, in *mula bandha*, you should engage the middle or the back portion of these tissues. Far be it for me to jump into this one too deeply, other than to say that my Guruji (Sri K. Pattabhi Jois, father of Ashtanga Vinyasa Yoga) always talked about controlling your anus. The translations I have seen of the *Hatha Yoga Pradipika*, which has an entire chapter on *bandhas* and *mudras*, often say the same thing. That is, *mula bandha* is a contraction of the anus, sometimes referred to as *aswini mudra*.

Recall that the PC muscles are part of the levator ani group, which technically means "elevator of the anus." This is pretty close to

Footnote: For the purposes of this discussion, I consider the lumbar vertebrae as a single joint as their function or movement is tied together.

what we're after when contracting the muscles for *mula bandha*. Thus it makes technical sense to use the PC. But, that's just me. In the end, what matters is that you have the experience of what is created, not the technical details.

If the *bandha* is an energetic component of who we are, what role does the actual muscle play? I describe the pelvic floor and the contraction of it as the pathway towards *mula bandha*. In other words, the physical contraction does two things. First, it creates a conscious mental relationship with *mula bandha*. It seems that *prana* (energy) follows thoughts. So if you are thinking of a part of your body, you are sending energy there. Second, the contraction of the PC muscles sti*mula*tes the energetic center, creating *mula bandha*. Its purpose is to prevent the escape or downward movement of energy through the pelvic floor.

Physical changes occur when contracting the pelvic floor muscles. These changes often fit into descriptions of the core muscles. There are debates about what the core muscles are. The pelvic floor is almost always part of that conversation. Remember, the pelvic floor muscles are at the base of the spine. They fill the circular hole at the bottom of our pelvic bowl. The back portion of the bowl is created by the sacrum, which links to either side of the pelvis at the SI joint. Just off to either side of the sacrum, filling in the sides towards the back of the bowl, are the piriformis muscles.

Think of the spine rising up out of the back of the pelvic bowl, towering above its foundation at the pelvis. There are other muscles that help stabilize this column as it rises, but at its base are the PC muscles. To see the balancing effects of these muscles on the spine, imagine for a moment that you tightened your PC muscles so much that the coccyx started to touch your pubic bone. (This is not possible,

by the way.) If the coccyx and therefore the sacrum move towards the pubic bone, there will be movement at the SI joint. The spine will fall backwards above the SI joint (counter-nutation). If the muscles let go completely, the opposite will happen. If there is no tension to hold the sacrum in place, the towering column of the spine will start to fall forwards and the coccyx will move away from the pubis.

My point is that the PC muscles help to stabilize the pelvic bowl and the spine. Of course no muscle (or in this case group of muscles) exists in a vacuum. There are other muscles and ligaments that help to maintain integrity of the pelvic bowl and stability of the spine. However, the PC muscles are at the root of it. Thus it is no surprise that they play a role in *mula bandha*.

You will recall what happens when we tighten the pelvic floor: it causes the lower abdomen to also contract. People experience it slightly differently. Some even feel a contraction in their lower back as well between the top of the pelvis and ribs. This is most likely a result of a contraction of the transverse abdominis (the deepest of the oblique muscles) as it connects to the vertebrae in the lumbar spine.

There is still one more factor at play in the connection between the subtle and gross aspects of *mula bandha* and the pelvic floor. What better force to interlink them than breath? You could even say that breath is the ultimate link between the subtle and gross in yoga. At its most subtle, the breath is the *prana*, or life force, that animates our physical bodies. It feeds us energetically. If we wish to contemplate this concept in gross terminology, *prana* presents itself in the form of oxygen molecules that nourish and sustain all of our nervous, muscular, and skeletal tissues. Everything in the body relies upon it.

When the diaphragm contracts, it compresses the abdominal contents and puts a downward pressure on the pelvic floor. If unrestricted, it will also push the abdomen out. You can give it a try yourself. Close your eyes and take a deep breath. The more deeply you inhale, the more your abdomen moves and the more pressure moves into the pelvic floor.

The diaphragm above puts pressure on the diaphragm below (PC). The energetic purpose of *mula bandha* is to prevent the escape of energy, specifically *prana vayu*, or downward flowing energy. By contracting the pelvic floor muscles, you prevent the downward movement of these muscles when breathing. In addition to stopping the downward flow of energy, you are literally stopping a downward physical force. This is the gross side of the subtle purpose of *mula bandha*.

Uddiyana

How do you know if someone is engaging or using their *bandhas*? The answer is that you see the results. You see the qualities created by *mula* and *uddiyana* in the individual as they move in their practice. What are these visible qualities? *Mula bandha* is the root lock, which means you would observe a grounded quality to the *asana* being performed. *Uddiyana*, on the other hand, means upward flying and is often observed as an overall ease and a particular lightness in the practice. The very famous, floating aspect in advanced practitioners is a sign of *bandha* use and control. This is not to say that there is no muscular effort from other areas of the body; there most definitely is. One must also have strength in order to make these movements happen. But to look effortless requires the support of the subtle aspects of our being.

Although we normally draw our abdomen in while performing *uddiyana*, anatomically speaking, this alone does not account for all the lightness of limb that we perceive. We may want to distinguish that a full *uddiyana bandha* is not possible when breathing. A full *uddiyana* is done on a held breath during *pranayama* and is known as a *kumbhaka*. During *asana* practice, if you are performing *uddiyana*, you are doing a sort of "half" *uddiyana*. As I mentioned earlier in the *mula bandha* section, the mind and our intention precedes the physical anyway.

Because we are discussing functional anatomy, we are looking for a muscle that has the functional capacity to create the lightness in our practice. This doesn't make "the *bandha*," however; at best it makes it a gross representation of the *bandha*; it supports and reflects the energetic intention and quality created by the *bandha*. Which muscle is located in this area and has the ability to create the lightness that we're talking about? The psoas muscle gets my vote.

The iliopsoas (the combination of the iliacus and the psoas major) is the strongest hip flexor in the body. Hip flexion is an essential movement for us humans. It takes us forward in our daily life as the primary muscle for walking. (This is actually a simplification. Walking is much more than flexing the femur so that one foot goes in front of the other. Many other muscles are required to carry out this complicated and coordinated action.)

When we walk, we are essentially controlling and moving our center of gravity forward in space. We are balancing ourselves on those two long sticks that we call legs. Our physical center of gravity is near the top of the sacrum. It is slightly different for men and women, but not much. Fundamentally, all types of movements (think of the graceful movements of dancers or the powerful changes in direction of football players) are manifestations of controlling the center of gravity in our body. The psoas is perfectly positioned to make this happen. It is bilateral (one on each side) and is a more or less tapering, tube-shaped piece of myofascia on either side of our center of gravity. It is intrinsically linked with the control of this area of the body and, in my eyes, the functional core of the body.

When you jump backwards or forwards or lift up into Handstand, you are controlling your center of gravity over, or in relation to, your foundation (in this case, the hands). In short, learning to control the *bandhas* is learning to have a physical and energetic connection to your center. Awareness of and ability to use the psoas seems to trigger the resultant effect of *uddiyana bandha*, flying upwards with control and lightness. At the very least, you should feel the beginnings of *uddiyana* and the lightness created, which will be refined over time. Performing *uddiyana bandha*, even if it's just the "half" version that we use while still breathing, requires that we engage the transverse abdominis to draw the abdomen in. This in and of itself provides certain stability in the area. This "functional *uddiyana*" is created by the relationship we have to the psoas.

To make a direct connection to this muscle in movement, let's look at the simple act of jumping forward and backward into High Plank or *Chaturanga Dandasana*. I choose this as an example because many people use these two movements as a place to observe one's ability to use their *bandhas*. Again, we're discussing the functional and anatomical component of the *bandha*, which we've established will be represented by the psoas. When we jump back from *Uttanasana* to a High Plank or *Chaturanga* the primary joint to change position is the hip.

If the hands are on the floor when we jump, they remain there until our feet hit the floor. Essentially we have extended the hip joint. The psoas does not extend the hip, nor do we need it to execute this movement. But something big has shifted with this movement: we are now horizontal. This has a major effect on how we interact with gravity. Because we are horizontal, gravity sends the body mass of our pelvis and hip joints towards the floor. Well, everything is heading towards the floor, but the change occurs here. As this particular area of mass moves down, the psoas controls the rate at which the hip joint moves into extension. It does this using isotonic eccentric contraction to slow down the rate at which the pelvis falls through the hip joints. How many of us had trouble preventing our pelvis from sagging when we first started jumping back? The abdomen stabilizes as well, but with a strong

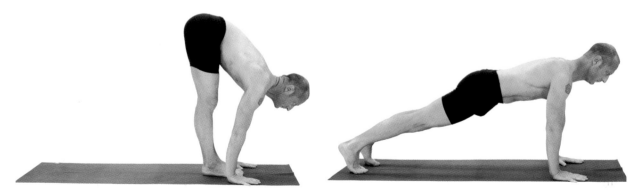

Figure 5.13: *The hip joint extends and the psoas does an eccentric contraction to slow it down.*

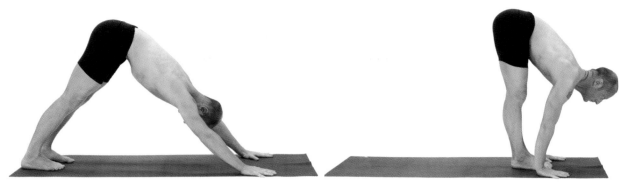

Figure 5.14: *The hip joint flexes and the psoas does a concentric contraction against the resistance of the hamstrings to pull the feet in.*

psoas muscle, the hip joint itself and the pelvis are stabilized. The pelvis is prevented from moving into hyperextension by the strength of the psoas muscle, a hip flexor. This act of "prevention" makes it look like the movement is occurring in slow motion.

When we jump from Down Dog to place the feet between the hands, we also take advantage of the psoas. In this case, it functions more like we expect—as a strong hip flexor.

To get our feet between the hands we need to flex the hip joints. What does this better than the psoas? In this case, it is not fighting gravity as much as it is fighting the tension of our hamstrings without the benefit of gravity. Because we are essentially "in the air" while this is happening, it is pure hip flexion versus hip extension.

This combination of functional movements while controlling your center of gravity is very powerful. Add to this a stable foundation through the hands and the shoulders and you will find a slow and controlled movement that fits the expression of being both grounded and light.

This function of the psoas merges together with the abdominal muscles and the pelvic floor. This is the same thing that happens with *mula* and *uddiyana bandhas*. They have a relationship with one another. They work together. Now there is one more element that must be added to the equation of *bandha*: the breath.

Breath and *Bandha*

Without breath, there can be no cultivation of *bandha*. From breath comes *bandha*. The control and use of energy in our body has a direct relationship to the breath. In yogic philosophy we use breath control, or *pranayama*, to both cultivate and interact with the energy in our body.

John Scott directed me to my first personal experience of the connection between breath and *bandha*. When I met John, I had been practicing Ashtanga Yoga for about one and a half years. I was in the UK for the very first time and I had decided to study with John for two weeks. At the end of the first week, he said to me something like, "David, you have shown up with a full primary series, but no breath and no *bandha*." Needless to say, I was crestfallen. At that point I thought I understood what breath and *bandha* were. I guess I knew intellectually what they were, but I hadn't experienced them in the way that he was describing. He sat down next to me and put my hand on his abdomen while he was breathing; I continued to hold it there while he did a few different types of *asanas*. Whatever I had been doing, it wasn't what John did in that moment. As John began to breathe and move, I could feel the way he was holding his lower abdomen and the kind of tension it was: it was as if there was *no* tension in his lower abdomen. It felt like it was magically held in. With my present understanding, I know that the transverse abdominis pulls the abdomen in this way.

I had one more week of practice with John and then I headed home. At home I gave every ounce of my effort to holding my navel in the way that he had. I purposely did not focus on the depth of my *asana*, only on trying to breathe correctly while holding my navel in the way I had witnessed John do it. Over the course of the following three months, practicing six days a week, I slowly started to understand. The breath led me to understand *bandha*. Slowly but surely a lightness and ease came to my practice that I hadn't experienced before.

There is plenty of debate about the "right" type of breathing in yoga. The more classical yoga practices, such as Sivananda, use a belly breath. The more vigorous styles of practice keep the belly in during breathing. Other methods don't pay much attention to the breath at all. My understanding at this point is colored by the method I have used and the experience I have gained as an Ashtanga Yoga practitioner. I am not claiming that the way it is done in Ashtanga Yoga is the "right" way; I see it as one technique to elicit qualities in the practice. There are many techniques in yoga.

Let's see if we can tie together *mula bandha*, *uddiyana bandha*, and the breath using anatomical terms. Remember that *mula bandha* refers to the root lock, which is associated with the pelvic floor. Its purpose is to prevent the downward flow and escape of energy through

the bottom of our torso. *Uddiyana bandha* is translated as "upward flying" and is the energetic lock responsible for the lightness we see in an advanced yogi's practice. The main muscle of respiration (breathing) is the diaphragm.

The diaphragm is shaped unlike any other muscle in the body, somewhat like a dome or a parachute. As far as attachments go, the diaphragm stands alone. Most muscles attach from one bone to another and move those bones relative to one another. The diaphragm attaches in its posterior part onto the spine and then circles around the bottom of the rib cage until it gets to the xiphoid process at the bottom of the breastbone. The fibers of the muscle run up and down and attach at the top of the dome to what is called the central tendon. When the diaphragm contracts, it shortens those fibers and one end moves towards the other. There are two ways that the diaphragm functions and these determine whether we breathe into the belly or into the chest. This functioning of the diaphragm is critical to understanding how *mula* and *uddiyana* function anatomically and the physical effect they create in our torso.

Everyone believes that a "belly breath" is the deepest breath. In belly breathing, people feel as though their diaphragm moves down between three and six inches and forces the abdomen out almost the same distance. As much as it might feel like this, it isn't happening. In fact, on our biggest belly breath, the top of the diaphragm isn't moving down much more than an inch, if that much. This will seem obvious when I tell you that the heart is sitting on top and is connected to the diaphragm via connective tissue. If the diaphragm moved down that far, what would happen to the heart?

As we breathe, the diaphragm contracts. As its surface moves down, it pulls on the connective tissue bags that surround the lungs. As a result, negative pressure is created in the chest

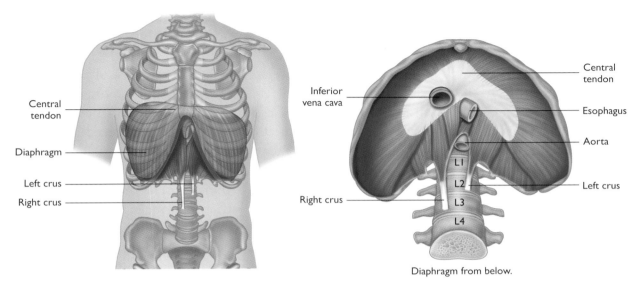

Central tendon

Diaphragm

Left crus

Right crus

Inferior vena cava

Central tendon

Esophagus

Aorta

Right crus

Left crus

L1

L2

L3

L4

Diaphragm from below.

Figure 5.15: *The diaphragm.*

cavity and the lungs fill. Movement of the diaphragm, even just an inch, pushes down on the abdominal contents below and forces the abdomen down. In belly breathing (take a couple of breaths with your abdomen moving out), the abdomen pushes out on the inhalation first and then towards the end of the breath, the chest fills. In addition, at the very end of the inhalation, you may feel a slight pressure on your pelvic floor as it stretches or is pressed down by the abdominal contents.

In the second type of breathing, the sequence of events change as the diaphragm works in a completely different way. A couple of things are required in order to make this happen. We change the tension in different areas of the "abdominal container." By abdominal container, I mean the container created by the diaphragm on top, the pelvic floor on the bottom, and the abdominal muscles around the sides and in front. To change this tension, we first contract the muscles of the pelvic floor. Tightening the pelvic floor means that when pressure comes down from the contracted diaphragm, it won't push the tissues at the base of the body downwards. The tension of our contraction prevents it. This is the purpose of *mula bandha*! It prevents the downward

movement of energy. In this case, we prevent the literal downward movement of the pelvic floor.

The second way we change the tension in the container is by pulling the lower abdomen in and holding it there during both inhalation and exhalation. If you hold the abdomen in and take a breath, you will quickly notice that the breath goes into the chest right away. The diaphragm no longer has the ability to push down and the abdomen is restricted from moving out. The force gets redirected upwards into the chest. Isn't this the purpose of *uddiyana*? That is, to direct the energy/breath/*prana* upwards?

When we hold our abdomen in, the diaphragm is forced to produce a different action. Instead of the top of the diaphragm moving downwards as it did in the first type of breath, the top of the diaphragm remains still. Because the abdomen is in, the abdominal contents are holding the top of the diaphragm in place. The fibers of the diaphragm are then forced to pull the lowest ribs upwards. Keep in mind that the ribs are not parallel to the floor of our abdomen. Instead, they angle down. As the diaphragm contracts in this way, the front of the ribs lift, making space in the chest cavity (just in a different way). With the space made, negative pressure is created and air rushes in.

Let's review. If you do nothing but take a big breath, the abdomen and pelvic floor (to a much lesser degree) are pressed outwards. If you tense the muscles of the pelvic floor and abdomen to prevent them from going out (as one does when applying *mula* and *uddiyana bandhas*), then the diaphragm functions differently. The breath is re-directed upward. This stimulates the more subtle aspects of the *bandhas* as energetic components for practice. Both ways of breathing are correct, depending on the method one practices. But physically creating *mula* and *uddiyana bandhas* during an *asana* practice literally and physically changes the way our breathing happens. That literal and physical change seems to mirror the energetic intentions of the *bandhas*, one of which is to provide us with a focal point in our practice that will support the body. From a gross physical perspective, when we engage the *bandhas*, we also contract the muscles that we associate with our core. This helps integrate movement and stabilize our spine. Therefore, the physical component of the *bandhas* alone impacts how we move through our practice.

Restrictions to Breathing

In addition to the interconnection of breath and *bandha*, we need to address another important component of breathing—the ribs. There are twelve pairs of ribs. The last two pairs are known as "floating" ribs. This means that, unlike the others, they do not attach to the sternum via cartilage. Each of the pairs of ribs is associated with one of the twelve thoracic vertebrae. They have a relationship with the spine that goes beyond

just attaching to it. They add support and stability to the spine.

Between each rib are three layers of muscles: the external, internal, and innermost intercostal muscles. These three layers of muscles assist respiration, especially when forced inhalation or exhalation is required (for example, when the cardiovascular system is taxed during exercise). If these muscles are tight, however, they will restrict movement between the ribs. As in any other muscle, we want the intercostals to have a balance of flexibility and strength. You can observe what happens when tension is placed on these tissues (and therefore the ribs) in your practice.

In what types of postures do you find it most difficult to breathe? For me it's during backbends and twists. Beginners will definitely have the hardest time breathing in these two types of postures. Why is that? What's happening? In both backbends and twists, pressure is being placed on the ribs and the tissues between them because they are being stretched. Stretching tissues increases their tension, just like lengthening a rubber band increases its tension. As a result, it becomes harder to separate the ribs from one another. If you can't separate the ribs from one another, how will the lungs be able to fill inside of the rib cage?

Interestingly, yoga always shows us where to focus and where we need to work. It guides us to the edge of comfort or sensation and then plays with that edge, coaxing it to go a little further. This is how we benefit from that interaction. Breathing while in a twist is an example of going to our edge. It is at the edge of our comfort zone that change is created. Change in the tissues occurs when we are at the edge of our perceived capacity, when we arrive there with the breath and then *breathe*.

6
THE SPINE

The spine is a fascinating structure. When we practice yoga, we spend a lot of time and energy finding our center, as we need this to move efficiently and effectively on the mat. The spine is our centerline.

My dear friend Fran quotes Alistair Shearer from *The Yoga Sutras of Patanjali (Sacred Teachings)*: "Yoga, when you boil it all down, is about the nervous system." What contains the nervous system if not your spine? It is the spine—its health and flexibility—that we're unknowingly working with in our *asana* practice. The depth of our backbend is only the tip of the iceberg. These physical goals extend far beyond the mat and into our daily lives, for example, our ability to sit up straight and stay there for any period of time! How can we free our spine from the forces of gravity and our slouchy posture?

In order to honor this amazing structure, we must dissect and study it in the same way that we have studied other parts of the body. We will approach it from the perspective of structure, movement, mysofascia, function in *asana* and a handful of dysfunctions that you may run into as a teacher or within your own practice. Each perspective adds a piece to the puzzle that we call our spine.

LANDMARKS: A REMARKABLE DESIGN

The design of the spine is a work of art. It consists of stacks of short, round bones with a thicker type of cartilage between them like a rubber bushing. These fluid-filled discs of cartilage are the real miracle of the spine. They provide shock absorption and allow for movement by maintaining space between the bones. The space is also for the nerves coming off of the spinal cord to fit between the vertebrae so they can feed their associated tissues and organs. These joints are referred to as anterior intervertebral joints.

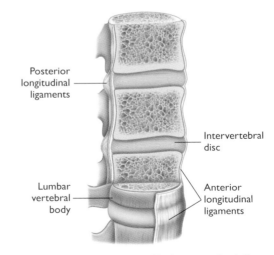

Posterior longitudinal ligaments

Intervertebral disc

Lumbar vertebral body

Anterior longitudinal ligaments

Figure 6.1: *Vertebrae separated by intervertebral discs.*

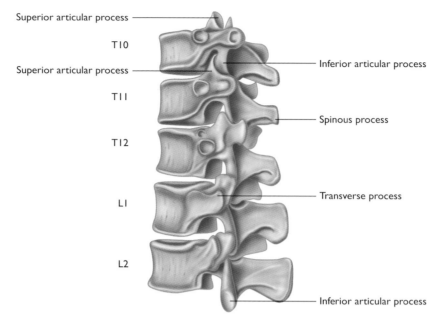

Superior articular process ——————
T10

Superior articular process ——————
T11

T12

L1

L2

—————— Inferior articular process

—————— Spinous process

—————— Transverse process

—————— Inferior articular process

Figure 6.2: *Vertebral foramen as well as the spinous processes and the transverse processes.*

In addition to the round flat part (or body) of the vertebra, there is also an awkwardly shaped area that sticks out in many directions behind it. These oddly shaped bones form the amazing ring that protects the critically important spinal cord. The bits of bone that shoot off sideways and backwards provide attachment points for the muscles. They also allow for or restrict movement in certain directions.

The articulations between the posterior parts of the vertebrae are called facet joints (also known as posterior intervertebral joints, or the zygapophyseal joints). Flat surfaces (two on the bottom and two on the top of each vertebra) join the vertebrae and help control spinal movements. We will go into more detail on these in a moment. The vertebrae articulate in two places: anteriorly, where the discs sit between the two bones; and posteriorly, where the bones meet one another at the two flat surfaces found between each vertebra. These posterior intervertebral joints are gliding or plane joints, which allow for movement in every direction along its surface. The catch with this type of joint is that each bone can only move a relatively small distance. Each of

these junctions between each vertebra adds a relatively small amount of movement to the overall range of motion of the spine.

TENSEGRITY AND THE STRUCTURE OF THE SPINE

You should understand how the tensional members (the myofascia) of the spine hold the bones in place. As much as we might think that the bones hold themselves in place because they're hard, this isn't the case. The overall health of the spine and associated discs is intimately related to how much pressure the various tissues surrounding the spine place on the vertebrae. Imbalance of tension adds stress and strain on the spine. Nowhere else in the body is the concept of tensegrity displayed more clearly and more beautifully than it is here. With any tensegrity model, the compression members cross one another and are tied together with tensional members. This is precisely what we find along the posterior intervertebral joints.

Each vertebra has two compression members (if you will) that stick out to the sides. These

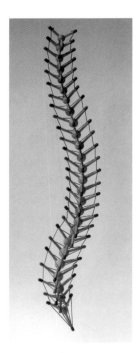

Figure 6.3: *We see a tensegrity mast arranged somewhat like a spine. An essential element to this kind of mast is having a strut from the compression member (bone) above stick down below a strut coming up from the compression member below, with a tension member (wire, elastic or connective tissue) joining the two. You can see that arrangement in the model, and we see it in the anatomy also.*

are known as the transverse processes. In addition, one compression member sticks straight out from the posterior of the vertebra. This is called the spinous process. All of these parts that stick out interact with the deepest layer of our musculature and create tensegrity.

The deep rotatores muscles attach from the transverse process to the spinous process below. Here we can see tensegrity quite clearly. If we include the other muscles that attach onto the spinous process from other places, such as the ribs in layers, we see how each vertebra is suspended in its own web of tension. When we step back and view the spine as a whole, we see that the entire spine has the potential to be suspended in the tension and not in the compression of bones.

This is critical to understanding the uneven pressures that may impose themselves on the vertebrae of the spine. When we look at disc

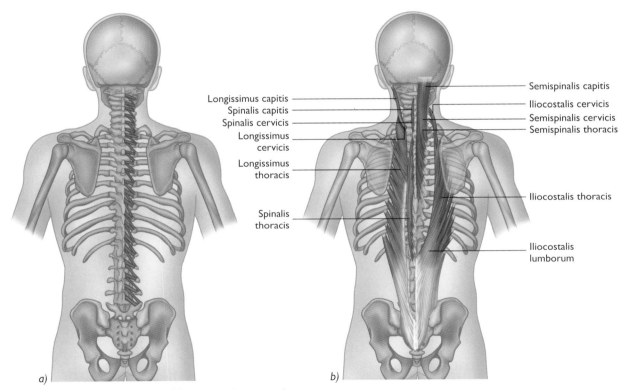

Figure 6.4: *a) Rotatores muscles, b) erector spinae muscles.*

problems, we can't ignore the possibility that the web of tension in which these discs and bones exist impacts how pressure is placed and distributed through them. Long-term tensional patterns in these tissues can lead to uneven pressures on the vertebrae and, therefore, the discs that sit between them.

HOW THE CURVES OF THE SPINE ADD TO ITS STRUCTURE

Let's look at the fundamental structure and shape of the spine. Seen from the front and in anatomical position, the spine is a column. From this point of view, it is a straight line of bone connecting the pelvis to the skull. If we look from the side, however, we see something quite different. The spine isn't a column in the pure sense of the word: there are natural curves running through it. These curves are important and add ten times more strength to the whole structure than if the spine was truly a column.[24]

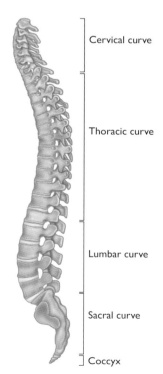

Cervical curve

Thoracic curve

Lumbar curve

Sacral curve

Coccyx

Figure 6.5: *Lateral view of the spine.*

These curves are sometimes referred to as primary or secondary curves. The primary curve is associated with the thoracic and sacral regions; this is what we call the kyphotic curve. It is considered primary because it's the first curve created in gestation and the fetal position. Although there is some genetic coding for the secondary curves to evolve in the lumbar and cervical regions, these curves are created when we begin holding our head up and arching our back as babies. The secondary curves are referred to as the lordotic curve. The later formation of these spinal curves is a result of tension of tissues created by our activities. Our life experiences take our genetic code a step further developmentally.

Interestingly, a similar thing happens with the arches of the feet. You could also consider the arches of the foot (primarily the medial arch) as a secondary curve; it is not inherent in newborns. It requires stimulation and action to further the basic genetic coding. I often say that we are all born flat footed. The arches develop when we start crawling and pushing off with the toes.

THE SPINE AS THE CORE OF THE BODY

The spine is literally the "core" of the body. It is the deepest, most centrally located structure. Various structures attach to it directly and indirectly, including the ribs, lungs, heart, organs, diaphragm, pelvic floor muscles, psoas, and other myofascia. All of these attached parts have a symbiotic relationship with the central tent pole that is the spine. They rely on it for a certain amount of stability and strength. At the same time, they add to the stability and strength much like canvas does for the tent pole. The tension of the fabric helps to strengthen the overall structure.

Ideally, the spine would divide the body equally into right and left sides. However, reality shows that very few people are so well organized in their walking, talking, and moving tensegrity model. Because so many tensional members (myofascia) connect to and around the spine, the imbalance of these tissues pulls the central pole out of alignment. The resulting imbalances have the potential to affect many other structures.

In addition to the myofascia, the skeletal structures can also pull the spine out of balance. If, for example, the pelvis is off kilter, it puts pressure on the sacrum, thereby forcing it off at an angle. When this happens, the spine naturally tries to correct itself to keep the head and eyes even with the horizon.

BONES OF THE SPINE

There are 24 (33 if you view the sacral and coxal vertebrae individually) individual vertebrae: 7 in the cervical spine (neck), 12 in the thoracic spine (upper and middle back), and 5 in the lumbar spine (low back). Below that is the sacrum, which is normally a fusion of 5 vertebrae and the coccyx (tail bone), which is normally a fusion of 4 vertebrae attached to the bottom of the sacrum. I say *normally* because

it is possible to have an extra vertebra in any of these regions.

Boney Landmarks

Spinous Process

The spinous process is the part of the vertebra that sticks out posteriorly. We can feel this part of the vertebra beneath the skin when we touch our own spine on our back. It is a location for muscles to attach to. It also impacts the ability of the vertebrae to move in different areas of the spine.

Transverse Process

This is the part of the vertebra that sticks out to either side, with one transverse process on each side. They are only palpable from the outside in the cervical and lumbar regions of the spine.

Body of the Vertebra

This is the part of the vertebra that sandwiches the disc along the front of the spine. The body of each vertebra is designed to support weight, as the vertebrae stack on top of each other.

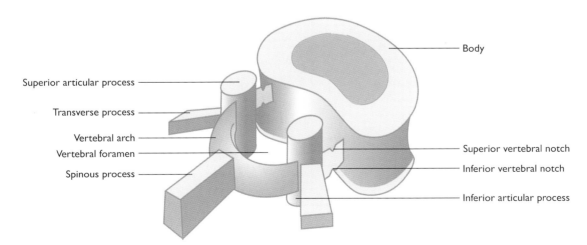

Figure 6.6: *Boney landmarks of a vertebra.*

Vertebral Foramen

Behind the body of the vertebra is the vertebral foramen. Foramen literally means "hole." In this case, it is a hole created by all of the elements and landmarks of the vertebrae. In other words, the body of the vertebra is continuous with the transverse process, which then turns into the spinous process. Together they create a ring of bone known as the vertebral foramen, which encases the spinal cord.

LUMBAR STRUCTURE AND MOVEMENT

Sitting on top of the sacrum is the last lumbar vertebra: L5. If we look at the size of the vertebrae, particularly the big, round, boney bodies of the vertebrae that sandwich the disc, we notice how much larger the vertebrae are at the bottom of the spine. The lumbar vertebrae are both wider and thicker from top to bottom relative to the cervical vertebrae. This is an indication of the weight-bearing nature of the spine and the lumbar vertebrae, in particular at the base of the structure. That is, the lower

you go on the spine, the larger the vertebrae in order to support the vertebrae above.

The spinous processes illustrate the differences in vertebrae as they run from the neck to the pelvis. These boney parts also change shape and size as you make your way up the spine. In the lumbar section, they have a good amount of space between them and are large and rounded. In the thoracic spine, the processes point downwards slightly and in the neck they are rather small. These variations are part of what allow for or restrict movements in different sections of the spine.

The posterior (back) intervertebral (between vertebra) joints (or facet joints) in the lumbar region differentiate the lower spine from the other regions. The facet joints of the spine are referred to as plane joints or gliding joints. Each vertebra has two of these flat spots sticking up just behind the body of the vertebra and two more flat spots going down just behind the body of the vertebra. When you stack the bones on top of one another, the flat spots above one vertebra meet up with the two flat spots coming down from the vertebra above it.

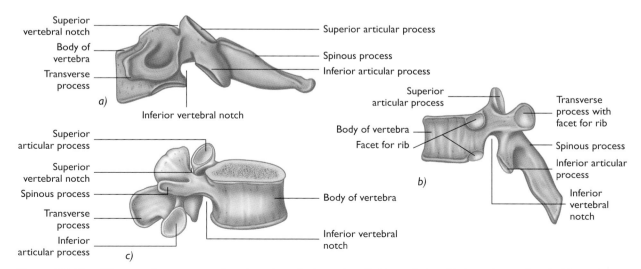

Figure 6.7: *The differences between vertebra size; a) cervical vertebra (C5) lateral view, b) thoracic vertebra (T6) lateral view, c) lumbar vertebra (L3) lateral view.*

Each vertebra is connected to the next with two synovial joints.

The position of the surface of the lumbar vertebrae facet joints is significantly different from the position of the joints in both the thoracic and cervical sections of the spine. In the lumbar region, they are essentially parallel to the midline of the body (the sagittal plane). This allows the more abundant range of movements found in the lumbar spine. From a structural point of view, it allows for the flexion and extension that the lumbar spine is designed to do.

The bones of the lumbar spine move relative to one another at both joints, where the bodies of the vertebrae come together at the disc and at the facet joints. Because of the orientation of the flat areas, there is plenty of glide in flexion and extension at the facet joints as the surfaces slide against and with one another. However, if we try to rotate at these vertebrae, the flat areas of the facet joints bump into one another. Rotation causes them to press into one another instead of sliding past.

The last movement of the lumbar spine is lateral flexion or sidebending. In this case, the orientation of the facet joints allows for gliding. The ribs are what hit the top of the pelvis and stop movement in this section of the spine. You can feel this for yourself if you stick your fingers into your side between your lowest ribs and your pelvis and then bend sideways (laterally). Your fingers should get pinched.

Most people are surprised by the amount of curve in the lumbar spine. It looks much more flat than curved in most people, because thick muscles fill in the curved part of the lower back. The curve is set up in such a way that lumbar vertebrae 4 and 5 are almost hanging straight down towards the ground. L4 and L5 are at such

an extreme angle that they actually have extra ligaments on their posterior part that attaches to the pelvis. These are called the iliolumbar ligaments and are an extra support mechanism for keeping these vertebrae in place.

THORACIC STRUCTURE AND MOVEMENT

The top of and the bottom of T12 form what is sometimes referred to as the lumbodorsal hinge. It is definitely a key place in terms of change in structure and function of the spine. All of the individual structures we have discussed in the lumbar spine apply to the thoracic spine as well. As you might have guessed, what changes are the size, shape, and resultant function of the vertebrae.

The bodies of the vertebrae from the lowest lumbar to the cervical region of the spine continually get smaller. The difference between L1 and T12 is not that significant in terms of size of the vertebral body; however, the difference between the size of T12 and T1 is quite significant. There is also a marked change in the range of function in this section of the spine as there is less need for size because weight-bearing is reduced. The thoracic region is basically twice as long as the lumbar and the cervical regions. There are 12 thoracic vertebrae, slightly more than double the 5 lumbar and slightly less than double the 7 cervical vertebrae. The small movements at each joint combine to make the whole range of motion of the spine greater than the range at each individual vertebral joint. Nowhere is this more true than in the thoracic region. Certain movements appear structurally inhibited; yet larger movement is possible due to all of the smaller movements "adding up." For the sake of simplicity, let's say that the average amount of movement between each vertebra is only 1 degree of flexion; if you multiply that by

12, you have 12 degrees of overall movement in the thoracic spine.

Let's go back to the spinous processes that you can feel along the back of your own spine. If you look closely at the thoracic spine and the shape and alignment of the processes sticking out, you will notice some variation as you make your way up towards the neck. The spinous processes near the bottom of the thoracic section are a little bit longer than in the lumbar region. Instead of sticking out more or less straight from the body, they start to point slightly downwards. As we continue to move up the spine, they point more and more downwards until we get to the thoracic region, where the spinous processes are almost on top of one another. Above this part of the thoracic spine, the spinous processes shorten slightly, and once again you see space between them. The angle of the processes here is similar to what we found near the bottom of the thoracic spine. The spinous processes alone have something to say about which direction of movement they will allow.

Another element found only in the thoracic region impacts the functionality of this part of the spine. Each thoracic vertebra is associated with a pair of ribs. One rib attaches to the vertebra on either side. At the very bottom, we find two sets of floating ribs. They are called floating ribs because they do not attach to the breastbone (the sternum) in the front of the body as the other ten pairs do.

From their connection to the thoracic spine, the ten pairs of ribs wrap around to the front and connect directly or indirectly (through cartilage) to the sternum. It is important to keep this in mind when we consider the way the thoracic spine moves. Because the rib cage protects vital organs, namely the heart and lungs, it is rigidly built by necessity.

I've been saving the biggest difference between the lumbar and the thoracic cavity for last. The facet joints, as you may recall, allow or restrict movement in different directions. The shift happens on T12 itself. The bottom two facet surfaces on T12 are aligned with the joints of the lumbar region (parallel to the midline). The top two surfaces change direction completely. Instead of being parallel to the direction that the spine is facing, the flat areas are now essentially parallel to the surface of your back (the coronal plane). This creates a

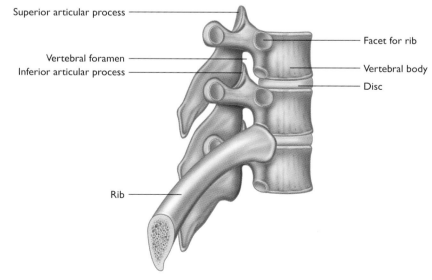

Figure 6.8: *Thoracic spine segment.*

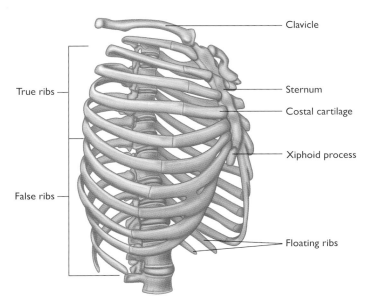

Figure 6.9: *Ribs and sternum.*

huge functional difference between the lumbar and thoracic regions.

In the lumbar region, if you take the vertebrae and move them forwards and back (flexion and extension), the facet joints easily slide past one another. If you did those same actions here in the thoracic region, instead of sliding past

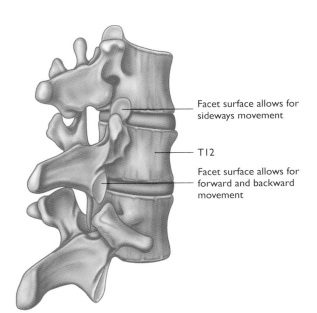

Facet surface allows for sideways movement

T12

Facet surface allows for forward and backward movement

Figure 6.10: *The change in angle between the facet joints lends itself to the movements that are possible at each section of the vertebrae.*

one another in extension, the vertebrae bump into each other, allowing very little movement. Still, there is some movement between them, and this region is more flexible than you might initially suspect.

In addition to the orientation of the facet joints, remember that the spinous processes in this region are pointed down and almost touching. Getting extension in this section of the spine is difficult because of the combination of facet orientation and spinous processes working against one another. Towards the top of the thoracic spine there is more space between the spinous processes, and as it turns out, the orientation of the facet joints changes to allow more movement. By the time we get to the cervical region, the change in facet joint orientation is more of a progression than the abrupt change we saw between the lumbar and thoracic sections.

Before we get too far ahead of ourselves, we need to deal with the other movements of the spine as they relate to the thoracic region. We have said that extension and hyperextension of the spine are restricted by both the facet joints and some of the spinous processes in this area.

In flexion, the spinous processes themselves do not really restrict movement, although they are not optimally oriented for it. The main restriction of flexion in the thoracic spine is the sternum in front of your spine. Just imagine for a moment what would happen to your heart and lungs if you flexed too far at this area of your spine. The excessive compression would make it difficult to breathe and possibly put excessive pressure on your heart.

The thoracic region really shines in rotational movement. The orientation of the facet joints is such that there is no facet or spinous process restriction to this movement. But there are limitations to the rotation from the joints themselves and the ribs. In terms of the joint, remember that the facet joints are synovial in nature, which means they have a connective tissue-based joint capsule. These 24 little capsules restrict rotation. The twisting force in the ribs loads them with pressure and force. You also have the small intrinsic layers of intercostal muscles between these ribs. The tighter they are the more restricted a twist will be.

Last but not least is lateral flexion or sidebending. There is minimal restriction (if any) of this movement at the level of the facet joints. Once again, the main restriction here is from the ribs. On the side that you are bending towards, the ribs eventually compress or bump into one another. On the opposite side, the flexibility of the intercostal muscles will to help determine how far apart the ribs can go from one another.

CERVICAL STRUCTURE AND MOVEMENT

The cervical region of the spine lacks the outer support of the ribs. The orientation of the facet joints have slowly changed from the mid-thoracic region until they are almost horizontal in the cervical region. With the exceptions of C6 and C7, the spinous processes have shortened considerably, allowing more space between the vertebrae. This allows for spinal extension in the cervical spine. The transverse processes in this area become narrower in the neck, with the exception of the top two cervical vertebrae (C1 and C2). Another major change in these transverse processes is that arteries actually run through the boney processes in the cervical region and eventually supply blood to the brain. The vertebral bodies in this region are significantly smaller compared to the lumbar vertebrae. The cervical vertebrae rely on the base of the solid thoracic vertebrae so that they can focus on supporting the head.

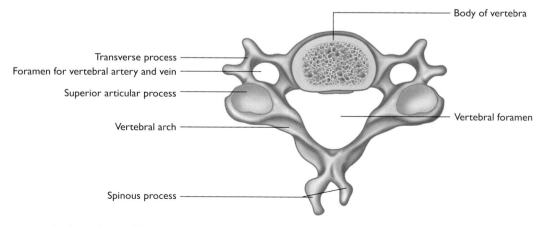

Figure 6.11: *Cervical vertebra and the facet joints.*

There is no strong resistance in movement at the cervical spine. Flexion and extension are basically unrestricted, though there is clearly an end to the range of motion. Rotationally, no boney restrictions show themselves, and lateral flexion (sidebending) happens pretty easily in the neck. Although we don't need to go into this in great detail, the standout change within the cervical vertebrae is between the first and second vertebrae. C1 is also called the atlas. Atlas, as you may or may not remember, held the world on his shoulders. Well, this atlas holds our own personal globe (the skull) on our shoulders. If you look closely, you will see that this vertebra has a wider base for the skull to be held upon. The atlas meets the bone called the occiput to support the skull. This atlanto-occipital joint allows the skull to tilt forward and back and side-to-side. Rotation at this one joint is limited.

C2 is named *axis* and is so-called because there is a little projection, the dens or odontoid process, that sticks up from it that sits in the middle of the atlas. This projection provides the skull with its great range of rotation. Functionally all of the vertebrae beneath it also rotate. If we were going to try and isolate rotation of the skull alone, however, we would look to the atlanto-axial joint.

MUSCLES OF THE SPINE

Posterior Spinal Muscles

The muscles of the spine that reside on our back are quite complex, but there are a number of ways to organize them according to depth and location on the spine itself. All of the muscles at the same depth share a similar goal: to maintain the spine in an upright and erect position. From the smallest of the muscles that attach from one vertebra to the thickest of them that span multiple vertebrae, the name of the game is keeping the spine upright. That is no small task.

Deepest Layers

The deepest of the muscles that directly attach to the spine are the smallest. These muscles interact with the vertebrae on a relatively individual basis and create the tensegrity-like structure at the spine itself. The first (that is, the deepest of these) are known as the rotatores muscles (see page 168). Technically there is a longus and a brevis that attach from the transverse process on one vertebra to the spinous process on the vertebra above. Because of the alignment of these tissues, they create

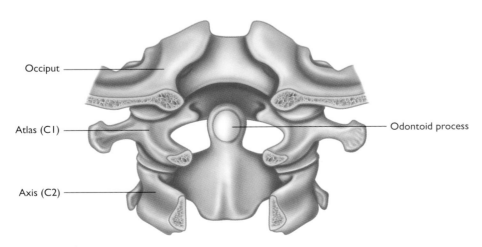

Occiput

Atlas (C1)

Odontoid process

Axis (C2)

Figure 6.12: *Atlanto-occipital joint.*

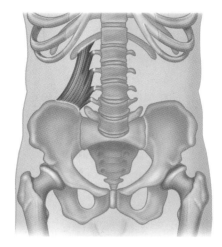

Figure 6.13: *Quadratus lumborum (QL).*

The next layer of muscles moving away from the spine includes the multifidus and semispinalis. They traverse their way through different sections of the spine. The multifidi span two to four vertebrae and are quite thick in the lumbar section. The semispinalis muscles have attachments in both the thoracic and cervical regions and continue the work of maintaining an erect spine.

We are generally familiar with the most superficial group of muscles: the erector spinae. These spinal erectors, whose name implies their function, span even greater distances than their deeper synergists. Three muscles comprise the erector spinae group. From medial to lateral, these are the spinalis, longissimus, and iliocostalis muscles. Their ropey bands span from the sacrum to the cervical vertebrae. They begin spanning more than four vertebrae in places and the two most lateral, the longissimus and iliocostalis, actually attach onto the ribs and use them for leverage to extend the spine.

that essential crossing of the compression members needed in tensegrity.

It is also at this depth that we find the ever-popular quadratus lumborum (QL) muscle. The QL is lateral to the spine but has attachments from the top of the pelvis to the lowest rib and to the transverse processes in the lumbar spine. It does assist in spinal extension and lateral flexion but is mostly used as a stabilizer, linking together the pelvis, spine, and rib cage.

Knowing that they all play a primary role in extension, these muscles activate around the

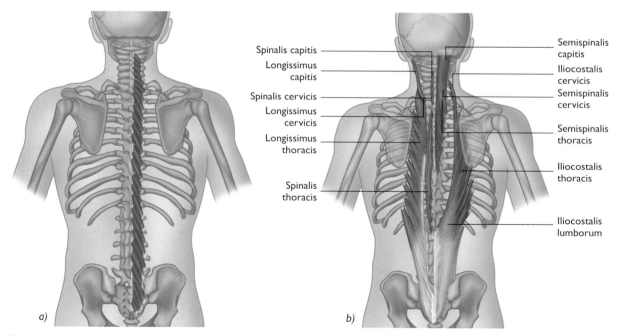

Figure 6.14: *a) Multifidus muscles, b) erector spinae muscles.*

spine when doing backbending postures. They are working in the most isolated fashion in postures like *Salabhasana* and its variations. Instead of maintaining the spine in an anatomically erect position, they actually lift the body off the floor when lying face down.

When we flip ourselves over for a Full Wheel Pose, or *Urdhva Dhanurasana*, the erector spinae group works to get us off the floor. During movement, they work in opposition to the abdominal muscles in postures like this. That is, the tension in the abdomen can restrict our ability to further extend the spine. At the same time, the erector spinae group works together with the abdominals to help stabilize the spine. The abdominal muscles move the spine; they just do it from a distance, or a more indirect location.

Abdominals

Tissues that form the abdominal cavity also affect the spine. The muscles on the front of this container are generally known as the abdominals, of which there are three layers. The most superficial is the external oblique, which lies on top of the internal oblique. Beneath these is the transverse abdominis. They create a girdle around our waist and are tied together in the front with the rectus abdominis, which is what we have come to know as the "six pack."

In general, the abdominals attach along the bottom of the rib cage, extending back to the transverse processes of the lumbar spine. They then head down to the top of the pelvis, along the iliac crest and to the inguinal ligament. They merge together with the rectus abdominis in the front. Collectively, the abdominals form the front and sides of the abdominal cavity and, because of their attachment points, are associated with stability and movement of the trunk. Another way of saying this is that the abdominals, though they may seem far away from the spine, both stabilize and move it.

All three layers assist in flexing the spine as they pull the ribs down towards the pubic bone. The obliques are on the sides, so they also help bring the ribs sideways towards

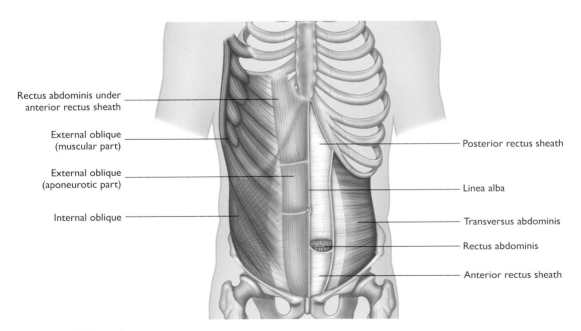

Rectus abdominis under anterior rectus sheath

External oblique (muscular part)

External oblique (aponeurotic part)

Internal oblique

Posterior rectus sheath

Linea alba

Transversus abdominis

Rectus abdominis

Anterior rectus sheath

Figure 6.15: *The abdominals.*

the pelvis (lateral flexion or sidebending). Because of the orientation and angle of the oblique fibers, they also have the ability to help rotate the spine. As you know, when a muscle has the ability to create a movement, it also has the ability to restrict a movement. Based on the actions listed above, the abdominal muscles can resist spinal extension, as in backbending. They can also resist sidebending and rotation of the spine.

The abdominals also have the ability to move the pelvis. We don't often think about these muscles as movers of the pelvis, but if the rib cage is sufficiently stabilized, the pubic bone can be lifted upwards, creating a posterior tilt of the pelvis. This is a common instruction given in *Utkatasana* or *Virabhadrasana II*.

The abdominals are also quite active in stabilizing the pelvis relative to the spine. Take a simple Plank Pose and hold it for a minute or so. Not only will you feel all of your muscles working, but before too long, you will become extremely aware of your abdominal muscles. They are stabilizing the trunk and keeping your bottom from sagging. Now think about *Navasana*, which requires hip flexion. In order for this flexion to occur, the pelvis is stabilized by contraction of the abdominals. Many postures, whether standing, seated, or reclined, rely on the abdominals to maintain a particular position between the pelvis and the spine.

Our abdominal muscles also play an important role in breathing, acting as secondary muscles of respiration. Because they create the abdominal cavity, a change in their tension can influence the amount of pressure created in the cavity, for example when we cough or forcefully exhale. The abdominal muscles add pressure to the cavity, which pushes on the diaphragm and compresses the lungs to push the air outwards.

LIGAMENTS

In all joints, ligaments stabilize, support, and allow for or restrict movement in varying degrees. The joints of the spine are no different. *How* that happens, however, is another story. We normally talk about two bones coming together to make a joint. But in the spine a long row of joints needs to be stabilized and supported. Thus the main ligaments of the spine often run its entire length.

The first and strongest of these ligaments is called the anterior (front) longitudinal (lengthwise) ligament (the ALL). This ligament is thick and dense and attaches to the front of the vertebrae, where the fibers of the ligament weave themselves into the fabric of the connective tissue, both on

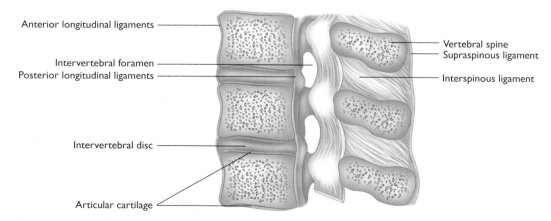

Figure 6.16: *Sagittal section of vertebrae.*

What is the body's mechanism to try and alleviate this constricted blood flow? As far as I know, there is only one thing that a muscle can do: it contracts. This is the opposite of what the injured area needs. It needs to relax! Relaxing is more of a lack of function than it is a function. In other words, lack of stimulation by the nerves is relaxation. When you ask your muscles to relax, you are actually asking your system to reduce the nervous system stimulation to the muscle. There is no nerve that tells a muscle to relax. Instead, the nervous system reduces the amount of signal telling the muscle to contract.

A great misconception about the disc is that it can somehow move between the bones, or that it slides out of place or out from between the vertebrae. This is how most people envision a "slipped" disc. Unfortunately, the words used here do not accurately describe what is actually happening between the two vertebrae. Instead, the discs are held in place pretty securely between the bones via connective tissues, particularly the thick ligaments that surround them in the front and back. In addition, the periosteum (the outermost layer of connective tissue) of the vertebra itself is well-integrated into the discs. In other words, it is difficult for the discs to move.

Ruptured Discs

A ruptured disc takes things to another level. They often cause extreme pain. It is possible for a ruptured disc to progress from a herniated disc. It is also possible that a ruptured disc can happen on its own without beginning with a herniation. It all depends on the situation and circumstances.

In a ruptured disc, the cartilaginous ring or disc itself tears from its outer wall to the center, where the nucleus and fluid are. The fluid then leaks out from the disc. As a result

of fluid loss in the disc, the space between the bones is reduced. The purpose and function of the discs is compromised, which can result in compression of the nerve roots, not only by the disc but also by the vertebrae themselves.

Because of the loss of space between the bones and the compression of nerve roots, a ruptured disc often leads to surgical intervention. Surgeons take metal hardware and bolt the vertebrae together so that the space between them is maintained. With the space maintained, compression on the nerve roots is alleviated. The latest remedy for this disc problem is to replace the disc itself. Depending on the situation, different types of prosthetic discs can be placed between the bones. Sometimes it is as simple as another piece of bone. It is even better when the replacement is able to move and adapt to the stresses placed on the spine.

The problem with fusing the vertebrae together is that you create a kink in the chain of movement running through the spine. If there are two links in the middle of that chain that don't move, you have a new place for stress to build. Often people who have had their vertebrae fused experience dysfunction in the disc above the fusion; for example, that disc may herniate or rupture and also need to be removed and fused with the vertebrae above. Sometimes this process is repeated a few times.

INTEGRATING ANATOMY INTO YOUR PRACTICE

Feeling a Spine

Grab a partner for this one if you can. What I would like you to do is feel the parts of the spine that are most accessible. Have your partner get on the floor on their hands and knees. Place your fingertips right on the spinous processes that stick up off of their spine. Start in the lumbar section and spread your fingers apart. Have your partner do all of the movements of the spine—flexion, extension, lateral flexion, and rotation. You should feel the spinous processes moving under your fingers, and from that we can infer movement at the vertebral joints inside. Move your fingers up to the thoracic region and do the same thing. Notice the differences in movements between the sections.

Connecting Hip and Spine Movements

Stand up for a moment. You may have noticed this before, but let's focus our attention on the interrelated movements of the spine and the hip joint. Using internal awareness, slowly take one leg back from the standing position (keep it in the air) and notice the point at which the spine begins to move as your leg moves back. See if you can do the same for flexion of the hip joint. Now do abduction of the hip joint. It is possible you will feel your pelvis move, which is a good clue that your spine is also moving.

Fluidity of the Spine

I'll share a little intention that I use in my own practice. It stems from my work with John Scott and has played a huge role in my understanding of integrated movement. Ideally we want to have a strong and flexible spine. We also want to have a relationship with each part of our spine.

Sun Salutations are a great place to explore the intention of integrating the movements of all parts of the spine. Look for the spine to undulate through the forward and backward movements in Sun Salutations. Try to loosen the movements a bit and even exaggerate them

to see if you can assess which parts move and do not move in your spine. Then you can place a bit more emphasis on any areas that don't move so easily.

Feel Your Twist

When you next practice, pay close attention to how you twist. Close your eyes and feel what's going on. Have the following questions in mind: Do my hips move as I twist? If so, how much do they move? Do I initiate my twist from the lumbar part of my spine? Am I doing most of the twist through the thoracic spine? Depending on your answer to some or all of these questions, explore your twist in a different way than you normally do. See if you can emphasize your thoracic spine if you tend to twist mainly from the lumbar. Or focus the twist through your lumbar spine if you tend to emphasize the thoracic. Perhaps you can create more stability in your pelvis, or have noticed a need for greater freedom through that area?

Backbending

No conversation about the spine would be complete without covering backbending. The first thing we ought to do is change the way we use that word, *backbending*. It gives the impression that this movement is all about the back, or the spine. But we have to consider what body parts must open to allow the spine to be more comfortable in a backbend.

I have seen a lot of people doing backbends and consider them in relation to my own experience. I've watched people do a backbend, then walk their hands towards their feet, grab their ankles, and even grab their knees or higher. Watching a "super backbend" like this while my anatomical mind does its calculations

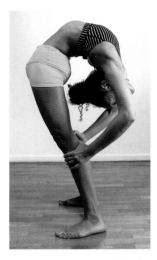

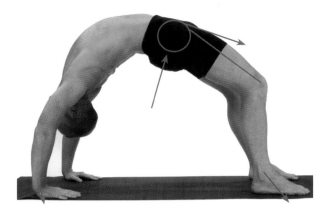

Figure 6.22: *The stronger I push up into a backbend, the hip flexors, if tight, pull my pelvis into an anterior tilt.*

Figure 6.21: *Notice where the pubic bone is pointing. Photograph supplied by, and the copyright of, Alessandro Sigismondi. Model Laruga Glaser (larugayoga.com).*

and sleuthing is always interesting. It asks the obvious questions, "How is this even possible? What are those vertebrae actually doing? Don't the spinous processes bump into each other at some point?" And then I saw it. The spine, although flexible and bending, stopped bending after a certain point. Instead, the pelvis moved. After the vertebrae hit their end range of motion, the pelvis has to rotate on top of the femurs to enable these "super backbends." This is a combination of posterior tilt of the pelvis and extension of the hips. I could see it in these backbends. The pubic bone was pointing up much more than it would be if standing in neutral while the legs are essentially in a neutral position, meaning that the pelvis has changed position along with the spine.

This single observation drove me into the laboratory of my own body. It also forced me to answer the following question: what tissues restrict the pelvis from moving in this way? The simple answer is, the tissues that anteriorly tilt the pelvis, which are also the tissues that flex the hips. These include the adductors, a quadriceps muscle, and the psoas. This epiphany led me to switch from thinking about which muscles needed to contract for the movement to occur

to thinking about which muscles needed to release for the movement to occur.

As we press up into a Full Wheel or other backbend, the spine goes into extension. You are now also trying to extend the hip joints.

This movement naturally stretches the hip flexors, which are basically the muscles that also cause the anterior tilt. Here we find a conundrum. The hip flexors are in a state of tension from their need to lengthen as the hip joint extends (not tension from contracting). That tension then pulls on the front of the pelvis, taking it in the direction of an anterior tilt that is more associated with hip flexion. As a result, the harder you press up into the backbend, the harder tight hip flexors will pull on the front of the pubic bone. This is probably the cause of 80 percent of people's sensation of compression in their lower back while doing a backbend. The tighter the hip flexors are, the more anteriorly they will tilt the pelvis. The more anterior the tilt of the pelvis, the more the lower spine has to bend. When the hip flexors do not restrict the pelvis, the pelvis can rotate backwards (into a posterior tilt) more easily, which is much more accommodating to the spine. If the hip flexors are open already, then the pelvis is less likely to be pulled in the direction of an anterior tilt.

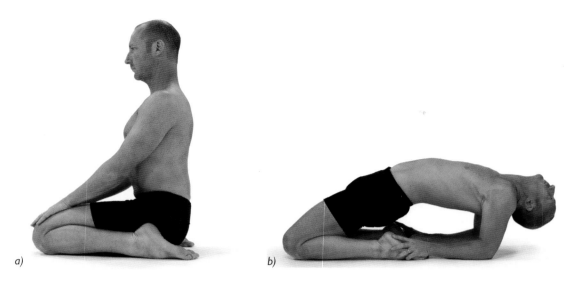

a)   b)

Figure 6.23: *Reclining and lifting the hips up puts pressure on the hip flexors, especially the quadriceps; a) Virasana, b) Supta Virasana.*

I put this to the test by focusing on the hip flexors before backbending. Although you can build a long sequence to prep yourself for a backbend, I was being more scientific about it. I asked the question, "How little do I need to do to make a difference? How can I be sure that there is a direct relationship between the amount of pressure I feel in my low back and my hip flexors?" To test my hypothesis, I did some research. First, I did a backbend to feel how much pressure and tension was in the hip flexors and the lower back. Then I stretched my hip flexors by coming into *Virasana*, which stretches the knee end of the quadriceps.

I moved into a modified *Supta Virasana* to increase the pressure on the hip end of the flexors. Then I pushed my hips up into the air to put even more pressure on the hip end. Guess what? When I lifted into another backbend, I felt less pressure in my lower back.

I am sure there are many ways to prepare the body for backbending. You should experiment to determine how much your hip flexors are involved in your lower back compression. It can bring a new level of awareness of where you want to focus your energy.

Spinal Dysfunction

Because the spine is so complicated, several conditions and injuries may be associated with it; so it is helpful to get some clarity about what is actually being affected (a disc, nerve, or vertebrae) and what the most common complaints and symptoms are. I don't wish for you to diagnose anyone. Instead, I hope you will more fully understand (or at least have heard of) some of the more common conditions associated with the spine. This way you can feel more confident working with someone with these concerns or referring him or her to someone who is more qualified.

Yoga and Disc Dysfunction

It is hard to give advice as to what individuals need with any or all of these situations in their yoga practice. The first step is to spend time doing a good evaluation of anyone who has any of these issues.

We have already discussed the basic anatomy of what happens when the discs are bulging, herniated, or ruptured. Generally speaking, flexion of the spine puts more pressure on the front of the vertebrae. This naturally sends the force into the disc in such a way that the fluid inside is pushed back and off to one side, where the original weakness already is. Therefore, excessive forward rounding of the spine can bring about more problems or further herniate a disc.

If I am working with someone who has a disc problem, I'll often keep his or her spine long and straight. I might even accentuate the lumbar curve and not have them fold as deeply in their forward bends. I find that backbending postures can alleviate pressure on the front of the spine, so I may create a sequence for them that includes simple backbending poses.

If a student has fusions in their vertebrae, I try to avoid having them move deeply in one direction and then the other. My theory is that too much back and forth starts to create pressure on the vertebrae above and below the fusion.

Sciatica

Sciatica is a condition often associated with disc problems and low back pain. Individuals have pain in the buttocks and/or down the back of the leg. This pain usually comes from one of two places. One place may be the spine. If something such as a bone or disc compresses a nerve root, sensation in the sciatic nerve further down will eventually occur. When this is the case, the individual would have pain or other sensation somewhere along the path of the sciatic nerve, including the buttocks and down the back of the leg. Sciatica can also come from the piriformis (one of the deep six lateral rotators of the femur and located in the buttocks). If it is tight and compressing the nerve, the piriformis can also create pain or other sensations in the buttocks and down the back of the leg.

Depending on which of these two is the cause, you could have two entirely different approaches for your student. Without going too far off into yoga therapy, the basic difference would be to either focus on restoring balance in the spine or work toward releasing the soft tissues of the buttocks, particularly the piriformis. If the student has had an MRI scan that shows there is something compressing the nerve root, then the focus would be spinal. If an MRI scan shows no problem with the spine itself, then you may want to proceed as if it is the piriformis.

There is a simple way to tell the difference between nerve root compression at the spine and tension in the piriformis. Ask your student to lie down on their back with both legs straight. On the side where the buttocks and back pain presents, have them try to raise that leg, keeping the knee straight. Although this isn't totally accurate, those that have a nerve compression near the spine will usually only be able to lift their leg between one and two feet off the floor. When we lift our leg, our sciatic nerve needs to stretch, but if a bone or disc is compressing the nerve, the student will have a sharp shooting pain when they lift their leg this high. In this case, you might work towards reestablishing the lumbar curve as previously discussed.

If they can lift their leg beyond a couple of feet with no major discomfort, it is more likely that there is compression from the piriformis muscle. In this case, Pigeon Pose or other postures that stretch the piriformis would be appropriate.

General Back Pain

Back pain is a common complaint. There are a million reasons for and causes of general back pain, and they won't be the same for everyone. Often the underlying cause is complex and influenced by many factors, such as postural patterns, muscular tension, mental stress, lack of exercise, too much exercise, job requirements, or injuries from years earlier. The list could go on and on. The only thing more complex than determining an underlying cause is trying to unravel it in a way that provides a clear plan of action for helping a person understand and even resolve their pain. Applying the tools of yoga to do this can be challenging and requires a good understanding of both anatomy and the effects of the *asanas*. An assessment of the pain that is thorough, precise, and without bias is key to successfully using yoga to resolve back pain.

Back pain has the highest rate of occurrence in people aged 45 to 64 years and is:

- The second most common reason for a doctor's visit.
- The third most common reason for surgery.
- The fifth most common reason for hospitalization.

If we are going to work with someone with back pain, we should take the time to do a proper assessment, take the history of the individual, and research their specific problem. It is beyond the scope of this book to teach you those skills, but the following examples are a good start to understanding some of the different causes for back pain that go beyond what is most commonly talked about.

I have gained a lot from observing people and trying to understand whether their pain is generally coming from postural distortions, a disc problem, or more systemic life stressors. Oftentimes it is a combination of the three. Instead of giving everyone with back pain the same advice, I try to figure out which general category predominates. This classification will determine which postures a student should or should not be doing. I am not proposing that you follow a protocol for each of these types. Because it is you who will be working with the student (or yourself), you should apply your own skills of observation and assessment and make decisions based on what you see, hear, or find in the moment. All I can do here is provide you with a general guideline and some basic direction.

The first category is postural distortions. These arise from repetitive movements or habitual patterns, such as sitting or slouching. Because the activity is repeated so often, the body will naturally develop imbalances in strength and flexibility in either the front, back, or sides. This is exactly what creates postural distortions: an imbalance in the tissues around a given area or the entire body. Some examples include scoliosis, leg length discrepancy, uneven pelvis (one side rotated forward or backward), and tight hip flexors that create a strong lordotic curve.

One of the most popular assertions is that a weak core causes lower back pain. At the heart of this claim is the transverse abdominis. It is common for people to advise someone with back pain to strengthen their core. I'm guessing most of you have heard this advice along the way? Maybe you have even given this advice?

While strengthening the abdominals can be an effective way for people who are not dealing with back pain to add support to their spine, in reality, the exact opposite might be more suitable for people with certain causes of back pain. For example, doing abdominal crunches or psoas-strengthening exercises with a herniated disc can exacerbate the problem. Abdominal work shouldn't be (nor was it meant to be) a panacea for back pain.

Core-strengthening exercises do help a number of people with back pain. General exercise and weight loss have also been shown to significantly reduce episodes of back pain. It seems to me that in the process of working the abdominals and basically getting into better shape, people tend to reevaluate stressors, foods, and other general health questions relative to their life. To alleviate back pain due to postural imbalance, a comprehensive approach to health that establishes an overall balance of strength and flexibility can work wonders. In other words, do yoga *asanas*.

Perhaps the most common advice I give to people with back pain is to reestablish their lumbar curve, stretch their hip flexors, and practice more backbending types of postures. This advice is grounded in some basic assumptions about the average person who shows up to a class and what constitutes the majority of their day—sitting. A series of anatomical problems arise from the average person's lifestyle. We commute to work, sit for most of the day at a desk, commute home, and then sit on the couch. Being seated for so many hours often leads to tight hip flexors; it can also cause compression of the front of the vertebrae, which removes the lumbar curve, and can eventually contribute to a herniated disc.

These people need to focus on opening their front body. These are the students who, when asked to do a backbend, look something like a coffee table. This shows how tight and restricted the front of the body can be. These students might start off in a passive backbend on a bolster. Others may be able to do more advanced postures such as Camel and Full Wheels, depending on their overall health and strength. You will have to determine for yourself where to start them off. You also must consider what type of stress people have going on in their life. (Back to those Converging Histories!) There is plenty of evidence relating stress and trauma to physical pain.

When working with students with back pain, I begin with a broad approach and slowly narrow it down as I observe, listen, and respond to what a client or student is saying and feeling as we go through different postures. Be willing to explore and change as the condition and circumstances require.

7
COMPARING THE UPPER AND LOWER EXTREMITIES

I've decided there is a need for another way of looking at what constitutes anatomical position. (That is, standing with feet hip-width apart and palms facing forward). This is the basis for anatomical terminology and for the named movements that we do, but it feels limited, particularly in reference to a body in motion. It assumes that we are standing and beginning our movements from anatomical position. I'd like to add a new perspective, derived from my observations of the functional similarities between the upper and lower body. To show how similar these are, I lie on my back, knees and elbows bent, almost as if preparing for a backbend except that my hands are turned such that the fingers point away from my head. It is easier in this position to see how

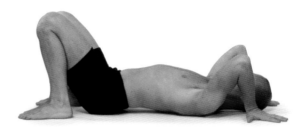

Figure 7.1: *This is a functional anatomical position for being supine on the floor.*

the upper limb and lower limbs actually mirror one another.

If I straighten my left arm and left leg, the movement is the same in both. If I move my elbow and knee towards each other simultaneously, then again, there is a mirroring effect. Let's look at how this mirroring begins in the structures of the skeletal system first.

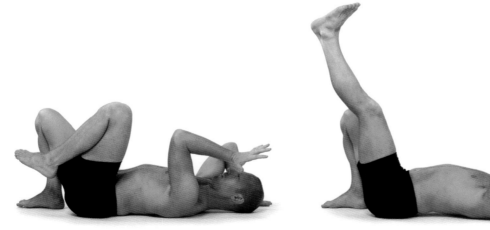

Figure 7.2: *Movements of the upper and lower limbs then mirror one another.*

I am still amazed by the similarities between the arm and the leg. Upon casual observation, they seem totally different. After all, they have completely different purposes, so their functions must be different, right? But if you look at the structures themselves, you will see they are strikingly similar in a number of ways.

We'll start at the bottom of each limb. As we've said, the foot is made up of 26 bones: 14 phalanges (toes), 5 metatarsals, and 7 tarsals. The hand is made up of 27 bones: 14 phalanges (fingers), 5 metacarpals, and 8 carpals. The ankle joint flexes, extends, abducts, and adducts. These movements are called dorsiflexion, plantarflexion, eversion, and inversion, respectively. The wrist moves

in these same directions: flexion, extension, abduction, and adduction.

Moving upwards, there are two bones in the foreleg and two bones in the forearm. The knee and elbow are both hinge joints. Even the pointy part of the elbow (the olecranon) correlates to the kneecap. The knee has the ability to rotate in either direction once it bends ten degrees or more. The radius and ulna also rotate relative to one another. Technically this rotation does not happen at one joint; instead our forearm rotates and moves our hand. We call these movements supination and pronation of the forearm.

As we move up to the femur and humerus, we find that both are long bones that end at the top

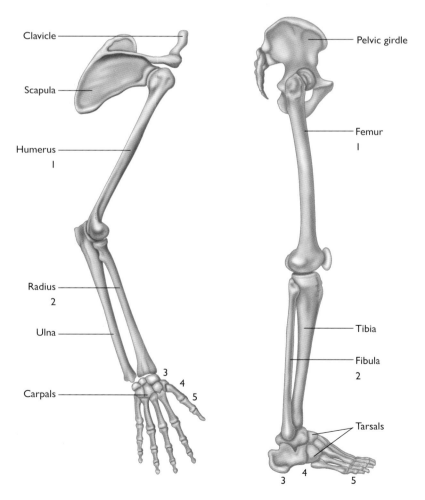

Figure 7.3: *Ntotice the similarities between the extremities.*

with a ball and socket joint built for mobility. Of course the socket for the femur is much deeper than the one for the humerus. The femur is built to handle weight and movement while the shoulder is built for mobility.

The similarities don't end there. If you look at one side of the pelvis compared to one scapula, you will find they are both flat, irregular-shaped bones. Take it one step further and compare the clavicle to the pubic bone. Their shapes and functions are quite similar as well. They each connect the pelvis and shoulder girdle together in the front. The two pubic bones meet each other at the pubic symphysis and the two clavicles attach to the sternum.

In addition to these obvious structural similarities, there are several muscular similarities as well. Think of the flexors of the forearms, which are much larger than the extensors. They are similar to the large calf muscles, which move the ankles and are significantly larger than their opposing muscles.

In the upper leg we have the quadriceps, which is a muscle divided into four sections. On the upper arm we have the triceps brachii, which is a muscle divided into three sections.

Both have a common tendon that crosses their respective joints (the knee and elbow, respectively), and both are dedicated to extension of the knee and elbow. Both the upper leg and upper arm have one muscle that crosses the joint. In the quadriceps, the rectus femoris crosses the hip joint. In the triceps brachii, the long head crosses the shoulder joint. Both of the muscles cross the joint above it and create the same action at their respective joints. Unfortunately, based on anatomical position, these movements are referred to as "opposite movements." But from our "new" anatomical point of view, the movement is similar and both move towards the torso. The rectus femoris lifts the leg towards the torso. The long head of the triceps brachii brings the upper arm towards the torso as well.

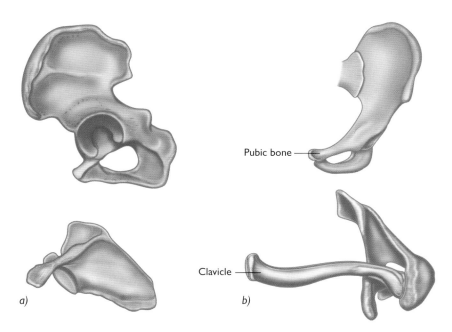

Pubic bone

Clavicle

a)   b)

Figure 7.4: *More similarities; a) comparing pelvis to scapula, b) clavicle to pubis.*

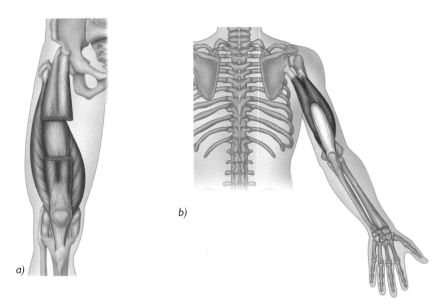

Figure 7.5: *Comparing; a) quadriceps, b) triceps brachii.*

On the other side of the femur we have the hamstrings, which are a group of three muscles with a portion of one of them (biceps femoris) having a short head that only crosses the knee joint. In the arm we have the biceps brachii, which is a two-part muscle. Lying just underneath the biceps brachii is the brachialis, which is similar to the short head of the hamstrings: the brachialis only crosses the elbow joint. The hamstrings (except for that short head) affect the hip joint and extend it.

The biceps brachii also crosses the shoulder joint and assists in flexing it. This mirrors the movement of the leg when the hamstrings contract. Both muscles move their respective limbs away from the torso. In addition, the hamstrings rotate the lower leg both internally

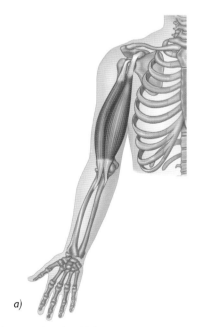
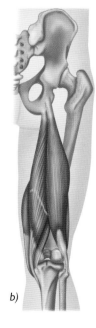

Figure 7.6: *Comparing; a) biceps brachii, b) hamstrings.*

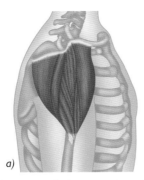
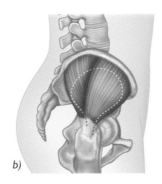

Figure 7.7: *Comparing; a) deltoid, b) gluteus minimus/medius.*

and externally. As it turns out, the biceps brachii is a powerful supinator (rotator) of the forearm. Although it only rotates the forearm in one direction, I find the similarity curious. We have a similar pattern of one less portion or muscle on the upper arm than on the lower arm. This makes sense, considering that the lower arm is smaller.

Even the gluteals of the hip joint have their counterpart at the shoulder joint. The deltoids are primarily abductors of the shoulder, as are the gluteus minimus and medius abductors of the hip. In addition, the front sections of both the gluteals and the deltoids pull their respective limb forward and rotate it internally. The back portions do just the opposite; they extend and externally rotate the limbs.

Even the infraspinatus and teres minor (two of the rotator cuff muscles) remind me of the deep six lateral rotators found in the hip joint. The subscapularis (another rotator cuff muscle) fits inside the scapula the way the iliacus fits inside the pelvis.

Looking at these similarities can help deepen our understanding of each of these limbs, based on what we know about the other. The most powerful and important mover of the lower extremity is the psoas muscle. Is there an equivalent in the upper extremity? We don't have an exact fit for the psoas of the upper body, but as we look closer at the shoulder girdle, you will see there are enough similarities in function and design to fit this comparison. Before we move to the "psoas" of the upper body, let's review the geography and some of the tissues that surround the shoulder girdle.

THE SHOULDER GIRDLE

Three bones come together to create the shoulder girdle. They are the upper arm bone (humerus), the shoulder blade (scapula), and the collarbone (clavicle). The movements at the shoulder are complex, which is fitting, as it is sometimes referred to as the shoulder complex. It is much

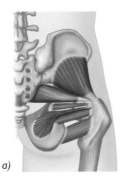
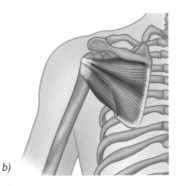

Figure 7.8: *Comparing; a) deep six lateral rotators, b) infraspinatus/teres minor.*

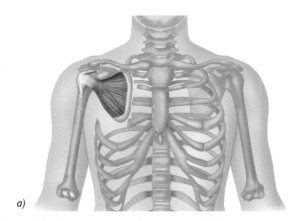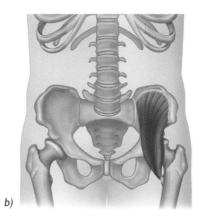

Figure 7.9: *Comparing; a) subscapularis, b) iliacus.*

more intricate than the pelvic girdle because the scapula and clavicle are not attached to the stable structure of the spine via the sacrum. Instead we have an independent scapula on each side of the spine. The clavicles attach to the sternum (somewhat similar to the pubic bones) but they are much more free to move around than their counterpart in the pelvis. In fact, the movements of each of these parts contributes to the overall functionality of the shoulder complex.

LANDMARKS AND GEOGRAPHY

One end of the clavicle attaches to the sternum. This is the only place that a bone from the shoulder girdle attaches to the center component of the body called the axial skeleton. A small cartilaginous disc between the sternum and clavicle helps mitigate the forces that naturally run through it. The other end of the clavicle heads out to the shoulder

itself and attaches onto the scapula at the acromion process.

At this juncture, the clavicle and the scapula are bound together by ligaments. There is not much range of movement here. Depending on the forces created at this joint, there may be some give, but no remarkable movement is possible. This is the acromioclavicular joint, or the AC joint; it is the bump we feel on the top of the shoulder. If these ligaments tear, we have a "separated shoulder." Since we have already connected to the scapula, let's do a quick tour of the bits and bumps on it. The scapula itself does not sit flat on the back as we might suspect. The rib cage is more round or circular in shape. If anything, the scapula sits at about a 45-degree angle relative to the body's orientation.

Our association with the shoulder blade (scapula) as being part of our back is so common that students are often surprised to

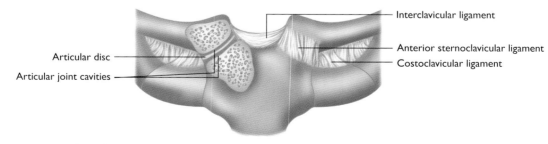

Interclavicular ligament

Anterior sternoclavicular ligament
Costoclavicular ligament

Articular disc

Articular joint cavities

Figure 7.10: *Sternoclavicular joint.*

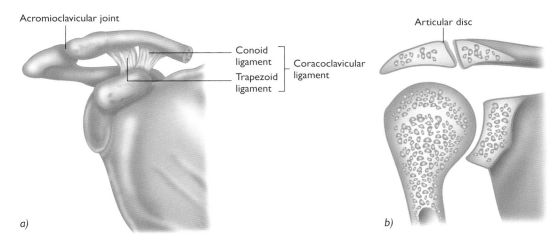

Figure 7.11: *Acromioclavicular joint; a) anterior view, b) coronal view.*

feel their scapula on the front of their body. There is a beak-like projection under the lateral part of the clavicle called the coracoid process. If you walk your fingers just under your clavicle toward your shoulder, you come across a bit of a depression in the tissues. Just on the outer part of this little depression is the pointy bit of bone I am referring to. It tends to be a little tender, as three different muscles attach to it. This is part of your scapula.

The acromion of the scapula is like a ledge that juts out over the top of the humerus. If we follow it around the back of the scapula, it is part of what is known as the spine of the scapula.

This boney ridge runs almost horizontally with a small angle down towards the center of the body. You can feel this relatively easily by placing one hand on the top of the other shoulder and moving your hand up and down.

There are points at the top and bottom of the scapula referred to as the superior and inferior angles. Between them is the medial border. On the outer edge is the lateral border of the scapula. At the top of the lateral border and under the acromion process is the glenoid fossa. (A fossa is a depression in a bone.) The glenoid fossa is the depression in which the head of the humerus sits. This is called the

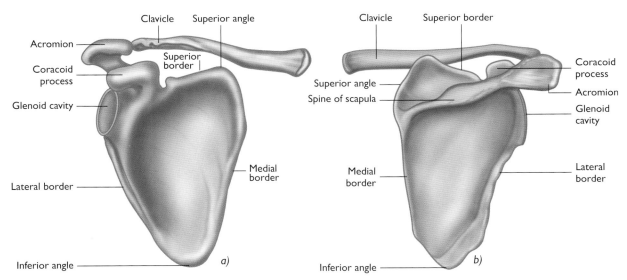

Figure 7.12: *Clavicle and scapula; a) anterior view of right scapula, b) posterior view of right scapula.*

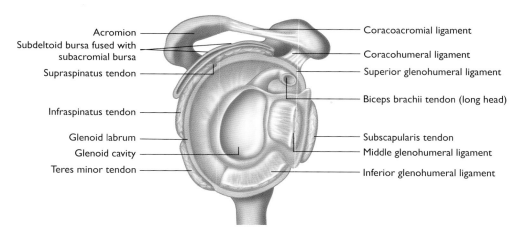

Figure 7.13: *Glenohumeral joint, right arm, lateral view.*

glenohumeral joint, a more technical name for the shoulder joint.

The humerus, because it is attached to the scapula, also heads off from the body at about a 45-degree angle. Go back to your coracoid process, under your clavicle, and keep heading laterally. You will end up on the humerus.

MOVEMENTS OF THE HUMERUS

Movement in the shoulder joint mirrors what we found in the hip joint. It flexes, extends, abducts, adducts, and rotates both internally and externally. This part is straightforward. When the humerus reaches its end range of motion for the ball and socket joint, it triggers movements of the scapula. In other words, when you raise your arm over your head, the humerus moves at the shoulder joint until reaching its end range of motion. When the head of the humerus bumps into the shelf-like acromion process sitting above it, the muscles that move the scapula kick in to get the arm the rest of the way over the head. However, this shift does not happen until the end of range of motion for the first joint is reached.

The humerus only abducts to 90 degrees at the shoulder joint in the average person.

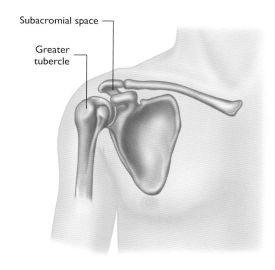
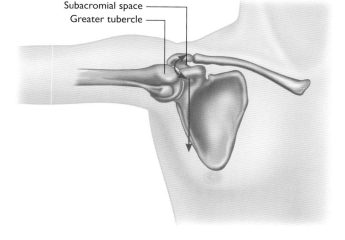

Figure 7.14: *Glenohumeral joint functions.*

If you were to place your hand on the opposite shoulder and pull it down so that it can't move, you will find you can only lift your arm to the side (abduction) about parallel to the floor. The same thing happens if you maintain the pressure on your shoulder and lift your arm in front of you. This means that every time you have ever raised your arm over your head, your bones have bumped together. This is normal and isn't painful unless something else is going on. There are ways to slightly increase the amount of abduction or flexion that you get at the shoulder joint before it hits the acromion. If you rotate your humerus externally before you abduct or flex at the shoulder joint, you will normally pick up between two and five degrees of movement. If you rotate the humerus internally as far as it will go, you will normally lose between two and five degrees of movement.

MOVEMENTS OF THE SCAPULA

The scapula, relative to the rib cage, is not a typical joint. Its movements are sometimes referred to as scapulothoracic movements. In most articulations, the bones touch one another and have some type of cartilaginous connection. Not here. The scapula floats along the ribs as it moves.

When the scapula moves, the humerus must move with it because they are connected. The scapula has six named movements. It moves up and down, which is referred to as elevation and depression. It slides around towards the front of the rib cage and also slides back so that the two scapulae move closer to each other on your back. These actions are called protraction and retraction. The scapula also rotates upwards and downwards. There are different ways to measure this movement. The bottom tip of the scapula is called the inferior angle. When it moves sideways and up, we're doing upward rotation. Another way to measure movement is by looking at the depression that the head of the humerus fits into, the glenoid fossa. When this points upwards, the scapula is upwardly rotating. When it points downwards, the movement is downward rotation.

There is at least one more action that we could talk about at the scapula. It isn't commonly discussed in anatomy books, but we see it and talk about it in relation to yoga. The movement I am referring to is the tilting of the scapula sideways. In yoga we see this in High Plank and sometimes in Chaturanga. When this tilt occurs, the inner or medial border of the scapula sticks up under the skin as opposed to being held down close to the rib cage.

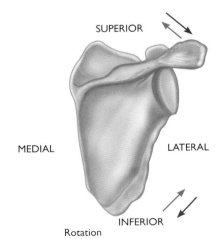

Figure 7.15: *Scapular motion.*

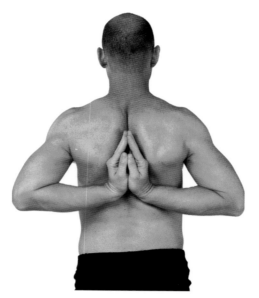

Figure 7.16: *Reverse prayer requires movement at the clavicle, scapula, and humerus.*

MOVEMENTS OF THE CLAVICLE

Finally we have the clavicle. The clavicle follows the scapula in most of its movements; it elevates, depresses, protracts, and retracts. Unlike the scapula, however, the clavicle can also rotate. This is not a particularly large movement, but it's enough that when your arm reaches behind your back (as in reverse prayer position) the clavicle rotates downwards and forwards along the axis of the bone itself. Clearly because it rotates in this direction, it must also rotate back.

When the movements available at all of these joints are combined, we get the incredible range of motion of the shoulder complex. With the arm abducted to 90 degrees, the hand can rotate almost 360 degrees!

THE SHOULDER AND BONE SHAPE

As we mentioned when discussing the body's other ball and socket joint (the hip), there are variations in bone shape from person to person. The shoulder offers its own variations between the two bones that fit together at this joint. In *utero* the arms bud out and then fold and twist into the fetal position, making for the natural twists that run through the humerus.

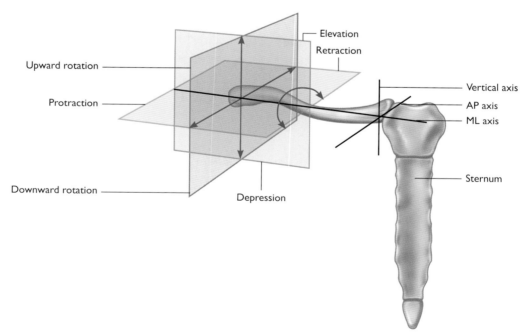

Figure 7.17: *Movement of the clavicle.*

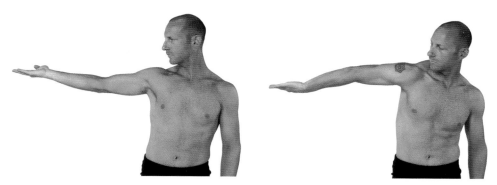

Figure 7.18: *All combined we get almost 360 degrees of rotation through the entire arm.*

There are three types of scapulae.[27] Anatomists look at the acromion in particular to describe these three types. A Type I acromion sits behind the glenoid fossa and sits at an angle though its bone shape is straight. In Type IIs, the acromion is curved over the top of the glenoid fossa. Type IIIs are curved as in Type IIs, but part of the acromion (at the front) hooks downwards slightly. Along with these different shapes, we can look at how far out the acromion is relative to the glenoid. Sometimes the acromion sits way out over it and sometimes it does not stick out very far.

When you combine these varieties of shapes, it gets even more complicated. If the acromion is more like Type I and doesn't stick out very far, the humerus will have more space as it abducts or flexes in the shoulder joint. If it is shaped more like a Type III, and

the acromion sticks out quite far over the humerus, abduction and flexion will be more restricted. Of course, these are the edges of the norm. The most common type is Type II—an acromion that sticks out in the middle range. The average amount of abduction and flexion at the shoulder joint is therefore 90 degrees for both. Those people with a Type I acromion can both abduct and flex their arm completely without the scapula moving.

MUSCLES THAT MOVE THE HUMERUS

The flexibility and mobility of the shoulder joint bring with it demands not seen in the hip joint. The hip has a deep socket and more stability, but it lacks the range of motion found in the shoulder. The increased flexibility at the shoulder demands stability. What we really

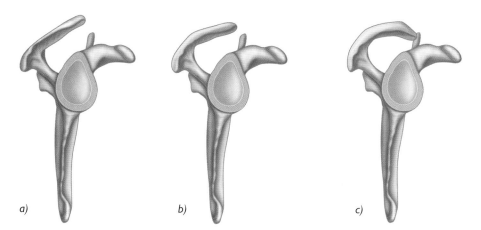

Figure 7.19: *Three types of scapulae; a) type 1: flat 17%, b) type 2: curved 43%, c) type 3: hooked 40%.*

need at the shoulder is stability with a certain amount of flexibility built into it. There is a joint capsule and ligaments that support it, but do these structures alone fit the demands I describe?

There are two layers of tissue in the shoulder joint. The large movers of the humerus, such as the pectoralis major and latissimus dorsi, are closer to the surface. Deeper and more intrinsic are the rotator cuff muscles. I refer to them as dynamic stabilizers of the shoulder. By this I mean that they stabilize the joint to make up for the lack of structure. At the same time, the rotator cuff allows for flexibility because it is made of muscles, which have more elasticity than the denser ligaments at the hip joint.

The Rotator Cuff

Four muscles comprise the rotator cuff. They are the supraspinatus, infraspinatus, teres minor, and subscapularis. The unfortunate reason these muscles are so well-known is that rotator cuff tears are rather common. The frequency of these tears is indicative of the high demands placed on this group. The name rotator cuff derives from the movement

they create, as well as from their common attachment. Because the head of the humerus is round and ball-like, fitting into a shallow depression, all of the movements including flexion and extension are a rotation in terms of the function of the joint. All of the muscles attach into a common tendon that is like a shirt cuff lying over the top of the humerus.

The first of the four muscles we will talk about is the supraspinatus. "Supra" means above and "spinatus" refers to the spine of the scapula. The area above the spine of the scapula is called the supraspinous fossa (depression). This muscle fills in that depression and then runs laterally to the top of the head of the humerus. As it does so, the supraspinatus runs under the acromion process through a space between the acromion and the top of the humerus. Because of this location, its action initiates abduction of the humerus. I say initiates because it abducts the arm about ten degrees or so. Then the much larger deltoid muscles have leverage to lift it the rest of the way.

The supraspinatus is one of two commonly torn rotator cuff muscles. This injury often occurs while lifting a heavy bag on one side. The movement requires that the arm abduct

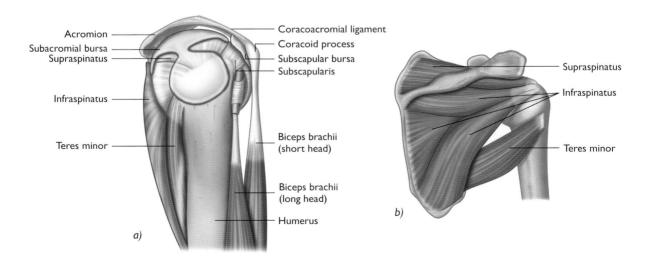

Figure 7.20: *Rotator cuff muscles; a) lateral view, b) posterior view.*

slightly while holding significant weight. There may be circumstances that lead to weakness in the tendon before an event like this happens, such as different physical activities and even age, but because the muscle runs through a relatively narrow space under the acromion, it is susceptible to a few additional factors. If there is overuse and swelling in the joint in general, this muscle can become compressed under the bone and impingement syndrome may develop.

A combination of other elements or factors makes such a narrow passageway tricky for this muscle. A fluid-filled sac (bursa) sits above the tendon and under a ligament. This can become inflamed. Bone spurs can develop in the area as well, irritating the bursa (leading to bursitis) and adding pressure to the muscle tendon. The pain associated with this can be in the front and side of the shoulder. This does not, however, mean that all pain in this area is related to the supraspinatus.

Although repetitive movements while weight bearing in yoga can contribute to shoulder problems, it is unlikely that specific movements will tear this particular muscle of the rotator cuff. It is the infraspinatus—the next of the rotator cuff muscles—that seems to dysfunction the most from yoga *asana*. Although tearing is a possibility, it is unlikely to result from general yoga practice. The most common dysfunctions in yoga practice are often in *Vinyasa*-style practitioners.

The infraspinatus is located under ("infra" means below) the spine of the scapula in the infraspinous fossa. This is a broader muscle that pretty much fills the entire surface of the scapula below the spine. Therefore, it is just under the skin on the bottom two-thirds of the scapula. Its tendon runs laterally and attaches onto the back of the head of the humerus.

This muscle works with two other muscles that externally rotate the humerus—the posterior portion of the deltoids and the small rotator cuff muscle called the teres minor. The infraspinatus muscle becomes the second most commonly torn muscle of the rotator cuff in its rotational capacity. We often see trouble from this muscle in baseball pitchers. The infraspinatus slows the arm after a pitcher releases the ball when throwing. It eccentrically contracts while its overall length increases as a braking mechanism for the arm. Because it is an external rotator, the infraspinatus resists and restricts internal rotation of the humerus. Many of the "binds" we do in yoga require internal rotation of the humerus (and of course scapular movement). For example, our humerus is internally rotated when we put our hands in reverse prayer position behind the back and when we bind the arm in *Marichyasana C* and other twists with a similar binding.

The teres minor works right along with the infraspinatus. It actually looks like a piece of the infraspinatus that has separated slightly. It attaches on the bottom of the scapula at the inferior angle and heads up to attach right below the infraspinatus; it contributes to external rotation of the humerus.

In keeping with the comparison of the upper and lower limbs, the infraspinatus and teres minor remind me of the deep six lateral rotators at the hip joint. It is common to find restriction at the shoulder joint when we try to externally rotate it. Only three small areas of tissue provide external rotation. Thus they must overcome restriction created by much larger, more powerful muscles at the shoulder joint, such as the pectoralis major, latissimus dorsi, teres major, anterior deltoid, and subscapularis. We will look at this more closely when considering how to set up the arms in backbends.

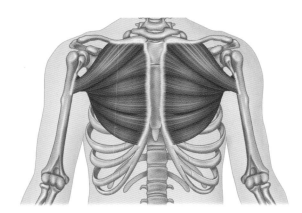

Figure 7.21: *Pectoralis major.*

Additional Movers of the Humerus

These other more powerful muscles are the second layer that moves the humerus. The pectoralis is situated on the front of the chest. It attaches from the clavicle to the sternum and then down onto some of the lower ribs. Its broad area of attachment converges as it heads towards the humerus and attaches onto what is called the bicipital groove. Here one of the tendons of the biceps lies between two raised areas of bone. The pectoralis functions as a flexor and extender of the humerus depending on the situation. It is also a powerful internal rotator of the humerus.

The large, broad latissimus muscle lies on the back of the body. Its attachments also begin broadly at the thoracolumbar aponeurosis (a common tendinous sheath in the lower back and sacral area) that is itself attached to the sacrum. It then attaches to spinous processes all the way up the spine to about T6. The latissimus dorsi also attaches onto the lower ribs (12-9) and then heads up to the humerus, usually draping over the inferior angle of the scapula. Like the pectorals, it attaches onto the humerus in the bicipital groove.

The latissimus dorsi is sometimes referred to as the "swimmer's muscle" as it is often well-developed in swimmers. That is because it

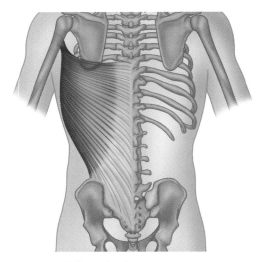

Figure 7.22: *Latissimus dorsi.*

is a powerful internal rotator, extender, and adductor of the humerus—all actions needed for swimming. We often associate its strength with adduction of the humerus, as in doing pull-ups.

The teres major is like the "little helper" of the latissimus dorsi in adduction and internal rotation. Although a small muscle, it is rather thick and dense for its size, making it quite strong. It attaches from the bottom of the scapula to the bicipital groove, in the same place as the pectoralis major and latissimus dorsi.

The deltoids are a small but powerful group of muscles. I refer to them as the gluteal muscles of the shoulder. Their attachment spans the lateral half of the clavicle, the acromion, and the lateral half of the spine of the scapula. It basically wraps around the top of the shoulder from front to back. Its fibers converge to attach to the deltoid tuberosity, a palpable bump near the center of the humerus. The muscle is divided into three sections—the anterior, middle, and posterior deltoids. The anterior portion assists flexion and internal rotation of the shoulder. The posterior section does the opposite; it assists extension and external rotation. The middle portion (assisted by the other two portions) abducts the shoulder joint.

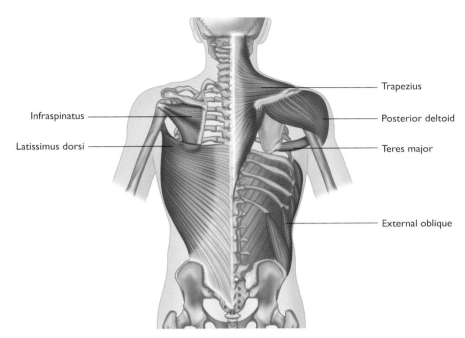

Figure 7.23: *Superficial back and shoulder muscles.*

All of these muscles work together to move the shoulder joint. We will pay particular attention to the latissimus dorsi in a moment. First, however, we need to look at the muscles that move the scapula.

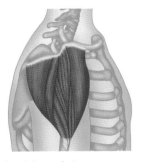

Figure 7.24: *Deltoid, lateral view.*

MUSCLES THAT MOVE THE SCAPULA

Closely coordinated with the movements of the shoulder are the movements of the scapula. Remember that when the scapula moves, the humerus also moves. The position of the scapula can affect which muscles are recruited to do a particular movement at the shoulder joint. If the scapula is not in the "right" position, it is possible that other muscles, particularly those that move the shoulder joint itself, have to work harder or differently than they are optimally designed to. *Chaturanga* comes to mind as an example. If the scapula is in the wrong place, it can cause shoulder muscles to strain. It is also true that if shoulder muscles are too weak, the scapula will adapt and move to compensate. This is a great example of how intricate the shoulder complex really is.

Most people are familiar with the large trapezius muscle that covers a notable portion of the upper back. It is divided into upper, middle, and lower sections. Although the upper section can elevate and the lower can depress the scapula, all sections seem to contribute to its upward rotation.

Other muscles move the scapula as well. The rhomboids sit between the shoulder blades. This muscle assists in downward rotation and retraction of the scapula and is thinner than most people imagine. There is also the levator scapulae, a downward rotator and (as its name suggests) elevator of the scapula. The pectoralis minor lives on the front of the rib

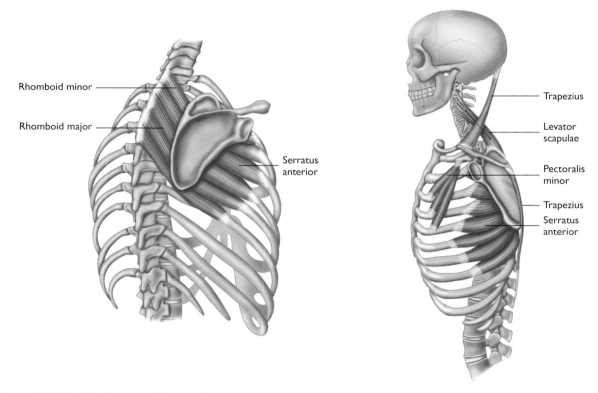

Figure 7.25: *Muscles that move the scapula.*

cage and attaches to the coracoid process. It is a downward rotator and depressor of the scapula, though few people are familiar with it.

All of these muscles really "assist" the more powerful movers of the scapula. You could say they need each other in order to make big and powerful movements happen. There is, however, one muscle that I have yet to mention—the serratus anterior.

The serratus anterior is named for its jagged-lined attachment on the side of the ribs in front of the scapula (*serratus*, like a serrated knife). From its attachment, the muscle heads back and between the scapula and rib cage to attach onto the inner (medial) border of the scapula. Due to this orientation, the muscle protracts (moves forward) and upwardly rotates the scapula. Its nickname is "the boxer's muscle," because an uppercut requires the combined movement of upward rotation and protraction of the scapula.

As it turns out, we do this movement in several yoga poses that require strength from the upper body. If you put your arms into the position for Down Dog, Handstand, Headstand, a forearm balance, or a backbend, you will find that your scapulae are protracted and upwardly rotated.

Of course, the humerus also moves to get into these positions. One particular characteristic about the serratus anterior is that it is also a powerful stabilizer of the scapula. If it dysfunctions and becomes weak (this can happen from nerve damage), you end up with a condition known as "winged scapula." The inner border of the scapula will stick up off the back of someone with this condition. We often try to avoid this winged position when doing arm balancing postures. Even in High Plank or *Chaturanga*, we are susceptible to the scapulae popping off the back. What keeps them on the rib cage? The serratus anterior.

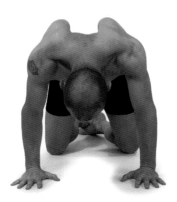 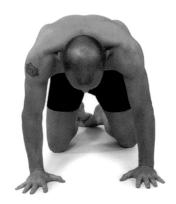

Figure 7.26: *Activation of the serratus anterior muscle causes the torso to be lifted between the two scapulae.*

This is yet another example of muscles sometimes doing the opposite of what we expect. I've already told you that the serratus anterior protracts the scapula. But what happens if we switch the origin and insertion around? Let's say I am in High Plank and my scapulae are sticking up.

I could think about moving my scapulae in a particular way to get them back down, but what actually happens is quite different. My scapulae are actually stuck relative to the floor because they are sitting on the head of the humerus, which is connected all the way down to the floor through my hands. This makes it difficult for them to move, although some rotation may be possible. In order to bring the scapulae back down onto my rib cage, I am actually going to engage the serratus anterior. Because my scapulae are connected to the ground via the arm and hand, the resultant action is for the rib cage to lift up between the scapulae. That's right, because of the positioning of the body and the scapulae, the chest moves instead of the scapulae, reversing the origin and insertion of this muscle.

Now, let's bring the functionality of two muscles together to create our "psoas" of the upper body. Although the serratus anterior it isn't an identical match for the psoas, adding another muscle will help to support my argument. First, what elements am I using to create a psoas of the

upper body? Size, position, strength, function, and resistance. In terms of size, the psoas of the upper body should span a large distance and be a strong shoulder extender. Shoulder extension would be the equivalent of hip flexion because both bring the limb closer to the torso. The muscle that best fits this bill is the latissimus dorsi. We have already described the large and expansive attachment of this muscle. It stretches from the sacrum, along the spine, and out to the humerus. It spans a large distance tying together the sacrum and pelvis to the humerus, just like the psoas major. The psoas connects the torso to the femur and the latissimus dorsi connects the torso to the humerus.

As for strength and function, we often assume the most powerful movement of the latissimus dorsi is adduction of the shoulders. This is definitely true in anatomical position (think of pull-ups). But what about the serratus anterior and its ability to protract the scapula around the front of the ribs? Once this happens, the same powerful movement (adduction) of the latissimus dorsi is now called extension of the shoulder. When the scapula is in a protracted position, the latissimus dorsi is the strongest extender. This also means it is the strongest resister of shoulder joint flexion.

This mirrors the resistance we get at the real psoas muscle in a backbend, for example.

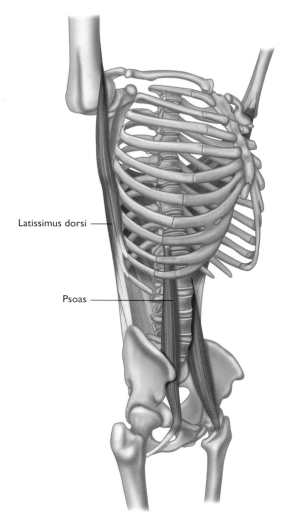

Figure 7.27: *These two muscles cross one another to create powerful movement toward the front of the trunk.*

Latissimus dorsi

Psoas

The psoas resists lifting the pelvis, or resists hip extension. The latissimus dorsi resists flexion of the shoulder in a backbend. We will look at this in more detail in the *asana* section.

INTEGRATING ANATOMY INTO YOUR PRACTICE

Shoulder or scapula? Take note where scapula movement comes into play when you are moving the rest of your arm. For instance, if you place your left hand on top of your right shoulder and "pin" it down and then try to abduct the arm (raise it to the side), you will

notice that it gets stuck at about 90 degrees (a few of you might be exceptions to this).

Position the scapula in a pose like *Chaturanga* (please modify for the purpose of exploration). With your knees on the floor, lower down to *Chaturanga* and with less weight being supported, move your shoulders from your scapulae towards your ears, down your back, around the front, and try to squeeze them together. Why? Use the extreme to help you find the middle ground in all of this and you will probably find your own "sweet spot."

You can also play with the position of the scapulae in your Down Dog. We are often told to externally rotate the upper arms while internally rotating the lower arms. There is nothing at all wrong with this, but notice how much of this action can come from and be supported by the scapula itself.

Do a Down Dog on your knees (basically a Child's Pose) and sit back on your heels. Let your elbows bend so that they just touch the floor, using the floor to push down into. Now see if you can sense the contraction of the serratus anterior as it brings your scapula around in protraction. Move into a real Down Dog and, for experiment's sake, bend the elbows slightly and try to move them towards the floor from the scapulae, as you did when the knees were bent. Can you sense the same contraction, maintain it, and then straighten the arms?

General Shoulder Pain and *Chaturanga*

Because of its dynamic movements, it can be difficult to figure out what is causing shoulder pain. For some reason, *Chaturanga* is often blamed. Although it is true this posture can cause shoulder pain, the pain is not really *Chaturanga's* fault.

After all, the pose doesn't exist until you do it. So the resulting pain must have something to do with the way you do the *asana*.

When we look at a movement like *Chaturanga*, we are not moving out of the normal range of motion of the shoulder joint. However, in order for the shoulder joint to function optimally, the rest of the girdle must be stabilized for efficient movement of the humerus. By efficient, I mean movement that doesn't over-burden or stress the muscles that control this joint. The great debate with *Chaturanga* is where to put those pesky scapulae. The more important question to ask before you try to make someone hold their scapulae in a particular position is, whether they actually have the strength to do it. If not, how will the shoulder joint have to function? What kind of stresses will it have to take on?

When you see a shoulder that is not in the "right" position in *Chaturanga*, it is not because of the shoulder. It is because the scapulae are not, or cannot, be held in the appropriate place. Why not? Because the muscles that stabilize the scapulae are either not strong enough or they don't have the correct neuromuscular pattern in order to hold this position.

Out of place scapulae in *Chaturanga* can strain various muscles at the shoulder, including the rotator cuff and biceps. There are other issues at play here as well, including where the shoulders line up with the hands. The further forward the shoulders are from the hands, the more strain there will be in the shoulders, because the bulk of the upper body is too far forward to be supported by the hands. Imagine holding a twenty-pound weight directly over your shoulder. This shouldn't be a problem. Now move it forward just a few inches and gravity starts to work on your shoulder in a different way. Therefore, do not apply yoga's general rule of stacking the joints to the wrists and elbows in *Chaturanga*.

There are always some exceptions to the rule, but most people will unnecessarily strain their shoulders doing this because they end up too far in front of the hands (the exceptions are usually people with proportionally short upper arms). This position also increases the wrist angle and can cause problems there too. Most people should have their elbows slightly behind their wrists. This brings the center of their chest and their weight closer to the line between their hands.

All of this assumes, however, that *Chaturanga* functions independently. But it doesn't. If you are working with someone who has shoulder pain in *Chaturanga*, you should also look at them in the posture that typically follows it, Upward Facing Dog. I often see a pattern where people are forward on their toes and in their shoulders in *Chaturanga*. During the transition into Up Dog, they tend to put the shoulders too far in front of the hands and wrists. This has a series of effects. It puts a lot

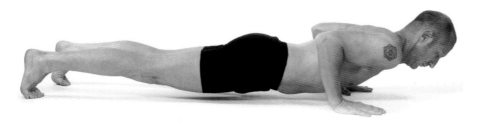

Figure 7.28: *Check your position in Chaturanga and find which position suits your body best.*

of stress on the wrists and also tends to stress the back as people try to make the backbending aspect of Up Dog happen. Additionally, the buttocks may be over tightened for the wrong reasons. And finally, it puts a load of stress on the shoulders.

Another potential risk for the shoulder is when students practice too much, too soon. This alone can inflame a number of areas in the body, especially the shoulders. This is especially true if they are practicing one of the myriad styles of Vinyasa Yoga. Depending on the beginner and the style, you may want to simply cut out some *Chaturangas.*

There are two basic options for beginners. The first is to put your knees on the floor before lowering into *Chaturanga.* The second is to move the hands slightly wider than what is traditional and let the elbows draw away from the body. This allows the larger pectoralis major muscle to get involved. Beginners often let the elbows stick out because their triceps alone are not strong enough to lower their body weight. Allowing the elbows to move wider grants the pectoralis major more leverage, and widening the hands a bit lessens the strain on the wrists.

This is a temporary adaptation until enough strength is created in the triceps.

If you have students with shoulder pain, take a moment to observe. Do not just try to make them do it differently because it doesn't look right; look at the bigger picture. Look at the line they're creating between the front of their shoulders and their hands. Also consider their general strengths and weaknesses in the practice and whether or not they are simply doing too much at the moment. There are many reasons why people exhibit pain in the shoulder. I often find (maybe partly because I am looking for it) trigger points in the infraspinatus muscle. The trigger point from this muscle has a strong referral pattern on the front and side of the shoulder and can trickle down into the biceps brachii and the rest of the arm.

The rotator cuff muscles work hard through *Chaturanga,* Up Dog, and Down Dog, and they work even harder if you jump forward, back, or through in your practice. Remember, these dynamic stabilizers steer the head of the humerus around in the shoulder socket. With all of this work, it is easy for them to tighten up and for trigger points to develop.

8

HAND, WRIST, AND ELBOW

We have discussed in great detail the kinematic chain that makes up the leg and its interlinking joints. We find the same dynamics in the upper extremity. The hand and wrist are on one end, the elbow is in the middle, and the shoulder girdle is on the other end of the kinematic chain of the arm. The interrelationship between the joints and structures of the upper extremity are even more adaptable than they are in the leg. Two key places are significantly different from the lower extremity with regard to possible movement.

First, the forearm has the ability to rotate in a different way than the lower leg. In the forearm, rotation happens at two joints where two bones (the radius and ulna) touch one another at the elbow and wrist. The movement at these joints is called pronation and supination of the forearm. The hand goes along for the ride but is also said to pronate and supinate. If you recall, rotation of the lower leg happens at only one joint, the knee.

The second place where there is a significant difference is at the proximal end of both kinematic chains. In the leg, we look at the mobility of the hip joint alone as the end of the chain. The arm, however, is more complex.

We certainly consider the shoulder joint itself, but we also have to include the mobility of the scapula and shoulder girdle as a whole. This means that changes in hand position not only affect the shoulder joint, but also impact the movement of the scapula and therefore the entire shoulder girdle.

You may recall that we discussed the idea of the leg being a kinematic chain, linking the ankle, knee, and hip. In both the arm and the leg, the central joints (the elbow and knee) create movement at both ends of the chain when they bend. In the upper extremity, the elbow impacts the shoulder girdle and the hand/wrist. This is especially true when the hand is on the floor in postures such as *Chaturanga*, Up Dog, and Down Dog, or arm balancing poses where we bear weight on our hands.

For instance, if you are in Downward Facing Dog and you bend your elbows, the rest of the arms are affected. Your wrists must bend and change shape to accommodate the new angle created from the elbows to the hands. If the elbows are pointing outwards, then this bend would create a stronger angle on the outer part of the wrists.

At the shoulder end, bending the elbow causes the shoulder joint to change position to accommodate the new angle created between the elbow and the head of the humerus. This almost always includes movement of the scapula, or at the very least requires the body to engage and stabilize the scapula.

HAND

The hand is an amazing piece of anatomy. Its fine motor skills and intricate design are, at this very moment, allowing me to type away on the keyboard. Its tissues and joints work harmoniously with my brain. The neuromuscular training I have done over the years allows me to type without looking at the keys. The tips of the fingers are loaded with sensory receptors and have the ability to sense subtle changes in texture and shape. Massage therapists use palpation skills to detect even the slightest tension in another person's body. Using their fingers, they have the ability to relieve that tension.

The entire upper extremity is designed to allow us to put our hand in almost any position we want it. When we consider the scapular movements, rotation of the shoulder, and forearm rotation, we can basically rotate our hands 360 degrees. In other words, if we abduct the arm with the palm up (external rotation), we can then rotate the other direction (internal rotation) and turn the palm to an upward position again (see Figure 7.18).

Of course, the last thing in the world we want is to injure or damage our hands. In yoga we use our hands to help bind postures, for support, and to transition our body weight. When the hand goes to the floor, it is easy to compare it with our foot. Should we treat our hand as a type of foot? Our hand does have arches running through it, though they aren't as tidy as the three we discussed in the foot. The arches

in the hand can be formed and shaped in a way that the arches in the foot cannot. If you look closely at your hand, you will find a part in the center that, no matter how hard you press into the floor, will not collapse. This is the most obvious arch of the hand and it is the part most like the arch of the foot.

When we place our hands on the floor, they do take on qualities of the feet. They often support some of our body weight. They can help maintain our balance in certain poses, and in arm-balancing postures, they are the foundation, just as our feet are in standing postures. When our hands go to the floor in our practice, we can create a rooting action similar to the one we create with our feet. In the foot section, we talked about *mula bandha* and *uddiyana bandha* relative to the arches and the quality these *bandhas* create. We can create the same qualities and keep a similar intention with the hands on the mat. This can easily be applied to poses such as Down Dog, *Chaturanga*, Up Dog, and any arm balance. This quality of intention activates the psoas of the upper body in most postures that require weight-bearing through the hands.

Structure and Movements of the Hand

From the comparison of the upper and lower extremity, you may remember that the hand has 27 bones in it. There are three phalanges (bones that make the fingers) in each finger except the thumb, which has only two. The fingers flex to make a fist and extend to return to anatomical position at the interphalangeal joints (between phalanges) and the metacarpophalangeal joints (joints where the metacarpals meet their respective phalanges). They also abduct and adduct away from and

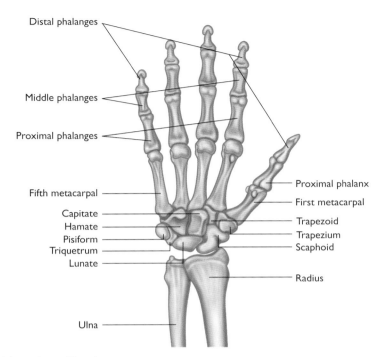

Figure 8.1: *Structure of the wrist and hand.*

towards the middle finger, which is the main ray, or centerline, of the hand. Perhaps this is why we're told to have the middle finger pointing straight forward when the hand is on the floor in yoga postures? The movements of the hand and wrist are coordinated and share many of the same muscles. These allow the hand, wrist, and fingers to move independently and/or together. The wrist moves in four directions. In wrist flexion, the palm of the hand moves forward at the wrist joint from anatomical position. Extension is the opposite action and returns the hand to anatomical position. Technically, we call the position of the wrist in Upward Facing Dog hyperextension.

The wrist also moves side to side. The hand moves away from the body in abduction and towards the body in adduction. The natural or relaxed position of the hand at the wrist joint is slightly adducted. This brings us back to my dangling question about the middle finger pointing forward as the centerline of the hand.

Muscles of the Hand and Wrist

The muscles that move the hand and wrist are a bit complicated, so we will do a basic overview here. Although there are some small muscles in the hand itself, most of the powerful muscles that move the hand, fingers, and wrist are actually located on the forearm.

Again, there are similarities between the lower leg and the forearm. In both cases the bulk of the muscles are not on the hand or the foot, nor are they bulky when crossing the ankle or the wrist, which would impede mobility. Instead, in both the arm and the leg, the stringy tendons from the bulky muscles cross the main joint and then attach to various places to move the very end of the extremity (toes and fingers).

Flexors

The flexor side of the forearm on the anterior (or palmar side) is larger, bulkier, and much stronger than the extensor side on the posterior

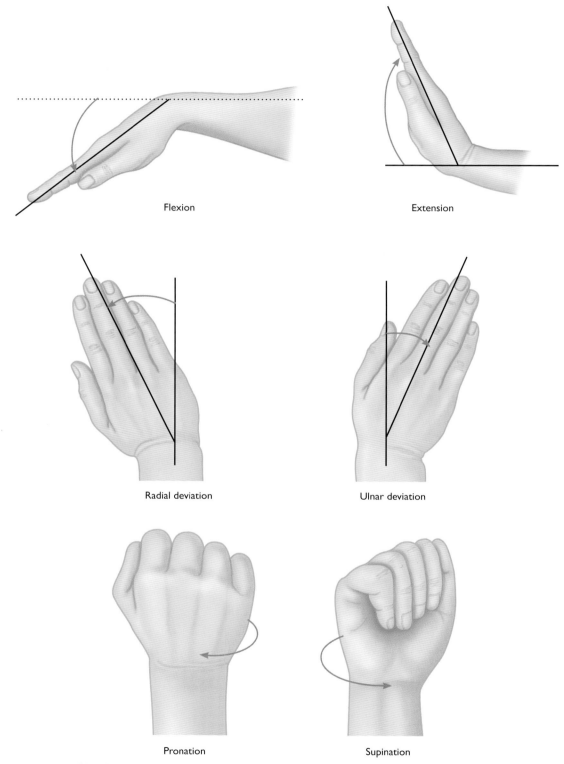

Flexion

Extension

Radial deviation

Ulnar deviation

Pronation

Supination

Figure 8.2: *Wrist and hand movement.*

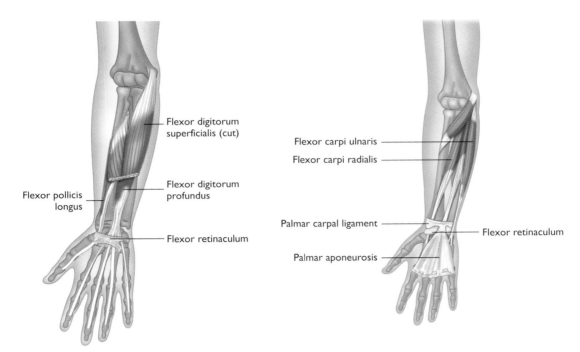

Figure 8.3: *Forearm and wrist flexors.*

forearm. This is comparable to the large calf muscles in the lower leg. The muscle names indicate what they do: flexor digitorum, flexor carpi ulnaris, and flexor carpi radialis. All are flexors and either move the fingers (digitorum), the carpals to the ulnar side (carpi ulnaris), and carpals to the radial side (carpi radialis).

The tendons of these muscles (including a few I have not named) pass through the carpal tunnel to get to their attachments on the hand and fingers, where they do their work. On their other end, these muscles attach close to or on the inside of the elbow above the joint on a bump at the very bottom of the humerus called the medial epicondyle.

Here's an interesting note about the strength of the hand and the flexors in particular. There is a position of the wrist that maximizes or takes advantage of the full strength of the forearm flexors. If you flex your wrist, that is, bring the palm of your hand toward your forearm

and try to make a fist, you will find it difficult. (Not to mention, it's not a very good fist!) If, however, you take your wrist and hyperextend it just slightly, you will find that the flexors are extremely strong and make a solid fist. In other words, a hyperextended wrist actually adds to the strength of the flexors.

Extensors

The extensor side of the forearm is generally smaller and not as strong as its counterpart. To keep things simple, we could say that the muscles on one side are mirrored on the other, where we have the extensor digitorum, extensor carpi ulnaris, and extensor carpi radialis. So they all extend the wrist and hand.

As far as attachments go, the distal end does not have a carpal tunnel like we saw on the flexor side. Instead, here we find only a tendinous sheath that no one has heard of. On their

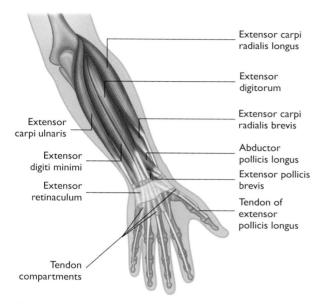

Extensor carpi radialis longus

Extensor digitorum

Extensor carpi radialis brevis

Abductor pollicis longus

Extensor pollicis brevis

Tendon of extensor pollicis longus

Extensor carpi ulnaris

Extensor digiti minimi

Extensor retinaculum

Tendon compartments

Figure 8.4: *Forearm and wrist extensors.*

proximal end, most of these muscles cross the elbow and attach to the lateral epicondyle of the humerus (it sits on the opposite side of the distal end of the humerus as the medial epicondyle).

Although these muscles oppose one another in flexion and extension, they work together to pull the hand to the ulnar or radial side. Of course, if we take a more sophisticated view of the two groups, we see that although their actions are opposite in flexion and extension, they work together to balance and move the hand and fingers in a precise and controlled manner. This is another example of the complex and beautiful integration of the body.

In fact, it is the delicate balance created by the concentric or eccentric contractions of the flexors and extensors that allows for such variety of movement in the hands. This interaction provides the speed, rate, and pressure of finger movements that enable us to type, play guitar, or play piano.

FUNCTIONAL UNIT AND MOVEMENT

To explore the function of the hand and wrist, we have to consider all the joints of the upper

extremity together. The upper extremity must be viewed as an integrated whole, just like the lower extremity. The leg, we now know, is a kinematic chain comprised of the foot and ankle, knee, and hip. The arm is no different. The hand and wrist, elbow, and shoulder complex must be viewed as an integrated whole. This is especially true when the hand is on the floor and we have a closed kinematic chain. In a kinematic chain, when the center joint moves (in this case the elbow), the surrounding joints also move.

Before we go further with alignment or positioning of the hand and wrist, it makes sense to look at the "knee" of the upper extremity—the elbow. In yoga we tend to look at the way the elbow is pointing more than we consider its function or dysfunction. For instance, we ask if the elbows are close to the body or far from it. Which way are they pointing? Are the creases of the elbows pointing in the right direction? Are they pointing towards each other, or straight forward?

The flexion and extension we find in the elbow is similar to what we find at the knee, with a slight difference in hyperextension. In hyperextension of the elbow, there is a strong bone-on-bone connection at the back of the elbow. This means that ligaments and muscles do not have to hold as much weight as they would if the elbow were shaped like the knee. In the knee, we do not have the same type of bone-on-bone connection to support hyperextension. Rather, the soft tissues prevent hyperextension. This means that you are less likely to damage the soft tissues in the elbow in hyperextension. However, this doesn't mean that if the elbows are hyperextending, you shouldn't try and bring the support out of the bones and into the muscles. You should.

Another difference between the elbow and the knee is that the elbow is divided into two joints. One of these joints is responsible for

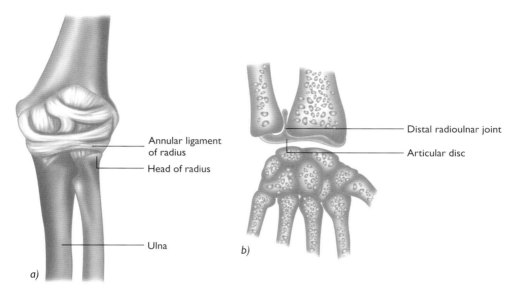

Figure 8.5: *a) Proximal radioulnar joint, left arm, anterior view, b) distal radioulnar joint, left wrist/hand, coronal view.*

flexion and extension. The other is responsible for rotation. This rotation does not just happen at the elbow, but also at the wrist. These joints are called the proximal and distal radioulnar joints and they pronate and supinate the hand and forearm.

This makes things a little more complicated than in the leg, where straight flexion and extension of a closed chain causes movement at the ends of the limb. In the arm, we add rotation into the mix at the central joint. This rotation impacts all the bones and joints in the kinematic chain. Remember, in the knee the effects of rotation are more or less purely in the knee joint.

Practically speaking, bending the elbows, especially when weight-bearing on the hands, often causes a certain amount of rotation. Because of bone structure and the two radioulnar joints, rotation at the elbow automatically creates rotation through both forearm bones and has an effect on the wrist. In the knee, rotation only happens when the tibia rotates under a bent knee. Rotation of the forearm happens at a separate joint than where flexion and extension occur; thus rotation can occur whether the elbow is straight or bent.

In anatomical position, the palms face forward in supination. If we rotate the palms to face backwards, this is pronation. This is a crucial movement for the hand and adds to the overall function of the upper extremity. Pronation and supination of the hand can impact the position of the elbow and shoulder. Unless you specifically create a different intention, pronation of the forearm is associated with internal rotation of the shoulder joint. Supination is associated with external rotation of the shoulder joint.

If we continue this chain of movement and raise the arms overhead, internal rotation of the shoulders is associated with retraction of the scapulae. In other words, the scapulae are squeezed together. External rotation of the shoulders is associated with protraction of the scapulae (they move apart from one another).

The position of the hand is related, through the chain of joints, all the way up to and through the shoulder and into the scapula. This relationship works both ways. Moving the scapula and shoulder joints can also place the hand in certain positions. So, although we may not focus on protecting the elbows as much as we do the knees, it is important to

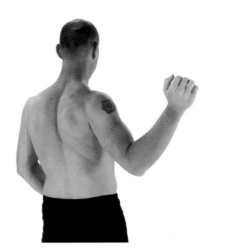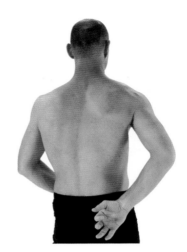

Figure 8.6: *Movements of the shoulder are tied to movements of the scapula.*

know where the elbow is and what it's doing. To fully understand this, we have to look at the surrounding joints. Having already looked at the shoulder, let's look further down the chain at the wrist and hand.

TYING IT ALL TOGETHER

When both hands are on the floor as in *Chaturanga*, Up Dog, and Down Dog, we are commonly instructed to align the middle fingers of each hand parallel to one another. This seems reasonable enough, considering that the middle finger is known as the "main ray" of the hand. If you hold your hand up in front of you and abduct (spread) the fingers, you will notice that the middle finger does not move. Instead, all of the other fingers move away from it. The middle finger is the centerline of the hand.

However, there are other components to the positioning of the hand. Let's look at the next major joint, the wrist. What is the correct alignment of the wrist relative to the forearm? If you let your arm hang by your side, you will notice that the wrist sits at a slight angle. It is a similar angle that I notice in my wrists while I sit here and type these words. Actually,

the angle is stronger when typing than when your arm is just dangling by your side. This is a slight adduction of the wrist. With slight adduction, the middle finger is not lined up with the centerline of your forearm; instead, the forefinger is more likely to be closer to parallel to the lines created by the forearm bones. We could use this as a reason to align our hands with the forefinger pointed forward in postures where the hands are on the floor. Which one is right? I look at both the wrist and the shoulder and allow these two areas to dictate the position of the hand.

The wrist and shoulder are generally more susceptible to getting injured. For people with tighter shoulders, I often favor using the index finger as the alignment guide. This allows the hand to turn out slightly, but not just from the wrist; it can also shift the position of the elbow and the shoulder. Typically, the tighter the shoulders, the more likely it is that the index finger will create the line that I am looking for in the wrist. This line shows the crease of the wrist to be parallel to the front edge of the mat.

If the shoulders are more open and flexible, then there is nothing wrong with the middle finger being the guide for alignment. The point is, as similar as we all are, we are also different.

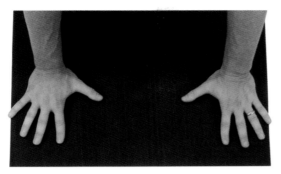 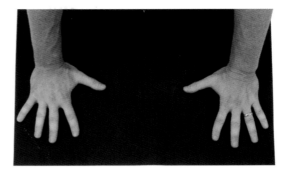

Figure 8.7: *Deciding whether your middle finger or index finger are pointing forward should be determined by the line of your wrist.*

Changing the alignment of the hands will impact the chain of joints further up the arm. I also allow alignment to change over time if necessary for a particular student. For instance, if a student's shoulders open up over time, then the hand might change from the index finger forward to the middle finger forward.

It is the nature of a good teacher to ask questions and inquire. This doesn't mean that one idea is right and the other is wrong; my intention is to encourage freedom from dogmatic thinking. Either of the above alignments can be argued for. What's more important is how the alignment of the hand can help or prevent a student from being comfortable and progressing in their practice. In this case, a lot depends on what's going on in the joints above the hand.

There is another underlying element to hand, wrist, elbow, and shoulder alignment that is important to acknowledge. We tend to apply the general rules of alignment from the lower extremity to the upper extremity. In terms of alignment in the knee, we often keep the knee over the ankle as a sure and safe way to avoid excess strain and to prevent injury. This same idea is often applied to the alignment of our elbow and wrist. I believe this is a mistake for most students. As I go against the grain on this one, I suggest that you allow your own experience to inform you. I only suggest that you inquire.

In *Chaturanga* we often hear that too much pressure can be placed on the shoulders, resulting in injury. Although it is possible to injure your shoulder in this pose, I suggest that it takes more than just the movement of *Chaturanga* alone to do it. It is how you do the pose that determines whether it will cause injury. If in *Chaturanga* your elbows are aligned directly over your wrists, you are doing two things. First, you are extending your shoulders quite far beyond their foundation (the hand and wrist). Second, you are keeping the wrist at a 90-degree angle in a potentially stressful, weight-bearing position. Remember, stress in one place tends to create stress at another place.

In this forward-leaning *Chaturanga*, you actually create stress in both the shoulders and the wrists. There are people with certain proportions that allow them to align their elbows and wrists in this manner. These people usually have a shorter upper arm (humerus) relative to the length of their forearm. As a result of this proportion, their shoulders are naturally closer to the line created by their forearms. This isn't the case for most of us. We can reduce the stress in both places by allowing the elbows to move back slightly in *Chaturanga*. This reduces the stress at the wrists by decreasing the degree to which they are hyperextended. In the shoulders, this moves the mass of our upper body more in line with its foundation, the hands.

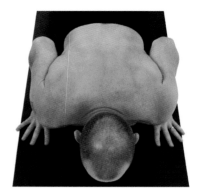 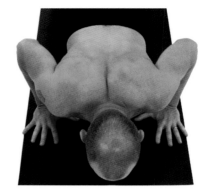

Figure 8.8: *Take note of the direction the elbows are pointing relative to my finger direction changing.*

INTEGRATING ANATOMY INTO YOUR PRACTICE

As discussed, many practitioners will notice that if their fingers point straight forward in *Chaturanga* as they lower down, the inner part of their hands lift up and their elbows naturally want to point outwards. Experiment with this: lie down on your stomach and set up your hands in preparation for *Chaturanga*. Rotate your fingers so that the index finger is pointing forward, and notice what happens to the hands and elbows. You may find it is easier to keep the elbows in with the hands rotated outwards.

Also notice the wrist angle and sensation created when you align your elbows over your wrists. What happens when you move your body back slightly and allow the elbows to sit just behind the line of the wrists? When you play with this, you may notice a change in the amount of pressure that travels through the shoulders.

Apply this same concept in a backbend (let's try *Urdhva Dhanurasana*). When you lie on your back to set up, instead of pointing the fingers straight towards the shoulders, experiment with rotating the hands and forearms so that the fingers point out towards the edges of the mat on either side of you. Notice what happens to the heel of the hands and the ability of the elbows to move towards one another. I am not suggesting that we want to keep the hands in this position through the whole of our backbend. But doing so reveals something about the relationship between hand position, elbows, and shoulders. I've recommended that students place their hands like this to get them up onto their head before going into the backbend. At this pausing point, they can rotate their hands back into the "correct" position for the pose. This gives the student more space to plant their hands firmly on the floor. As always, there are exceptions to the general rule.

Just as an experiment, do a few Sun Salutations with a focus on your hands. Whenever your hands meet, press them together, or when they go to the floor, press them firmly down, especially if you are about to put weight into them. See if you can make a connection between the hand and shoulder girdle stabilizers (the upper body psoas).

Wrist Pain

By far the most common topic concerning the wrist joint in yoga includes pain, particularly in a weight-bearing position. *Chaturanga*, Downward Facing Dog, and arm balancing postures can put a lot of stress and strain on the wrists. Because the most common condition at the wrist is carpal tunnel syndrome, people

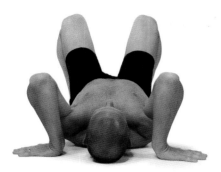 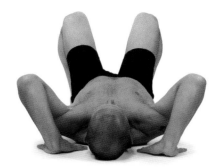

Figure 8.9: *Again notice how the direction of the elbows changes when I change the pointing of my hand.*

tend to assume that their wrist pain is caused by this condition. Of course, there are other reasons why your wrist may hurt.

As in all other joints, there is bone, cartilage, ligaments, tendons, and associated muscles that can cause dysfunction in the wrist. Any of these can be injured to varying degrees and therefore elicit pain in an area. One should not assume that pain in the wrist is always carpal tunnel syndrome.

Working Hypothesis

I have a working hypothesis on wrist pain for yogis. I haven't done any scientific studies to prove this, but I will share my thoughts and observations. One of the common precursors to carpal tunnel syndrome is overuse of the flexor muscles of the hand and wrist. These muscles are commonly tight simply due to the jobs we have and the tools we use in our daily life. Almost everyone uses a computer and types. If not, then you grab a pen to write. We are constantly grasping and grabbing things around us, because that's exactly what the hands were designed to do.

When the flexors are tight and we put our hands on the floor, the wrist is in a hyperextended position. Hyperextension in this case is not a bad thing. It's just the way we put our hands on the floor. Hyperextension of the wrist is a

normal and natural movement, but it does impact the flexors.

In order to hyperextend the wrist, we must work against tension that already exists in the flexors, the muscles that oppose hyperextension. We have postulated that most people have a lifestyle that requires them to use and often overuse these flexors, thereby making them tighter. When you stretch a muscle that is tight, you can feel it. When you stretch the flexor muscles through extension, you feel this tension at the wrist. I'm not suggesting that all pain at the wrist is caused by tight flexors, just as not all wrist pain is carpal tunnel syndrome. What I am suggesting is that overuse of the flexors creates an imbalance that has to be worked through.

This lack of balance can either be relative to the tension we have been talking about or the balance of strength around the wrist. Both strength and flexibility need to be in balance to support the wrist in hyperextension. Lack of balance can lead to over-compressing the top of the wrist in postures that require us to put all our weight in the hands. I suggest this is a root cause for much wrist discomfort while practicing yoga. Of course, if there are previous injuries, these can be part of the problem as well. The idea that bending at the wrist beyond 90 degrees is detrimental doesn't stand to reason. It is definitely more stressful on the wrist, but

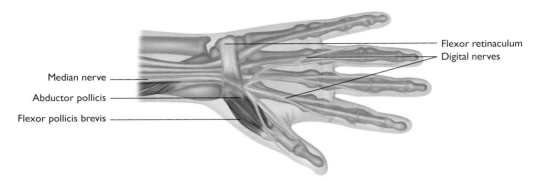

Median nerve

Abductor pollicis

Flexor pollicis brevis

Flexor retinaculum
Digital nerves

Figure 8.10: *Carpal tunnel syndrome.*

we just need to progress towards this level of flexibility and gradually build the strength to control the tension around the joint.

I have also observed that wrist pain is most common in people who do not maintain a consistent practice, or who only practice one or perhaps two days a week. It seems these people are far more likely to exhibit pain in the wrist if they do any kind of Vinyasa Yoga class.

Carpal Tunnel Syndrome

Carpal tunnel syndrome (CTS) is a serious complaint that describes a specific set of conditions. This is where the tendons of the muscles that move the fingers and hand on the flexor side compress the median nerve as it passes through the carpal tunnel. The carpal tunnel is created by bones and a piece of connective tissue that holds the tendons down at the base of the hand.

This seems simple and straightforward enough. Compression of the nerve by the tendons, which are usually inflamed and swollen, causes pain, tingling, and numbness on the thumb side of the hand. This condition often leads us to look closely at the wrist. But like all conditions, several factors can play into this condition. Good evaluation of the problem is always the most intelligent first step. We could (and perhaps should) first ask what has caused the

tendons to get inflamed and swollen. Is there anything we can do about it? Are there factors further up the chain of joints and tissues adding to the strain on these muscles of the forearm?

General posture and shoulder tension can cause strain as far down as the wrist. Remember, we need to look at things holistically. Most people won't develop CTS from practicing yoga. Instead, they will show up in your class with CTS. If they are in an acute stage of the syndrome, they might not show up to a yoga class at all.

There are two means of working with students suffering from CTS. One is to accommodate their hand and wrist by modifying angles of the wrist with props, a rolled up mat, or even gloves that have padding on them. Next, we need to consider how we can help alleviate the tension in their flexor tendons by stretching them, often without bearing weight. Putting the hands in Reverse Prayer position is a great strategy.

If you have the skill to recognize what the person actually needs, you can work with the whole of the shoulder girdle to release tension and/or strengthen areas of it. In other words, work with the micro but don't forget about the macro if they are in an acute stage of wrist pain. It may be more appropriate to spend time working with the bigger picture of how their wrist functions relative to the rest of their arm and shoulder girdle.

in our practice. Our difficulty can change the way we approach things, how hard we work, and our ability to let go of things.

Our initial inquiry is important because it gets us to take a close look at ourselves. This inquiry can take place in the moment (as we actually move into the *asana*) or it can be from a longer-term perspective (as we consider our path towards the *asana*). Both are equally important. We can almost always make specific changes to our technique, as it also lives within a continuum, shifting and adjusting as our experience of the posture progresses and our body changes over time.

We can work hard for a long time on a particular pose and not see any obvious change. Conversely, we can make one simple change and see a dramatic effect in a matter of days. If change doesn't happen right away, it is easy to slip into a compulsive "trying to fix" mode. This can have potentially harmful effects. Why? Because it takes us out of our "felt sense" and keeps us in our "thinking" mind.

This is where letting go is important. We know that change is a guarantee in life. There is nothing wrong with trying to change things for the better, but taken too far, this can negatively affect other areas of our practice. Our efforts to force change can lead us to focus exclusively on one thing. How we let go and accept things as they are is critical. The best trick I know to reach this level of acceptance is to remember that things (everything!) will most certainly change over time.

I don't intend for you to take this anatomical information and use it to obsess over the physical components of your practice. Instead, I hope it will inspire you to inquire about, contemplate, and explore the whole of your

yoga practice. This inquiry will force you to use your head; however, without practical experience and sustained effort, that intellect is useless. Be willing to accept where you are and that change may be slow. But change is a sure thing and anatomy and *asana* are powerful tools to help us evolve.

Understanding anatomy changes our *asana* practice just as *asana* practice changes our anatomy. Our physical practice is the doorway to a deeper understanding of ourselves on all levels. This self-knowledge is incredibly powerful. Although that introspective journey is one that I cannot take with you, I hope to get you started by deepening your understanding of your physical self as we explore the body in motion.

It is easier to look at a single pose as though it exists within a vacuum, perhaps as easy as it would be to observe the knee without considering its surrounding joints. So I've created little anatomical stories that weave their way through multiple postures and common patterns within those postures. As you read and explore these stories, please keep in mind that each posture within each story has more than one intention and works on more than one part of the body. To keep the "plot" of my anatomical stories as clear as possible, I consciously leave out some of the many benefits and effects of each pose in order to focus on a specific anatomical relationship. This will enable you to see the anatomical connections among postures. As you begin to see with these "new eyes", I hope you will also begin to see patterns in your students that reveal why they may be struggling with other postures. This new understanding might lead you to use particular poses to help your students open certain areas of their body and continue to evolve into trying more difficult postures.

9
ANATOMICAL PATTERNS IN FORWARD BENDS

When we think of a forward bend, nothing particularly fancy or awe-inspiring comes to mind. If someone says "forward bend," we naturally think of the simplest versions—standing or sitting with both hands making their way towards our feet while we fold at the waist.

I remember when I began practicing seriously and regularly. Forward bends were somewhat difficult for me. I can't recall exactly where I was with them, but I think I could just barely touch my toes. I have no doubt I did that with a well-rounded spine. Along the way my practice changed; I have had a number of opportunities to learn and grow from my experiences in forward bends. For instance, for some time I had pain at the sit-bone end of my right hamstring in a forward bend. Then one day it

stopped completely. Before I could celebrate, however, it switched to the opposite side. These experiences are lessons along the path of the process of transformation, a natural part of progress and change.

But there are deeper forward bends than this. There are places in the practice of *asana* that we take hip and spinal flexion well beyond what is required in a basic forward bend. In *Kurmasana*, or Tortoise Pose, for example, we will see how each *asana* builds upon another to bring our torso as flat as possible on the floor with the arms extended under straight legs. When we can move this deep into the pose, there is minimal pressure on the arms or elbows. I remember trying this posture for the first time and it seemed impossible, as though there was no chance my body would ever be

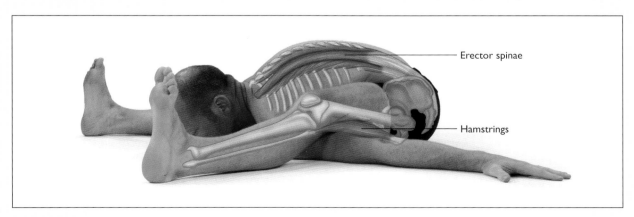

Erector spinae

Hamstrings

Figure 9.1: *Kurmasana.*

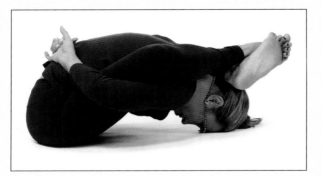

Figure 9.2: *Supta Kurmasana.*

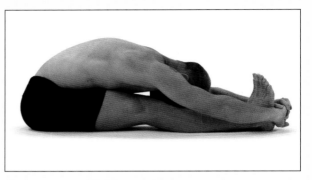

Figure 9.3: *Paschimottanasana.*

comfortable in it. I felt extreme pressure on my arms, elbows, and lower back. It hurt! Time and practice has definitely changed things.

I chose *Kurmasana* as our "pinnacle pose" because it requires that our tissues be open beyond what is needed in a simple forward bend. In it, we have to take our torso *through* the thighs, not just *to* them. *Supta Kurmasana* (Tortoise with the legs behind the head) takes this a step further, requiring the ability to externally rotate the femurs in addition to deep flexion. As it turns out, the hamstrings can also restrict our ability to rotate the hips, especially when in deep flexion.)

As always, there must be some postures along the way that help us get from a basic forward bend to the deeper or more complicated *Kurmasana*, right? Oh, there are! They are sometimes hard to see, but I'll do my best to build our way there after covering the basic forward bend that we are all familiar with—*Paschimottanasana.*

FORWARD BENDING

In Sanskrit, a forward bend is known as *Paschimottanasana*—the "western stretch" in English. Traditionally, the back of the body is referred to as the west and the front as the east. The very name suggests the all-encompassing

quality of the pose. It affects the entire back of the body. In addition to being all encompassing, a forward bend seems fairly simple, doesn't it? Just reach forward and grab your toes, feet, ankles, or whatever you can reach, right?

Wrong. The complexity of such a seemingly straightforward posture is that there are several joints that have the potential to block or impede our intended goal of folding completely in half. I am sure you are already well-acquainted with the most common restriction to forward bending, the hamstrings. As we will see, there are many other places where restriction can and does occur as well.

When I refer to *Paschimottanasana* as all-encompassing, I mean that it impacts the entire line of tissues associated with the back of our body. These tissues run from the feet, through the calf muscles, through the backs of the thighs, the hips, up the spine, and all the way to the head and neck. In his book *Anatomy Trains*, Tom Myers refers to this as the superficial back line of the body.

There is a direct fascial relationship connecting the bottoms of the feet to the top of the head through this line. From a fascial (connective tissue) point of view, tension anywhere along this line can create restriction in other areas. Even the feet can impact what a forward bend feels like. You have probably had this experience yourself already. If your feet are pulled towards you in dorsiflexion and your toes are extended, you'll notice a different sensation through the backs of the calves and up your legs.

If you straighten your feet completely (as if they were parallel to an imaginary wall in front of you) pressure is put into the hip joints. If you bend your knees, the dynamics and amount of pressure in the hamstrings changes, in addition to your ability to rotate the pelvis. It also allows you to bend further forward. If your hips are tight, the spine has to round more to help bring the head and chest closer to the legs. Even your spine's ability to move may impact how far we go in this pose.

Interestingly, the body is actually designed to flex. After all, in *utero*, all of our joints are in flexion. In the fetal position, our ankles, knees, hips, spine, arms, and even head are flexed. We are, in many ways, designed to forward bend; that is, until we start running, cycling, and doing other sports that tighten the hamstrings and hip muscles, which make forward bending at the hips more difficult.

I often say that an ideal or complete forward bend, where the chest is on the thighs, is the result of approximately two-thirds movement at the hip joint and one-third movement at the spine. More "classical" approaches to a forward bend purposely include a rounded spine. My personal experience is that a rounded spine doesn't impact all the muscles that are stretched in a forward bend. Thus I will describe a "flat-back" forward bend, which is what I practice and teach.

It turns out that flexion at the hip joint in a seated or standing forward bend is pretty much the opposite of how we normally think about hip flexion. (Remember, flexion of the hip happens at the junction of the pelvis and the femur. If either of these bones moves towards the other, we are doing flexion.) In other words, in both a standing and seated forward bend, the pelvis moves around the

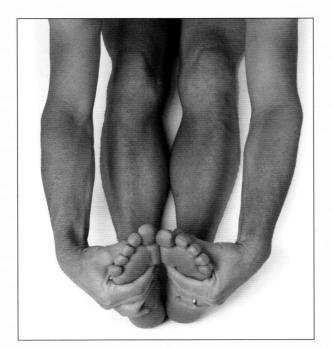 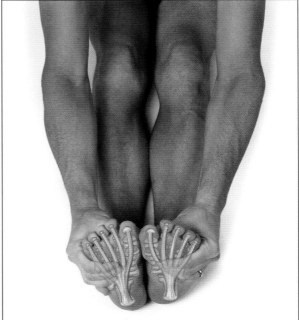

Figure 9.4: *Straightening the feet affects the pressure in the hip joint.*

head of the femur. Note that this differs from the typical version of hip flexion where the femur moves forward and up at the hip joint. Why is this distinction important? It can change our intention as well as the sensation that we seek in our forward bends.

As the pelvis rotates around the head of the femur in hip flexion, any or all of the hip extenders can resist this movement. The tissues with the most direct line of resistance are the hamstrings. These muscles are the ones most often "stretched" in a forward bend. Other muscles make up the group known as the hip extenders, including all layers of the gluteal muscles (the gluteus maximus and the posterior portions of the gluteus minimus and medius) and the adductor magnus.

Stubborn hip extenders are the simple part. The more indirect restrictors to forward bends are the bottoms of the feet, the calf muscles, and even the spinal muscles. All of the tissues in these areas are connected directly through connective tissue and function along the entire "western" side of the body. We will look at postures that work on these areas to further our ability to do simple forward bends. Because there are so many joints involved in forward bends, we'll look at many postures along the way. In the end, each will bring us to a deeper forward bend such as *Kurmasana*.

PUTTING THE PIECES TOGETHER

We often come across our first forward bend in Sun Salutations, usually at the beginning and end when we bow forward to salute the sun. This is usually done on just one exhalation and only begins the process of lengthening the hamstrings. These two forward bends are obvious; but there are

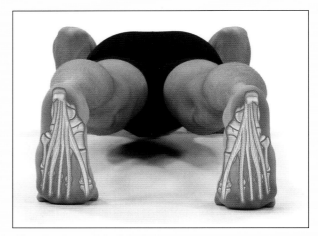

Figure 9.5: *The tension in the bottom of the feet can affect your hamstrings and back of your body.*

also a few not-so-obvious components of a Sun Salutation that further our journey to a deeper forward bend.

When we jump (or step) back from our first forward bend, we land on the toes (in a hyperextended position). This, along with the following *Chaturanga*, is our first opportunity to stretch and tone the bottoms of the feet. As mentioned, this layer of tissues is part of a long line of fascia, and a part of the chain of joints, that has the potential to impact our forward bend. How flexible are your toes? I bet you never even considered this could impact your ability to bend forward!

Not long after *Chaturanga*, we find ourselves in what is perhaps the most popular yoga posture in the world—Downward Facing Dog. It's interesting how many people sense that Down Dog is related to a forward bend, yet somehow this focus remains stuck at the hamstrings. And although the hamstrings *do* restrict Down Dog, this posture's relationship with forward bending (or stretching the back of the body) goes much further than that. The foot, ankle, and calf muscles also impact our forward bend. Down Dog is just as much about our feet, ankles, and calves as it is about our hamstrings. Lengthening these

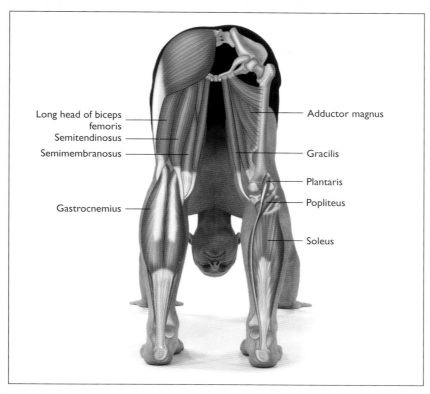

Long head of biceps femoris

Semitendinosus

Semimembranosus

Gastrocnemius

Adductor magnus

Gracilis

Plantaris

Popliteus

Soleus

Figure 9.6: *The calf muscles continue the line of tissue that affect your hamstrings and back of your body.*

tissues in Down Dog supports the forward bends that follow.

When our ankle joint is flexed (dorsiflexion) in Down Dog, we are placing pressure on the calf muscles, the gastrocnemius and the deeper soleus. The gastrocnemius crosses both the ankle and the knee joint and is therefore affected by the position of both of these joints. If the knee is bent, there is less pressure on the gastrocnemius. The soleus only crosses the ankle joint and is stretched regardless of the position of the knee. Therefore, tight calves in addition to tight hamstrings can cause some students to bend their knees in Down Dog.

These two calf muscles link to the bottom of the foot via the plantar fascia and Achilles tendon. They also connect upwards to the hamstrings. The reason these tissues are often forgotten is that, due to their size and general strength

(they easily lift twice your body weight), we don't really feel the amount of pressure placed on them in Downward Dog. What we do experience is the restriction.

Ideally, you will integrate this information by moving through Sun Salutations in a way that actually feeds the bigger picture of your understanding of your body, while focusing on the smaller picture, your legs. As you flow through the postures again and again, feel the interrelationship of the feet, calves, and hamstrings as they go through the movements of *Surya Namaskara*. When you arrive in Down Dog, mindfully encourage your heels towards the floor. (In some systems, it is taught to avoid wrinkles on the fronts of the ankles in Down Dog, essentially keeping the heels up slightly. I can't come up with any good anatomical rationale for this, unless of course the person has an ankle injury or other anatomical anomaly.) Your attention during this familiar series of *asanas* can increase the effectiveness of the Sun Salutations, furthering your journey to a more complete forward bend.

Standing Forward Bends

After Sun Salutations, many yoga practices flow into a standing series that includes various forward bends. The most simple of these has the legs hip-width distance apart, folding forward and grabbing the toes, feet, heels, or some other variation. I will also discuss postures such as *Trikonasana* (Triangle), *Parivrtta Trikonasana* (Revolved Triangle), *Utthita Hasta Padangusthasna* (Standing Leg Raise), and *Prasarita Padottanasana*.

In a simple forward bend, the line of tensional resistance in the back body is nicely lined up through the feet, hamstrings, and muscles of the spine. Almost everyone can experience restriction in the hamstrings here. But there is something more subtle going on. When we are standing, our legs have to engage to one degree or another to keep us upright. This means the hamstrings and calf muscles (both stretched in forward bends) are also slightly engaged for balance. This is a delicate balancing act.

Let's imagine we are looking at someone doing a standing forward bend from the side. Are their legs vertical? What happens when the hips move behind the ankles? What happens if the hips move in front of the ankles? Because of the balancing act required for stability we tend to lean back in the pose. Often we'll shift the hips behind the line of the legs to avoid the sensation of falling forward. This is a natural and instinctive thing to do, which means that more effort is required to change the tendency! Thus the flexibility of your hips and hamstrings partly determines where you place your hips, relative to the legs.

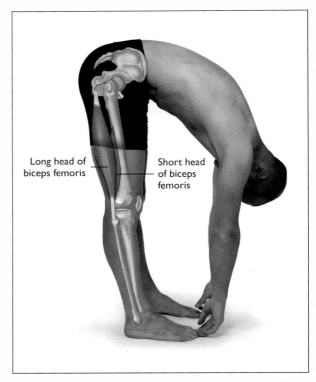

Long head of biceps femoris

Short head of biceps femoris

Figure 9.7: *Tight hamstrings affect the ability of the pelvis to move and increase pressure in the spine.*

For instance, if tight hamstrings are limiting your forward bend to the extent that your lower back is about 90 degrees from your legs, the further forward you go, the more likely you are to fall over.

This is because there is more weight in front of your gravitational line than there is for someone whose torso is flat on their thighs. So you compensate by pulling the hips back behind the legs and feet, which are the foundation of the pose. If you look (or feel) closely, you will notice that the joint that actually changes when you move the hips back is the ankle. The downside to this is that, by pulling the hips back, you avoid placing pressure on the very muscle that the forward bend is designed to lengthen (the hamstrings). To correct this, you need to bring the hips back in line with the legs. As you do, the sensation of falling kicks in. So now you're stretching the hamstrings, but you have activated other restrictors. The muscles that engage to keep you upright at this point are the flexors of the toes. The toes grab on for dear life if you go too far forward.

But it's not just your toes. You also feel a general tightening of tissues in the entire leg when you go too far forward or back. Going way back usually causes the front of the legs to engage. Going too far forward engages the toes, calves, and hamstrings. In a nutshell, to open the back of the body, we need to be in balance.

When we are able to stack the hips over the ankles, the compensating tissues can relax more easily. Your body becomes closely aligned with the gravitational line running up from the ankle and through the leg. In this balanced space, we can work on creating some length,

and not just in the hamstrings but also in the spine. And that, we know, is the real reason to practice any *asana*!

Triangle Pose

Many other standing postures further our journey in forward bending. Among them are Triangle (*Trikonasana*) and Revolved Triangle (*Parivrtta Trikonasana*). These two very different postures impact the hamstrings and hips in different ways. Both ultimately help our forward bend.

In Triangle, the angle of pressure placed on the hamstrings changes. The outstretched leg is both externally rotated and abducted relative to anatomical position. When we reach for

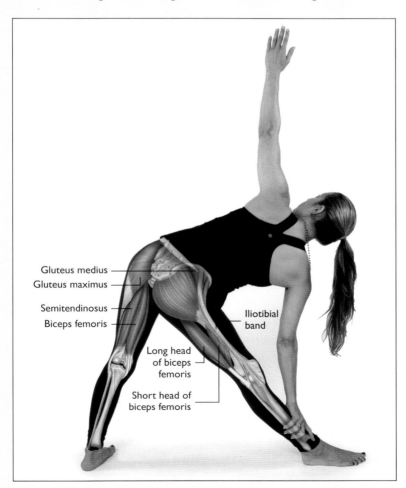

Figure 9.8: *Triangle places pressure on the hamstrings from a different angle.*

our shin or the big toe, the pelvis tilts over this leg sideways, the sit bone moves away from the knee, and we experience a sensation of stretching in the hamstrings.

But there is another element of Triangle Pose that deserves our attention and that is indirectly related to our forward bends. As anyone who has ever been in this pose knows, it's easy to get caught up in the obvious stretch in the front leg. The work in the back leg is not always so obvious and is even less so if you have particularly tight hamstrings. I remember what a revelation it was for me when the actual sensation of Triangle moved from the hamstrings of my front leg to the outer hip of my back leg. My hamstrings had (at last!) opened enough so that the posture could place pressure on the gluteals of my opposite (back) hip.

The opening we feel in the back hip in Triangle is a lengthening of tissues that potentially restrict both hip flexion in a forward bend and hip rotation. Because the hip is so complex, the pressure we place on it from different angles is important. Seeing how the different angles of pressure contribute to our simple forward bend evokes a more integrated perspective of the body and further clarifies how one *asana* can build on another.

Revolved Triangle Pose

This pose plays a dual role in forward bending. Not only does it require open hamstrings, but it also places pressure on the outer hips. We will return to this outer-hip work when we explore twists. For the purposes of this section, let's focus on the general tension around the hip that can reduce our ability to fold forward.

In Revolved Triangle, most of us try to keep our hips relatively even—both horizontally (from right side to left) as well as square (relative to the front or back of the mat). At least, this is the ideal we strive toward. In trying to reach this ideal we experience different sensations in both hips, not just one.

When you teach, you get to see *Parivrtta Trikonasana* expressed in many different ways. In some students, the hips are not even close to horizontal. Other students shorten the distance between their pelvis and their shoulder on the same side as the forward leg. Due to limitations, some students have no choice but to let their hips fly way out to the side, off of the midline of the posture.

All of these modifications reveal tension or lack of awareness. The first pattern (keeping the hips horizontal) is the most subtle and difficult to sense internally and therefore to deal with. It is natural for the pelvis to drop because we're twisting in the same direction already. It can be confusing and awkward to hold your pelvis completely steady. It is even more challenging to correct this pattern by rotating the pelvis in the opposite direction of the twist after being in the pose, although a teacher's guiding hands can help.

When a student shortens their torso, they have usually overreached when entering the pose. I see it over and over again. We reach out with the arm and hand that we're ultimately going to place on the floor to try and create length. What often happens is that we lengthen so much on the side of the extended arm that the other side ends up shortening. The result is that the hip and the shoulder are squashed together, unless you then correct this by pulling the hip back or opening the chest. This is a classic example of a good intention but poor execution. If this applies to you, try lengthening out of both sides equally without throwing that arm up in the air.

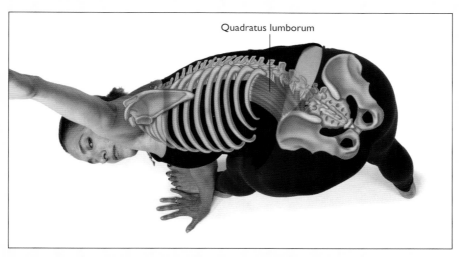

Quadratus lumborum

Figure 9.9: *In this image you can see the shortened distance between hip and shoulder as well as the hips at a strong angle.*

Depending on where your tightness lies in and around the hips in Revolved Triangle, you may feel more through the hamstrings, outer hip, or outside of the front leg. Both illustrate how tension can restrict us in the pose. The outer hip muscles are working against our hip's ability to rotate while in a forward bend.

Wide-Legged Forward Bends

Enter the adductors and their relationship to forward bending. Things change when we move the legs wider than hip-width distance apart. In this stance, we add tension to the inner thighs by also stretching the adductors. These thin flat muscles (except for the adductor magnus, which is not thin) flex, adduct, and internally rotate the femurs.

However, as you may recall from the anatomy section of this book, one of the adductors, the adductor magnus, is referred to as "the fourth hamstring." When we take our legs wide, we lengthen the adductors simply by abducting. When we ask our body to forward bend, the fibers of the adductors that restrict flexion, namely the posterior part of the adductor magnus, now adds to the amount of restriction that can be found in the hamstrings when folding forward at the hip joints.

The adductors restrict forward bending in another way. They are also internal rotators of the hip joint. When we take both legs into a posture like *Upavistha Konasana* and bend forward, we aren't doing pure flexion anymore. Now we are asking the joints to externally rotate. Recall that the pelvis is moving in a forward bend, not the femur. In *Upavistha Konasana*, when the pelvis anteriorly tilts around the heads of the femurs that are abducted, we are literally creating external rotation along with flexion at the hip joint.

This explains why, in a seated wide-legged forward bend, it is usually more difficult to keep the feet pointed straight up. It is quite common to find that as we draw forward, our feet roll forward and down towards the floor. This reveals any limitation we may have in the muscles that allow external rotation of our hip joints.

When we shift the position of the femur and the pelvis in a wide-legged forward bend, we change the dynamic of what will restrict the movement forward. Sometimes widening the legs allows students with tight hamstrings but flexible adductors to be able to do the pose

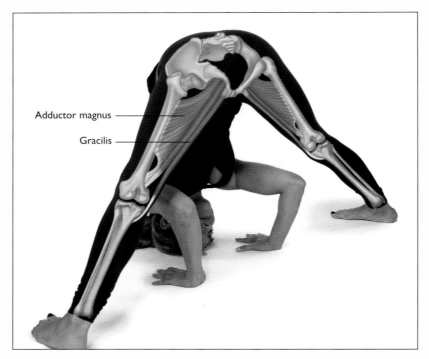

Figure 9.10: *The adductors are lengthened both in the abduction of the legs as well as rotation created.*

quite well, but they will struggle when their legs are closer together.

The reverse is also true. If you have relatively open hamstrings but tight adductors, it will be easier for you to fold forward with your legs together than it is when your legs are apart.

We see this in *Baddha Konasana* compared to *Upavistha Konasana* as well. If you can fold forward in *Baddha Konasana* but struggle in *Upavistha Konasana*, it is likely that your adductors are more flexible than your hamstrings. If you are the opposite, you are probably able to fold forward quite well in *Upavistha Konasana* but not well in *Baddha Konasana*. In other words, it is likely that your hamstrings are more flexible than your adductors.

The hip joint is surrounded by tissues from every angle, enabling it to move in all different directions. However, as much as these tissues offer mobility, they can also restrict movement

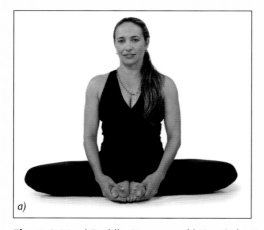

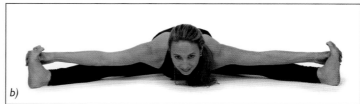

Figure 9.11: *a) Baddha Konasana, b) Upavistha Konasana.*

in various directions. This is enough to disprove the common assumption that a forward bend is just a hamstring stretch.

The entire back of the leg impacts the flexibility of the hip joint in a forward bend, and this is where we usually focus. Don't forget that muscles that are better known for rotation, adduction, and abduction at the hip also impact our ability to go into a forward bend. Lets elevate our awareness and observation of the whole.

The Spinal Portion of Forward Bends

I don't think most people really look at *Halasana* (Plow Pose) and its variations as a forward-bending pose. In fact, it is usually classified as an inversion or as a shoulder stand variation. For me, however, no other posture more effectively lengthens the "western side" of our body. We stretch the calf muscles in Down Dog, the hamstrings in forward bends, and the gluteals and adductors in wide-legged postures. What remains is the spinal part of a forward bend.

The main reason Plow is such an effective spinal stretch is that the neck is flexed more

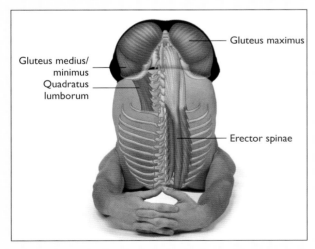

Figure 9.12: *Halasana.*

or less completely. This position lengthens the whole body of spinal muscles. Before I encourage students to take this pose, I make sure that their shoulders are open enough to support it (as well as the Shoulder Stand that often precedes it). This ensures that we don't end up doing a "neck stand."

With the neck and the rest of the spine flexed, when we roll up into Shoulder Stand and draw the legs back into Plow, the weight of the body through gravity places a great deal of pressure on the paraspinal muscles. You can mindfully increase or decrease the intensity of the stretch in this pose by repositioning the pelvis and feet. Walking your feet further away from your head brings the pelvis further over the head. This increases the amount of pressure you feel along the spine. (This can also place more strain on the neck, so be careful and make sure this would be appropriate for you.) If you feel too much strain on the neck, walk your feet closer to your head. This moves the pelvis in the opposite direction, diminishing the stretch in your back.

These paraspinal muscles are the same ones that attach at the sacrum and become part of the connective tissue that covers your sacrum. This same connective tissue becomes the sacrotuberous ligament (this ligament goes from the sacrum to the sit bone). This piece of connective tissue that we call a ligament becomes the tendons of the hamstrings. By lengthening these muscles above the pelvis, we indirectly affect all the tissues along the same line of connective tissues below the pelvis. This means that stretching the upper back muscles in Plow impacts how we fold forward in a seated forward bend.

Expanding our notion of a forward bend to include *Halasana* furthers our understanding of the whole-body experience of this type of pose. All our parts and pieces comprise a single whole. Now let's shift our focus from the hamstrings to these other parts to fully understand the totality of a forward bend.

ONE-LEGGED VARIATIONS

There are plenty of variations of both standing and seated one-legged forward bends. Some of the variations include *Supta Padangusthasana, Janu Sirsasana, Marichyasana A (1)*, or *Ardha Baddha Padma Paschimottanasana*. Any of these variations can potentially change the position of the pelvis in the forward bend. Changing the position of the pelvis puts pressure on different tissues at different angles.

By changing the pelvis, I mean shifting the direction that it faces. Is it facing straight forward as it would if you had both legs together in front of you like a standard forward bend? Are you going to allow the pelvis to turn so that it points anywhere from 10 to 45 degrees off of that straight forward direction? I won't argue that one of these is right while the other is wrong. They are just different and impact the tissues differently.

Reclined One-Legged Intense Stretch

Supta Padangusthasana is a great posture to begin exploring the way joints interlink in a forward bend. In this forward bend, the pelvis is essentially being pulled in opposite directions.

Interestingly, this pose illustrates the relationship between the hip flexors and the hip extenders, namely the quadriceps and the hamstrings. Both the hamstrings and the hip flexors have to open for a posture like this.

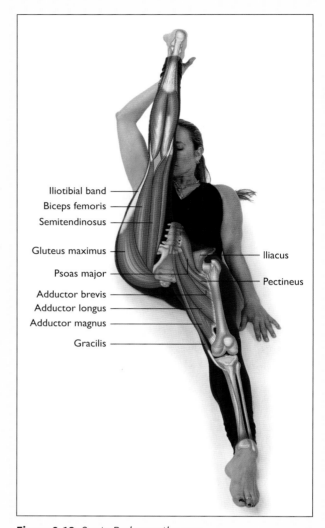

Figure 9.13: *Supta Padangusthasana.*

When we raise the leg we want to stretch, whether we are standing or laying on our backs, at some point the hamstrings will begin to hit their edge of flexibility. At this point the pelvis starts to tilt back and the pubic bone moves towards the ribs. We also come up against the tension in the hip flexors of the leg that is on the floor, as they will restrict the pelvis from tilting back. This typically causes the knee to bend, so that the hip flexors (the quadriceps in this case) soften and allow the pelvis to rotate and accommodate the tension in the hamstrings of the leg being lifted. To keep the knee straight and prevent the pelvis from tilting, we must balance the tension in our hamstrings with the strength of the quads.

The more we try to work the extended leg down if we are reclined (or straighten it if we're standing), the more pressure is placed on the hamstrings of the opposite leg. By straightening the leg, we keep the pelvis from accommodating the tension in the hamstrings of the opposite leg. It is forced to either stay in place or get pulled into an anterior tilt as we increase the tension in the front of the leg.

Seated One-Legged Forward Bends

Janu Sirsasana is a clear example of how the position of the pelvis can affect which tissues are lengthened in a forward bend. If you did this pose with the pelvis pointing straight towards the front of the mat, the hamstrings of the straight leg would stretch just as they would in a forward bend with the feet together. But that's not all that's going on here. The bent leg is abducted and externally rotated, which requires the pelvis to rotate around the head of the femur. This motion creates even more external rotation (sometimes I refer to this as "double" external rotation) and is similar to a wide-legged forward bend.

Moving the pelvis off the midline of the mat only impacts the alignment of the straight-leg hamstrings. Regardless of this angle, the bent leg is still in the same position relative to the pelvis. What changes is the hip joint of the straight leg. When we "forward bend" over the straight leg with the pelvis at an angle, we are more likely to experience restrictions in the lower back and side of the body of the bent knee just above the pelvis. These could include the quadratus lumborum, the iliocostalis lumborum, and the obliques. This is because now we have to rotate the spine.

Again, the same posture done slightly differently can completely change which tissues are being stretched. This is true of most one-legged forward bending postures. The position of the pelvis dictates which tissues are lengthened as well as which ones you are working.

ARM-BALANCED FORWARD BEND

Did I say arm-balanced forward bend? Yes, I did. Take a second to visualize it. Once you get past the fact that you're in an arm balance, the forward bend is obvious. Most poses fit in

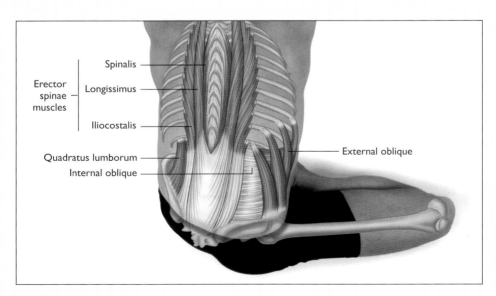

Figure 9.14: *Janu Sirsasana.*

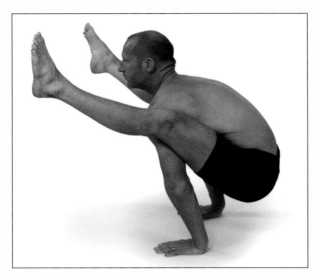

Figure 9.15: *Tittibhasana.*

more than one category, anyway. Think about Revolved Triangle; it is both a forward bend and a spinal twist. Let's look at *Tittibhasana* (Firefly Pose) as both an arm balance and a forward bend.

If our basic definition of a forward bend holds true (that is, the torso lies between or in front of the thighs), then *Tittibhasana* is definitely a forward bend. That said, it certainly feels different than a basic forward bend. This is a classic example of postures building towards one another. The work we have done in our basic forward bend should allow us to do *Tittibhasana*. If we still have work to do, *Tittibhasana* will remain out of reach.

If the hamstrings are open from our forward bends, it is easier to get our shoulders further behind the legs. This is imperative to lift into *Tittibhasana*. One reason this posture is more difficult is because we no longer have the resistance of the floor to work against. Without the floor, we must rely on the strength of the quadriceps working against the tension in the hamstrings.

Firefly Pose demonstrates what our unassisted range of motion is. It is unassisted because

the only leverage you have to straighten your knees and keep your hips flexed is the strength of the quadriceps and other hip flexors. As the strength of the quadriceps increases, or if the resistance of your hamstrings reduces, it is easier for your legs to straighten in *Tittibhasana*. If you can straighten the legs in *Tittibhasana* when there is no additional assistance, such as the floor, then when you *do* have the floor to work against, as you will in *Kurmasana*, you will be able to go even deeper into the pose.

THE MAIN EVENT: *KURMASANA*

Finally we reach our pinnacle of forward-bending postures. It is the pinnacle, not because we're perched at the top as in *Tittibhasana*, but because of the depth of the stretch. The difference between Firefly Pose and Tortoise Pose (*Kurmasana*) is that *Tittibhasana* doesn't allow for the resistance of the floor to work against as we develop the length in the hamstrings. The work we have done in our hamstrings and gluteal muscles in the preceding forward bends sets us up for this even deeper posture.

In *Kurmasana*, at the very least, our sit bones and hands are on the floor. In the fullest expression of the pose, our pelvis, thighs, hands, arms, and chest are all on the floor. Getting from the modification to the full posture primarily requires flexible hips. Secondarily, our spinal muscles must be able to accommodate the pressure that is often felt in the lower back in the forward bend. In fact, I would say that the two poses most potentially injurious to the lower back are *Kurmasana* and *Supta Kurmasana*.

Making our way into this posture can be precarious. It is important that you be at a level of practice where you are truly ready to work

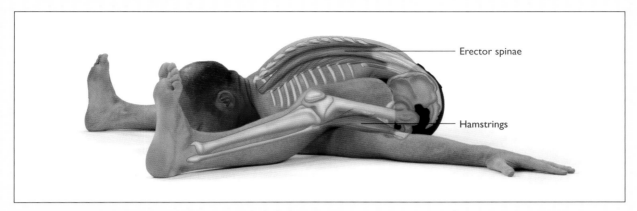

Figure 9.16: *Kurmasana requires open hamstrings, hips, and back muscles.*

on this pose. There are two ways of entering *Kurmasana*: from a standing position or seated on the floor. The first is more dynamic and in some ways easier because of the leverage available. Entering from a seated position is more appropriate for students just beginning to work on *Kurmasana*.

When entering from a standing position, we can see how flexible hamstrings help us fold forward and through the legs. Loose hamstrings also allow us to more readily take advantage of the leverage created by the hands pressing forward onto the backs of the ankles. This pressure sends the shoulders further behind the legs. At this point, the spine and hips are deeply flexed. If the back and hips still resist opening, we will feel excessive pressure and have a difficult time getting the shoulders far enough back to support the arm balance needed to enter this way.

Once the shoulders are far enough behind the legs, the adductors must engage to keep the thighs up against the sides of the body. If the legs slide too far away from the sides of the body, the backs of the knees will be on the elbows, and that can hurt. In order for the adductors to work effectively, they must be strong enough to overcome the resistance of the abductors, which can also restrict hip flexion. This is exactly what we have been exploring all along-how the tissues around the hips interact.

We have to bend the elbows and establish our seat next, all the while engaging the adductors to keep the legs from sliding away. From here, you have to resist gravity as everything slides down onto the floor. In order for the chest, thighs, and arms to get on the floor, we slowly engage the quadriceps and feel them working against the length of the hamstrings. The fact that we're in such a deep forward bend means that we're going to come up against the tension of the hamstrings as they are lengthened. Of course, the more tension in the hamstrings, the more difficult it is to straighten the knees. The more tension we find in the hamstrings, the greater the posterior tilt of the pelvis, which is partially why this is a precarious posture for the lower back.

We can also use the upper body to create sensations and forces that help us work more deeply into the pose. We tend to focus on the legs but adding in some work with the upper body can make all the difference in the world. I usually suggest that students press their upper arms back up against their legs. This does two things: it prevents excessive pressure on the clavicles and it creates some resistance that allows you to extend the spine even more in the posture. Extending the spine also helps to resist the posterior tilt of the pelvis created by tight hamstrings.

We do not want the sternoclavicular joint to go "pop" in this posture. Pressing the arms back

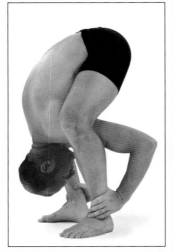
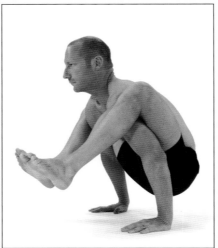
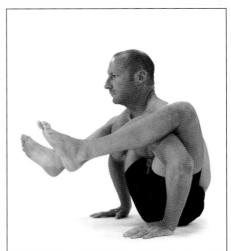
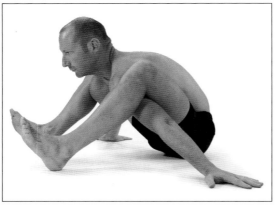
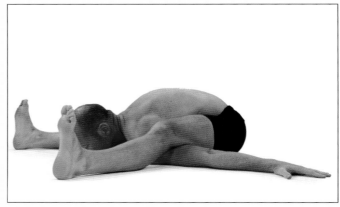

Figure 9.17: *Entering Kurmasana requires control and good technique when first approaching it. Tension in any of the places along the back line of the body can put a lot of force into the lower back.*

into the legs can prevent this from happening. Squeezing the legs in and pressing them down through the arms shifts the emphasis away from the sternoclavicular joint. As an added benefit, this will also teach you how to more strongly contract the quadriceps and change your perceptions and sensations in the posture.

COMMON PATTERNS

As always, when looking at a certain *asana*, I look for patterns and how they relate to other postures. I also look for patterns that negatively impact a student's progress, which I call "avoidance type" patterns. Avoidance patterns are not conscious. They are simply the body doing what it needs to do to arrive at its intended goal. These include turning the feet out, bending the knees, rounding the spine, rolling the thighs out, and even scrunching the shoulders. They each tell a story of what is going on in our forward bends.

Rounded Spine

The most common pattern that we see in forward bends is a rounded spine. This indicates a couple of possibilities. It is possible that you have a rounded upper or thoracic section of the spine. However, it is more common that the pelvis cannot rotate around the heads of the femurs. It can be a bit of a catch 22. If you do not forward bend, how will you lengthen the tissues that you need to stretch? If you put too much pressure on your spine in this way, you could injure the spine or its discs. What to do?

This is why I encourage students doing forward bends with a rounded back to maintain or intend a small amount of arch in their lower back. It doesn't mean that I can necessarily see the arch in their spine, but just the intention or effort of trying to undo some of the roundedness or flexion of the lower spine is enough to start the process of change. This technique helps students to stretch the hamstrings safely while gradually evolving to a flat-back forward bend.

Feet Turned In and Thighs Externally Rotated

Have you noticed how, when deep in a forward bend, the feet want to twist so that the soles start to face one another? Ever wondered why? In this case, the thighs rotate externally to unconsciously avoid the direct line of tension in the hamstrings; that is, if the legs are straight then there is a more direct line of tension created by the hamstrings. If the legs are rotated, that tension is diminished. As the thighs rotate, the knees often bend a bit as well. We see this expressed in the feet.

Remember, this type of pattern can be the body's way of navigating around its limitations. When we fold forward, we place pressure on the heads of the femurs. That pressure can cause the femurs to externally rotate, thus creating the pattern I am describing. To compensate for that, we need to work in the opposite direction by internally rotating the thighs. The easiest way to make this happen is to use the adductors, which are also hip flexors. Just squeezing the legs together helps reduce the amount of external rotation created by the pressure of the pelvis on the femur and helps keep them heading in the right direction.

Bending the Knees

There are several good reasons to bend the knees in forward bends. For starters, if we cannot sit upright, the abdominals must contract to keep us from falling backwards.

Bending the knees is a simple solution to this problem. It also reduces the force of the

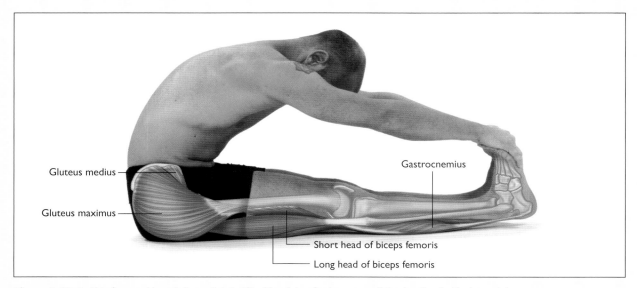

Gluteus medius

Gluteus maximus

Gastrocnemius

Short head of biceps femoris

Long head of biceps femoris

Figure 9.18: *In this forward bend, the pelvis is tilted back too far because of the tension in the hamstrings.*

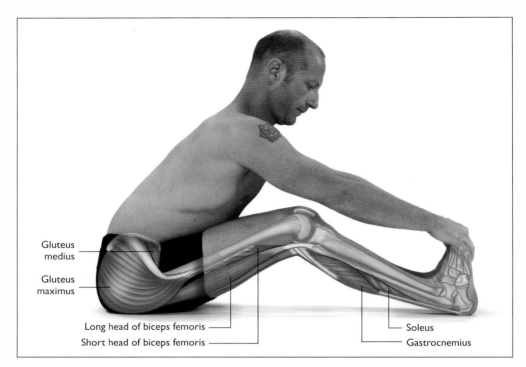

Figure 9.19: *In this forward bend, the pelvis is allowed to tilt forward more because bending the knees has reduced the tension coming from the hamstrings.*

hamstrings as they pull on the sit bones. This allows the pelvis to move to a more neutral position. If we're sitting on the floor, as in *Paschimottanasana*, then we might actually be able to sit upright with the knees bent.

There is a down side to this, though. Remember, one reason to take a forward bend is to lengthen the hamstrings. When we bend the knees, we reduce the amount of pressure on the hamstrings. This reduces the amount of length we can potentially create in them. So how do we strike a balance?

I always tell students that if they need to bend their knees in a pose (this assumes we're not working with an injury), once they are in the pose, they should at least *try* to straighten the knees. I'll often say, "Use 20 percent of your strength to try and straighten the knee(s)." The number 20 is not necessarily the "right" number. It is just an amount that directs students to work on straightening the legs

without causing strain. This puts pressure back into the hamstrings.

This small amount of effort helps to balance out the amount of pressure we get in our hamstrings. With the knees soft we can overstretch the sit-bone end of the hamstrings. We already discussed this relative to sit bone pain in the first part of the book. So certainly you can bend the knees, but then try to straighten them again to a reasonable degree. This way you redirect the stretch back into the whole of the hamstring muscle.

Hyperextended Knees

Hyperextension of the knees is a genetic issue that has to do with the shape of the end of the bones that comprise the knee. Because hyperextension happens at the boney level, it is much harder to change anatomically. What we really need to do is retrain hyperextended knees to not collapse into hyperextension. We're making a functional change. Basically, we want to create a new neuromuscular pattern that prevents potential long-term damage to the knee.

There are many people who have a slight hyperextension in their knees and who live a full and active life without any trouble. Thus I tend to focus on this issue when people show significant hyperextension. If the hyperextension is slight, it's often not a concern unless there is dysfunction or injury at the joint as well.

There are a number of potential problems in more extreme cases. The cartilage can wear away unevenly. The PCL can be overstretched, creating even more hyperextension; the tendons of the hamstring and gastrocnemius muscles can be overstretched. The simplest solution is to keep the knees slightly bent, which can undo the hyperextension and retrain the muscles to know how far to extend the knees. The joint becomes accustomed to maintaining that slight bend; over time and with awareness, the adjustment becomes automatic.

Overdoing with the Upper Body

It seems worth it to let the upper body enter the conversation here for a moment. The forward bend itself is mostly about the legs, hips, and spine, but we use the arms to grab onto something, be it the toes, feet, shins, or straps. This brings me to a shoulder pattern that all yoga teachers loathe to see: shoulders up in the ears with the back of the neck all scrunched up; it just rubs us the wrong way, right?

This pattern tells me the student is relying too heavily on arm strength in their forward bend. There's nothing wrong with giving a verbal cue to draw the scapulae down the back, but I use

this pattern as an opportunity to encourage students to really work into their forward bend. I ask them to let go of whatever it is they're holding onto with their hands.

Once they let go, primarily the hip flexors are required to maintain the pose. This is a good thing. We want to use the hip flexors and quadriceps as much as possible in forward bends, so that their inherent strength is working with/against the tension of the opposing muscles (the hamstrings). After they've let go of their support and connected to these muscles holding them in the forward bend, I invite the students to re-grip whatever they were holding; now it is simply assisting them in the forward bend, not making it happen.

If I want to redirect their shoulder movement, I use a correction I'm sure you're familiar with. I get them to move their scapulae, but not so much down their back as towards the front in protraction. When they do this, the elbows point more towards the floor. This naturally reduces the scrunching in the neck and shoulders and moves the scapulae towards the front.

These so-called "problem" patterns provide opportunities to help train new neuromuscular patterns that will be used in other postures. To be fair, it is not that the scapulae have to move in this direction in a forward bend at all. They don't. However, the more familiar our body is with a movement, the easier it will be to access the same pattern of movement later and in other postures that require the same pattern.

WHAT ABOUT THE ABDOMINALS?

Have you wondered why we haven't mentioned the abdominals as a hip flexor, yet. It's because they aren't. Does this mean we don't have to engage them to do a forward bend? That's right; we do not *need* them for that movement, though they are often used. The abdominals can function in two ways in a forward bend. They can help stabilize the torso relative to the pelvis, so that we can more deeply flex the hips. They can also contract to deepen the flexion of the spine. At this point, the abdomen can become like over-squeezed glutes in an Upward Facing Dog. That is, it can be unnecessarily overdone. This is another example of the body doing whatever it can to bring you closer to your desired goal. Can you relax the abdomen in your forward bend?

In fact, I would say that to elongate the spine in a forward bend, you have to relax the abdominals. If your abs are engaged, the lower back/spine will likely be rounded in flexion, and in order for the spine to lengthen (or flatten) it must be able to extend.

There is another common pattern relating to the abdominal muscles and the hamstrings. It is commonly seen in forward bending as well as in Downward Dog. Students with tight hamstrings often have a difficult time relaxing the abdomen in a forward bend. This has to do with the relationship between the hamstrings and abdominals relative to the pelvis. If you try to "tuck the tailbone," as many people do in postures like *Utkatasana*, both the hamstrings and the abdominal muscles shorten to create this movement.

Let's look at this relationship in a seated forward bend. When the hamstrings are tight,

they pull the pelvis towards a posterior tilt. As a result, the spine moves back relative to the position of the pelvis. To prevent themselves from falling backward, students automatically engage the abdominal muscles to stabilize the torso.

We see this same pattern in Down Dog. Tight hamstrings and contracted abdominals create a pattern of tension that leads to a rounded lower back. Tension in the hamstrings results in a posterior tilt of the pelvis and shortens the abdominals as well. Until those hamstrings open, it will be hard for the abdomen to let go, relax, and allow more length and space in the spine.

CONCLUSION

A forward bend is both simple and complicated at the same time. It is simple to bend forward and grab your toes or feet in some way. But it is difficult to coordinate various parts of the body to create a deep and rich forward bend. Naturally we take advantage of our strengths and avoid our weaknesses. This is possibly one of the larger lessons of yoga *asana*. Our work is to bring as much balance to our body as we can and to have faith that this will also affect our mind and other habits.

To begin to see your forward bends more holistically, pay attention to the parts of your anatomy that you tend to avoid. Re-pattern them. These little changes will add up to a nice and simple forward bend.

10
ANATOMICAL PATTERNS IN EXTERNAL HIP ROTATION

An externally rotated hip shows up in multiple places in any yoga practice. Postures such as *Trikonasana*, *Parsvakonasana*, *Janu Sirsasana*, *Baddha Konasana*, *Padmasana*, *Kapotasana* (Pigeon Pose), and *Eka* and *Dwi Pada Sirsasana* (leg[s] behind the head) all share this common theme.

As discussed previously, there is more than one way of looking at what is commonly described as external rotation at the hip joint. We can look at the femur to see how it is positioned relative to the pelvis. This, however, is just half of what external rotation is. In different postures we do exactly this. But we also need to see how we take that rotation further by moving the pelvis around the head of the femur after the femur has externally rotated.

I am going to set the bar high for our pinnacle posture of external rotation as we explore these patterns of movement. *Eka Pada Sirsasana* (Leg-Behind-the-Head Pose) can seem unattainable for many of us. It is one of those postures often placed on a pedestal, one of the "Holy Grail" postures in yoga. Other *asanas* in this lofty group include Lotus, deep backbending, and Headstand. These are the postures that everyone wants to do, but sometimes feels are impossible to attain. Good

news! Your enlightenment is not tied to your ability to get your leg behind your head. It sure looks impressive though, doesn't it?

Eka Pada Sirsasana is one of my personal challenges. I've spent a lot of time and energy working towards this pose and beyond in *Dwi Pada Sirsasana* (both legs behind the head). These are the postures that most quickly disappear for me if I travel too much or if my focused and dedicated daily *asana* practice slips. The point is, I am all too familiar with the ebb and flow of my ability to do these poses.

It bears repeating—difficulties are opportunities. These postures have led me through a winding road of discovery and surrender. Putting your leg behind your head is rather precarious and potentially dangerous if the right tissues are not already opened or strengthened. It is also anatomically complicated and requires patience when deconstructing.

It is vitally important to explore all the places where we can prepare for such a difficult pose. Where in our sequencing do we build to this posture? What anatomical patterns are we looking for?

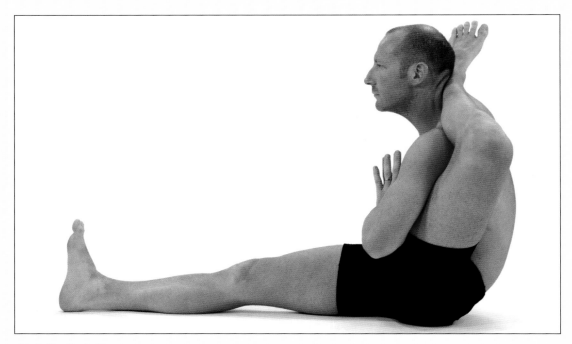

Figure 10.1: *Eka Pada Sirsasana.*

THE ANATOMY

In terms of anatomy, remember that two bones come together to make the hip joint, the pelvis and the femur. If either of these two bones moves while the other is stabilized, we're moving the hip joint. This seems obvious enough, but we often limit our notion of movement at the hip joint to movement of the femur. We are accustomed to thinking about movement beginning from the anatomical position.

Since the hip has tremendous range of motion in all directions, the tissues surrounding it can pull it in all directions. I mention this because it is especially important to realize that muscles of the hip often create more than one movement and different parts of the same muscle occasionally create opposite movements. The gluteus medius comes to mind. Its front portion flexes and internally rotates the hip joint while its back portion extends and externally rotates it.

To complicate matters further, the resistances we feel at the hip can actually change when we flex at the hips from anatomical position. We have explored this in the hip section, but I'll reiterate it here because it is exactly what happens as we head towards our pinnacle pose. In order to get the leg behind the head, we have to combine several movements at the hip joint, including flexion, abduction, and external rotation. This combination means that we will actually be stretching the external rotators (the deep six in particular) in external rotation because we have fully flexed the hip. The opposite is true in anatomical position. Normally in external rotation we stretch the internal rotators.

Because of the combination of actions required, we can think more holistically when working with the hip muscles. We don't have to limit our preparation to the exact movement we're trying to create in *Eka Pada Sirsasana* because the same muscles do more than one action. Personally, I think it's best to get as close to a desired pattern as possible when practicing, but changing the angles of pull on the same muscles is also beneficial.

The gluteus medius is a rotator and an abductor. If we adduct the hip, then we stretch this muscle. Now, consider that the same muscle also does internal and external rotation. In a way, stretching the abductors by adducting the hip joint will also improve its ability to allow rotation.

STANDING POSTURES

Standing postures provide our first inkling of how to work with the external rotation pattern. Sure, there are some standing versions of Half-Lotus, but the depth of work in that particular pattern is in the seated postures. Why? Because when we are in a standing pose, the legs are also being used to keep us balanced and upright. Thus the muscles in the legs are often loaded with tension from contraction in various ways. When we get to the floor, we're able to work more deeply with the patterns of Lotus. Our initial work on externally rotating the hips begins well before we arrive at standing Half-Lotus.

Trikonasana

Triangle is the first stop on the way to a fully externally rotated hip. We have two hip joints and two legs, so there are two potential areas where we can work on external rotation—the front and back leg. In Triangle, the front and back legs are in different positions, but both feed into this pattern. In the front leg, we are externally rotating. In the back, we are lengthening some of the tissues that we need to open in order to go further.

The Front Leg

External rotation begins in the front leg in Triangle Pose. Relative to anatomical position, the hip joint abducts, externally rotates, and flexes all at the same time. The movement that has the most impact on our journey of external rotation is abduction. This occurs as we work to bring the pelvis into a vertical position. Whether we manage to do so or not isn't as important as what happens as we try.

By working to align the pelvis in this way, we start to place pressure on the adductors. The more vertical the pelvis gets, the more pressure we place on the adductors and the more we increase the actions of both abduction and external rotation. Remember, the adductors are also internal rotators and can limit external rotation. The work we do in Triangle to open them will

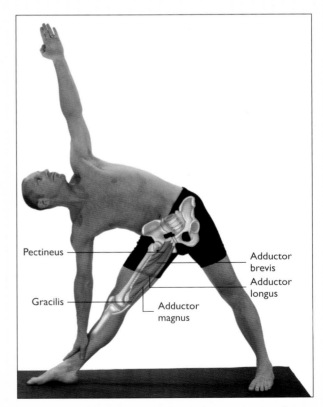

Figure 10.2: *Although a simple enough posture, Triangle gets the pattern of externally rotating the hip joint started.*

help us later when we get to the postures that require even more rotation.

In *Trikonasana* try to visualize the pelvis as it tilts around the femur as much as you visualize the work in the femur. Perhaps you can feel the rotation better now? It is also possible that you have been working with an intention that is different from what the literal anatomical position is. If you've been told to internally rotate the femur, don't think of it as wrong, we are being as anatomically literal as possible. This is the difference between the felt sense anatomy and the literal anatomy. Here the leg is literally externally rotated relative to the body being in anatomical position. From that externally rotated position we could intend to internally rotate. So is it internally rotated or externally rotated? Explore the sensations and feelings to understand the anatomical connections.

The Back Leg

In literal terms, the back leg of *Trikonasana* is adducted at the hip joint. This is much different from what happens in the front leg. Instead of putting pressure on the adductors (as in the front leg). The back leg of the pose places pressure on the abductors, namely the deeper gluteals. This includes gluteus medius and minimus. Both are internal and external rotators of the hip (depending on whether you're talking about the anterior or the posterior section), as well as being abductors. As we work with adduction in this leg, these muscles are lengthened.

Although the actions required by Triangle in the back leg are not strongly rotational, lengthening the abductors indirectly affects our ability to rotate the legs in other poses. This posture has changed over time for me. It started out as an intense hamstring stretch in the front leg. Eventually that stretch moved into the gluteals

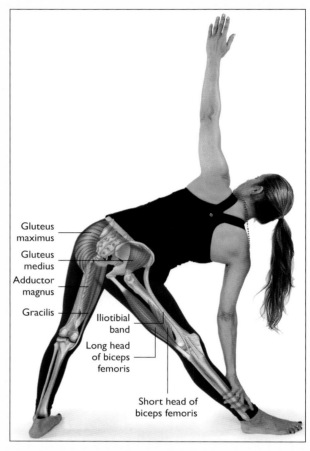

Figure 10.3: *The lateral part of the back leg indirectly relates to our ability to rotate the hip joint.*

of the back leg. Not only was I progressing in the pose, but I was also establishing connections to more advanced postures.

Parsvakonasana and *Virabhadrasana* II

Parsvakonasana and *Virabhadrasana* (Warrior II) continue the work in the front leg that we began in *Trikonasana*. A similar pattern of flexion, abduction, and external rotation is found in these postures. The most obvious change is that the front knee is bent to about 90 degrees. This may seem like a small change, but it makes quite a difference. Bending the knee adds pressure and stress to the front hip joint and deepens the amount of hip flexion. This can reveal our tendency for general hip tightness in similar postures. It also increases

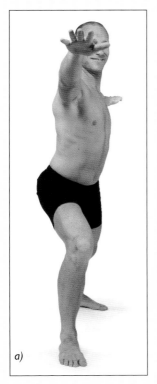 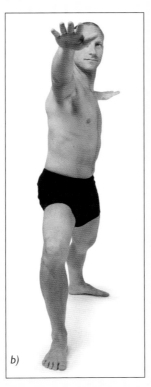

a)   b)

Figure 10.4: *a) it is common to see the butt sticking out in Warrior II, b) the correction is an abduction at the hip joint.*

the stretch of the hamstrings at the hip end while placing more pressure on the gluteals. Both of these groups impact our ability to rotate at the hip. The adductors get mixed in because they are also lengthened. With the added pressure in all of these tissues, we can see several patterns emerge.

One of the most common patterns in these two postures is that the hip of the front leg starts to stick out to the side.

Because in both poses, we want to abduct the hip, we are naturally increasing the tension in the adductors. In this case, the tension results not from contracting the adductors, but because we are lengthening them. Tight adductors won't allow the knee to move out and in line with the big toe, which coincides with the hip sticking out more than we want. Remember that the adductors can also impact the pelvis. In this case, tension from the adductors pulls the pubic bone down and forward, which causes

the pelvis to anteriorly tilt, further accentuating the hip being pushed outwards.

Because the joint itself is abducted, the gluteals have less impact on our ability to rotate the femur or the pelvis, unless they are particularly tight (in which case, they will have more of an effect). Anterior tilt in this position is technically external rotation at the hip joint. This is important because the most common correction for the hip sticking out is to tuck the pelvis. By tucking the pelvis, we internally rotate the hip by moving the pelvis instead of the femur.

The effort of keeping the knee in line with the big toe sends pressure back into the hip adductors, which are also internal rotators. Helping to lengthen the internal rotators allows for more external rotation in this and other poses. Although we do internally rotate the hip slightly, tucking the pelvis also allows us to work more clearly on abducting (which lengthens adductors) and avoids our potential for compressing the lower back.

Let's recap. These standing postures show us what external rotation looks like. They solidify the desired patterns in the hip joint. They also reveal our limitations. The tendency for the knee to fall inwards reveals the amount of tension in our hips. The more the knee falls in (or, conversely, the more the butt sticks out), the more tension there is. By aligning the knee over the toes, we place pressure on the adductors.

Janu Sirsasana and *Baddha Konasana*

When we move to the floor for postures like *Janu Sirsasana* and *Baddha Konasana*, the position of the pelvis relative to the femur changes. In the standing poses, we just explored, the relationship between the femur and pelvis was abduction and flexion in the front leg.

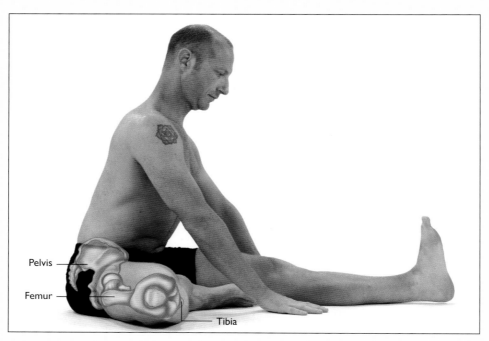

Figure 10.5: *Janu Sirsasana. Note the position of the pelvis relative to the femur.*

However, in seated postures like *Janu Sirsasana* and *Baddha Konasana*, for example, the pelvis has significantly changed.

The hip joint now rotates externally. Remember that movement of the femur or the pelvis is movement at the hip joint. Imagine a *Virabhadrasana* from above. In order to make the relationship between the pelvis and femur look similar to that in *Janu Sirsasana*, we would have to sit up at the hip joint. In this case, we are moving the pelvis.

Two components require our attention in *Janu Sirsasana*: the rotation of the hip joint and the forward bend. When working on hip opening, the primary focus should be on the bent-knee side of the pose. The forward bend is secondary. Let's take the time to focus on what it is we're doing here as we explore the pose as one component of a much larger pattern of external hip rotation.

One of the most common debates in this posture is where the knee should be pointing.

You typically hear that the knee should be out to the side at a 90-degree angle. However, there are different ways to measure what that 90-degree angle is and where the 90 degrees

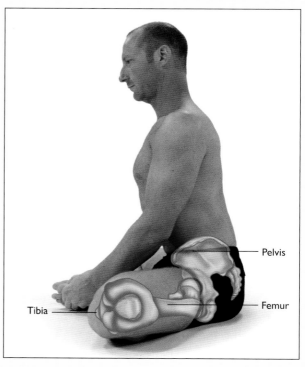

Figure 10.6: *Baddha Konasana. Note the position of the pelvis relative to the femur.*

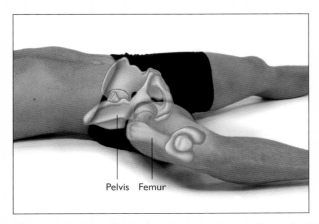
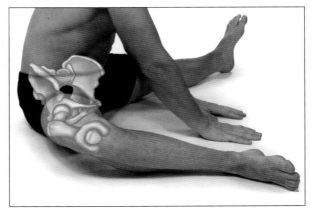

Pelvis Femur

Figure 10.7: *The pelvis is what changes when we flex and rotate the hip joint.*

is created. Is it relative to the other leg? Is it relative to the pelvis? How are we measuring the 90 degrees?

I prefer to focus on maximizing and working with the external rotation pattern and putting pressure in the hip joint. With this intention, it is more effective to look at the relationship between the femur and the pelvis as a measure of this 90-degree angle. The next great debate is whether the pelvis should be square to the front of the yoga mat. Does it even matter? The two debates are directly related to one another.

Let's say we take the right side of *Janu Sirsasana*. Our right leg comes back and we intend to

bring it to a 90-degree angle relative to the left (straight) leg. As we do, we will abduct, flex, and externally rotate the right femur relative to the pelvis. The question is how much movement will we allow from the left hip joint? Many times we include movement at the opposite hip joint when entering a pose like this.

If we are focused on the 90-degree relationship being established from the shin relative to the left leg, it is possible that we have moved our pelvis to make this shape. The alignment of the pelvis can muddy our understanding of the extent to which we're really externally rotating the right hip. It is not that moving the pelvis is wrong, but at the very least, it's good to

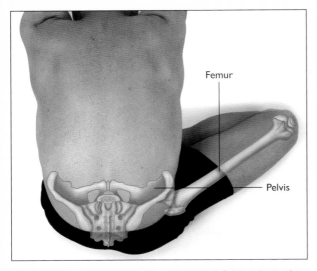
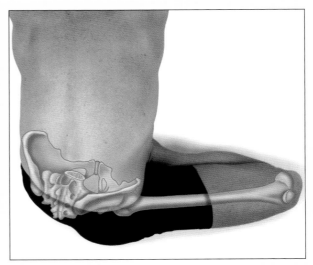

Femur

Pelvis

Figure 10.8: *The pelvis has moved at the left hip joint in the second image.*

know what we're doing! We may think we have abducted and rotated more than we actually have. If you focus on keeping the pelvis square to the front of the mat and you bring the right foot in without allowing the pelvis to move at the left hip joint, you will see the true range of motion of your right hip in this pose. It is easier to change the amount of movement at this joint when you actually know your starting point.

Because we work one hip at a time in *Janu Sirsasana*, the pelvis can adapt to the amount of abduction available in each joint. Let's compare it to *Baddha Konasana*. If your bent leg doesn't easily reach the floor in *Janu Sirsasana*, it is possible that the pelvis will tilt to allow the knee to drop lower. This can happen if we intentionally draw the thigh towards the floor (not a bad idea); it can also happen if someone presses our thigh to the floor. In both cases, the thigh reaches the floor because the pelvis has tilted to accommodate the movement; however, in so doing, we may not be exploring

the true range of motion in the hip joint. We want to pay attention to where the movement is actually coming from.

Baddha Konasana can be considered a two-sided *Janu Sirsasana*. It provides a more honest picture of what's really possible at each hip. Have you noticed that in *Baddha Konasana* the knees and thighs may be further from the floor than in *Janu Sirsasana*? If so, this means the position of the pelvis is compensating in *Janu Sirsasana*.

In *Baddha Konasana* there is no opportunity for the pelvis to compensate. With both legs folded into the same position, the pelvis does not change its angle relative to the top of the mat. It also can't tilt up or down to compensate, because the other side is in the same position. This increases the general intensity of *Baddha Konasana* compared to *Janu Sirsasana*. It is much easier to feel the intensity of the stretch through the adductors and their attachment at the front of the pubic bone.

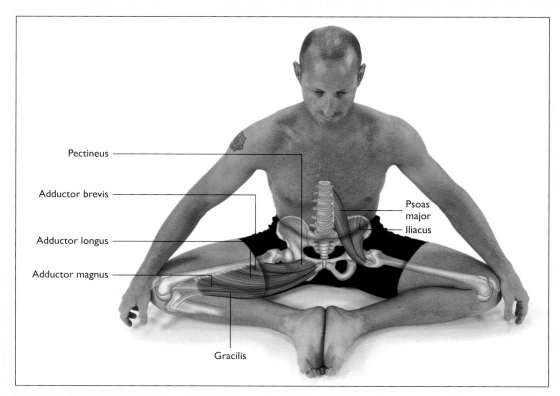

Figure 10.9: *A double sided Janu Sirsasana increases pressure on the adductors, since the pelvis cannot compensate.*

Is it possible to feel this same sensation in *Janu Sirsasana*? Not as easily, but yes, it is possible. In order to focus on the right hip in this pose, we need to direct some additional pressure into that joint. In bending the right knee to take the pose, the right side of the pelvis often moves back. We need to move it forward again relative to where we have placed the femur. There are two ways to do this. First, we can move it on the horizontal plane, which involves moving the right hip point (the ASIS) forward relative to the extended femur. We can also "rotate" it forward, either by tilting the pelvis or rotating the thigh back and down. You could also combine all of these movements into one. To play with this, open the knee slightly by moving the foot away from the extended

leg, a bit more than you would normally do in *Janu Sirsasana*. Depending on how strongly you do this, you can end up putting more pressure on the knee than you want. Moving the foot away from the thigh is just for exploration purposes and helps reduce pressure on the knee. Begin with a small amount of effort; don't push too hard too quickly. Enjoy the exploration.

PROGRESSING

It is time to evolve these postures. Now the pelvis takes an interesting turn, literally. The pelvis moves around the head of the femurs to take us into the forward bend in both of these

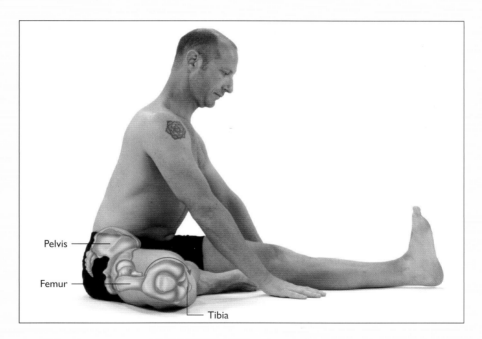

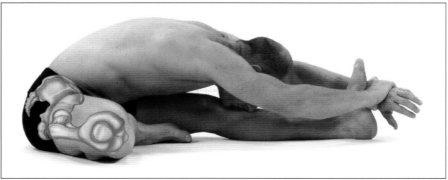

Figure 10.10: *The pelvis rotates forward at the hip joints as far as possible. It then finds movement at two other places, the left hip and the right knee joint. Notice in the second image that the right foot has not changed position.*

postures. At this point we see the hip's real ability to externally rotate. (Note that in the forward bend version of these postures, the knee can be affected by what happens in the hip.)

When the pelvis starts to rotate around the head of the femur, it will eventually meet its range of motion. At that point, even though the femur is externally rotated, it will start to move in the same direction as the pelvis. The femur will start to internally rotate because it is traveling in the same direction as the pelvis. Essentially the pelvis is pulling the femur along with it as it moves forward and down. When we talk about internal rotation at this point, the action is not happening at the hip joint as we might assume. So where exactly is the femur internally rotating from?

Remember, we have already maximized the amount of movement available at the hip joint. That's why the femur started moving in this scenario. The "extra" movement begins to occur at two other locations. The first place is at the opposite hip joint. While one hip has maximized its rotation, the other side can go further because it is only flexing. It hasn't arrived at its end of range of motion. This movement is also occurring at the knee. Here we need to be more cautious.

Placing the foot in front of the pelvis with the outer edge and top of the foot on the floor stabilizes the foot and shin. In a sense, it is stuck where it is. You may recall that the foot is solidly connected to the foreleg, which ends at the knee. When the femur starts "rotating inwards," this movement actually happens at the knee. This is potentially problematic and is exactly why we often hear the verbal adjustment to rotate the femur back and down. I couldn't agree more with this intention. Though the actual movement here is at the knee joint, the restriction is at the hip. This is evident because the pelvis can't rotate any

further. As the muscles around the hip open, the pelvis will be able to rotate further, thereby reducing the amount of rotation in the knee joint. This same principle applies to our next pose, Half-Bound Lotus Forward Bend.

Ardha Padmasana and *Padmasana*

We continue external rotation of the hip with Lotus Pose and its variations. When we look at a nicely-bloomed Lotus, both the lower leg and the upper leg have externally rotated like the petals of a lotus flower that have fallen out to the side. When this has happened, the bottom of the foot is pointing upwards to the ceiling and the thigh or knee is resting on the floor. When the hip does not allow for enough rotation, the knee pinches or we feel pressure in the ankle.

As with *Janu Sirsasana*, we must create as much external rotation in the hip joint as possible. But because of where the foot has to end up, *Ardha Padmasana* actually requires the foot to lift up as much as six inches higher than it is in *Janu Sirsasana* to get on top of that thigh. This means we need even more external rotation at the hip joint.

Therefore, in both Half- and Full Lotus, most of the problems we come across can ultimately be linked back to limitations in hip mobility. Problems include ankle pressure and pain, shinbones pressing too firmly together, and knee pain. It may be helpful to shift our perspective of Lotus Pose as being not so much a hip opener as it is a pose that requires one to have flexible hips.

In the West, it is less likely that we arrive in *Padmasana* with open hips. Our hips are typically stiff due to any number of activities we have done throughout our life.

Sports and activities that require running, jogging, cycling, and just sitting in chairs can

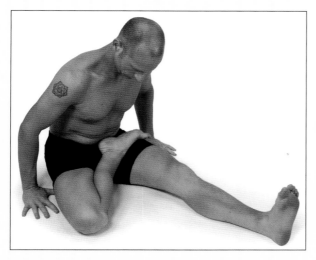 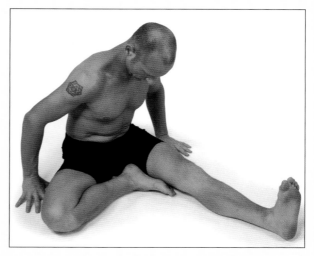

Figure 10.11: *The foot moving from the floor to the top of the thigh asks even more rotation from the hip joint. If it doesn't come from there, the knee will have to compensate.*

all lead to tight hips. But because Lotus is such an alluring posture, we'll investigate how to encourage external rotation in the hips in a manner that is both safe and effective. Along the way, I'll make some observations about what not to do and why. There is certainly more than one approach to getting into *Padmasana*. I'll share what has worked for me and how I teach my students. Naturally, the common thread running through all effective pre-Lotus techniques is that they focus on the hip joints.

We'll start with one of the most common patterns that beginners use to get into Lotus Pose. I often see students grab the foot and shin with their hands on top, palms facing down. They then begin to draw the heel in towards their abdomen. This method tends to internally rotate the lower leg at the knee joint. Generally speaking, this should be avoided. Advanced practitioners can sometimes get away with it because as they release their lower leg, it rotates externally to match the upper leg.

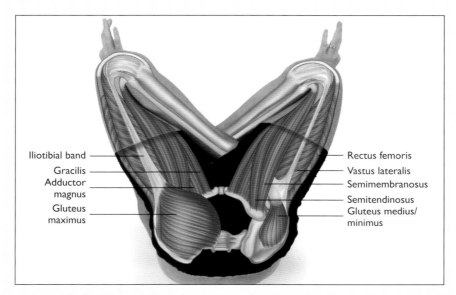

Iliotibial band

Gracilis

Adductor magnus

Gluteus maximus

Rectus femoris

Vastus lateralis

Semimembranosus

Semitendinosus

Gluteus medius/ minimus

Figure 10.12: *Restriction at the hip joint isn't limited to the deep gluteal muscles; hamstrings, and adductors can also play a role in preventing lotus.*

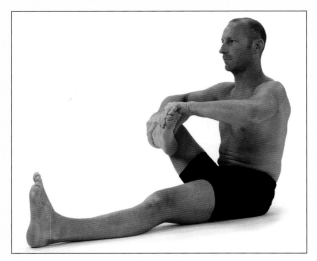

Figure 10.13: *By placing the hands on top, the lower leg internally rotates.*

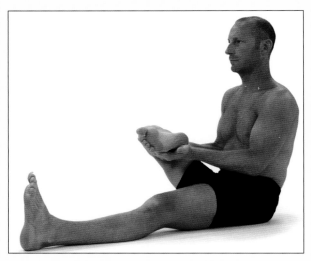

Figure 10.14: *By placing the hands under, the lower leg externally rotates.*

Rather than grasp the foot like this, I suggest we encourage external rotation of both the upper and lower leg. John Scott shared this method with me many years ago; I have used it ever since.

Instead of taking the foot from over the top, take it from underneath and let the foot and shin rest in the both hands. Allow the heel of the foot to rest in the heel of the hand (same side) and then let the hip joint relax. Because the heel of the hand is resting under the heel of the foot, when the hip relaxes, the knee drops slightly while the foot stays in place. This externally rotates the lower leg at the knee and hip joints at the same time. Just because we use a particular technique does not ensure that we get it right away and suddenly have the perfect Lotus. But it trains our tissues to move in a particular way, creating a new pattern.

Many people complain of pressure on the outside of the ankle in Half- or Full-Lotus Pose. There are remedies for this; one is to dorsiflex the ankle joint. This usually avoids the over "sickling" (inversion) of the ankle, but does it address the real problem? Flexion of the ankle is also used to "protect" the knee. We need to understand why the foot is in this

position in the first place and why the knee needs protection. There are two reasons.

Internal rotation of the lower leg at the knee usually causes sickling of the ankle, but this doesn't happen by itself. The hip is involved, too. General tension at the hip joint determines where the knee is. Where the knee is determines where the foot can be. This is the nature of a kinematic chain of joints such as the leg.

Another reason the ankle ends up in this position is that the upper leg is not externally rotated enough or is not flexible enough to allow the foot to end up high enough on the thigh. If the knee is too high and too wide, the foot cannot reach the top of the opposite thigh. These two issues can combine. Both will cause the foot to slide down onto the inner part of the thigh creating a sickled ankle.

It is also possible for the foot to come too far across the thigh. This is a different sign of tension in the hip moving into Half-Lotus.

When we have tension in the Lotus hip, it is possible to compensate by pulling the hip joint across (adduction). I've seen this many times. The first leg goes into Half-Lotus and as this

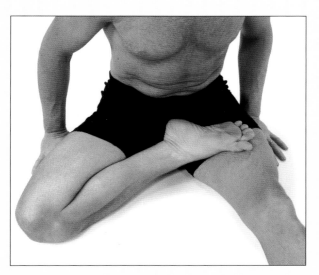

Figure 10.15: *When the foot sits this low on the thigh it is a reflection of the hip joint being tight.*

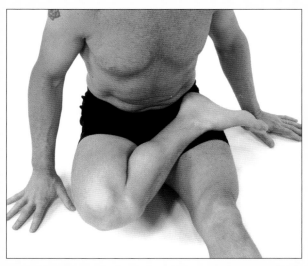

Figure 10.16: *When the foot is this far across the thigh, it stays elevated and can put the knee into a more vulnerable position.*

happens (let's assume we're talking about the right leg here), we actually adduct the hip joint. If we engage the adductors to make this happen, we are potentially adding to the internal rotation of the thigh. This can cause the knee to float above the floor, which brings us back to the idea of "protecting" the knee. If it is in a vulnerable place, then of course protect it. But we shouldn't ignore the root cause of either the pain or the vulnerability. What we really need to do is bring the work back to the hip.

When we see an elevated knee in Half-Lotus, it is easy to fall into assuming that the adductors are the issue. If we could open them up, we think, our knee would be lower. Our elevated knee can certainly have something to do with the adductors, but that may not be the only restriction. Other tissues can limit the leg's ability to abduct and drop towards the floor. External rotation is also restricted. Because the adductors are internal rotators, they can restrict our ability to externally rotate the hip joint. The biggest culprits in restricting this movement are the deep external rotators of the hip. These include the piriformis muscle, but also the fibers of the gluteus minimus and medius when the hip is flexed.

Full Lotus

When we add a second leg to our Lotus, we see some parallels to *Janu Sirsasana* and *Baddha Konasana*. We have discussed how the pelvis adapts in Half Lotus similar to its adaptation in *Janu Sirsasana*. If the hip is tight, the opposite side (especially the sit bone) will lift up in Half Lotus, with the knee close to the floor. In Full Lotus, there is little or no room for the pelvis to adapt in this manner. Lotus also requires the second leg to externally rotate more to get into position. If this doesn't happen, you end up with a Lotus Pose with the ankles crossed but the feet not on the thighs. This shows how far we still have to go in our hips.

MOVING FORWARD

When we fold forward over a Half- or Full Lotus, the movement is the same as in *Janu Sirsasana* or *Baddha Konasana*: the pelvis has to rotate around the head of the femur. If it can't rotate any further, it takes the femur with it. The consequences can be more serious when this happens in Half- or Full Lotus than in the earlier postures.

Because the leg is completely folded and the lower leg is deeply rotated, the possibility of injury is increased. I'm not surprised that Lotus is a common site for knee injury in practitioners, because two of the most common anatomical patterns converge in this asana—internal rotation of the lower legs and generally tight hips. This can be a recipe for long-term stress at the knee.

I'm not suggesting that you shouldn't try *Padmasana*. What I am suggesting is that we pay attention to where pressure is being applied in the pose. Our focus should be on the larger joints that can take the stress more easily. In this case, the hip, because the hip is a difficult joint to injure.

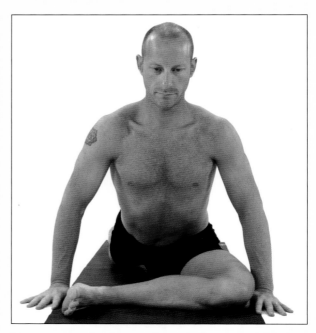

Figure 10.17: *The shin parallel to the front edge of the mat ensures pressure into the deep gluteals.*

Kapotasana (Pigeon Pose)

There are a number of *Kapotasana* variations. We'll focus on one that leads us to our pinnacle pose and that works well with our exploration of external rotation. It is also a preparatory pose for getting the leg behind the head. This prep plays off the same idea and principles discussed in preparation for *Padmasana*. The more classical way of doing this pose is to bend the front knee fully and point the toes back towards the extended leg. In that version we usually stay more upright, using the hands for leverage. In this variation, we draw the shin further out in front of us. In fact, we bring it far enough out that the shin ends up parallel to the front edge of the mat. This places the leg in a position similar to Double Pigeon or Firelog Pose, which we discussed in the hip section. This configuration can be used in several different places to put pressure on the key muscles that restrict external rotation of the hip. Here we are primarily after the deep six lateral rotators, the gluteus minimus, and the gluteus medius.

You may recall that, because we are flexing the hip first, we are flipping the fibers around at the back of the pelvis. As a result, our strong external rotation actually stretches the external rotators. This is opposite to how we normally lengthen a muscle. Typically we would do the opposite of what we know the muscle does when it contracts. If we wanted to stretch the external rotators, normally we would internally rotate the joint. Because the foreleg is out so far, it creates more pressure on the hip joint. It's important not to over-stress the knee in this position. Since we're using this pose as a segue into drawing the leg behind the head, we will look for the relationship of rotation and flexion at the hip. By approximating a similar leg position, we should be able to access the same tissues that are needed to be open to achieve our pinnacle pose.

As we fold forward, the pelvis once again begins to rotate around the head of the femur. This creates a strong external rotation at the hip joint, which in turn puts pressure on those deep rotators. This is why I consider this good

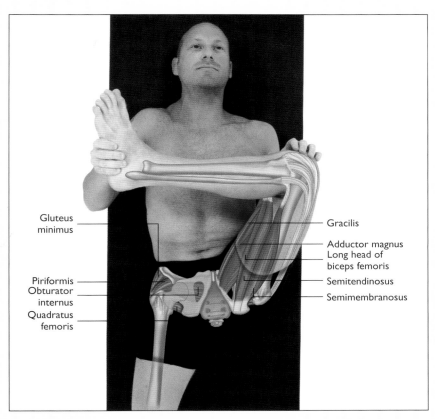

Gluteus
minimus

Gracilis

Adductor magnus
Long head of
biceps femoris

Piriformis
Obturator
internus
Quadratus
femoris

Semitendinosus

Semimembranosus

Figure 10.18: *Restriction at the hip joint isn't limited to the deep gluteal muscles; hamstrings, and adductors can also play a role in preventing lotus.*

preparation for the next posture, *Eka Pada Sirsasana*.

Eka Pada Sirsasana (Leg-Behind-the-Head Pose) and *Dwi Pada Sirsasana* (Double Leg-Behind-the-Head Pose)

Now it's time to move on to our pinnacle pose. All of our efforts in postures that create external rotation may or may not have paid off-yet. Just because you can do the other poses doesn't necessarily mean you will be able to do this one. Although our focus has been on external rotation of the hip, *Eka Pada Sirsasana* requires more than just this. So let's start by considering the chain of joints most directly involved in *Eka Pada Sirsasana*. The first is the leg itself and the relationship of the ankle, knee, and hip joints. The second chain is created between the

hip joint, the SI joint, the lumbar vertebrae, and the thoracic spine. Notice that the hip is in both chains. We naturally focus on the hip joint when attempting a pose like this. That intention is definitely correct. We need the hips to be as open as possible before moving towards this pose.

If the hips are tight, other parts of the body will have to compensate and adapt to that tightness. In this case, when you reach your end of range of motion at the hip, the pelvis will start to tilt back. And because it is connected to the spine, as the pelvis tilts the lumbar vertebrae begin to flex along with the lower thoracic vertebrae. This increases the pressure in the low back. In this situation, tight hips can potentially create injury in the low back.

In order for the femur to move back in the type of deep flexion where the leg actually moves to

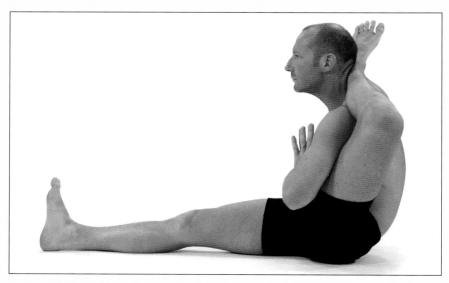

Figure 10.19: *The tighter the hip is in a posture such as this, the more the spine will have to compensate.*

the side and behind the torso, the hamstrings need to be open. Luckily the knee is bent in *Eka Pada Sirsasana*, which automatically reduces the amount of tension in the hamstrings. That said, they are also needed at the next stage of movement, external rotation of the hip. Although rotation of the hip joint is not one of the hamstring's main actions, they can definitely show up when putting the leg behind the head. People with tight hamstrings will often feel a line of pull or a burning sensation down the outside and back of the leg. Others feel a similar sensation along the inner part of that leg, essentially along the lines of the hamstring.

The most ardent restrictor of our ability to rotate the hip joint are the muscles we have been working with all along, the deep rotators. As we lift our leg up and begin to take it back, the hamstrings get involved. But as we add external rotation, we get pressure in the deep external rotators. The deep six lateral rotators, the gluteus minimus, and the gluteus medius are now in a prime position to prevent us from taking the leg back far enough that we can duck the head forward to slip the leg behind it.

A common problem in this pose is that the leg is not taken wide enough (it's not abducted enough). As a result, instead of the lower shin or ankle sitting in the curve of the neck, it will sit on the back of the head.

This small difference is important from the perspective of leverage. There is an inherent tension that is trying to undo that external rotation in this pose. That is, if your leg slipped over the top of your head, it would fling out, un-rotating (internal rotation) before it fell to the floor. Our head and neck resist this natural inclination. When the shin is up against the top of the head, the neck muscles have to work harder than if the ankle was in the curve of the neck. Why? If you think of the top of your head as the end of a lever arm (with the cervical spine as the lever), more pressure will create greater force. If, however, you add pressure closer to the fulcrum (the base of the neck), then less muscular effort is required to resist the leg's natural tendency to unwind.

There is just one more element to consider. This element can help keep the foot down behind the head and neck. It can't all be about flexibility, can it? No, it is definitely not. There are three

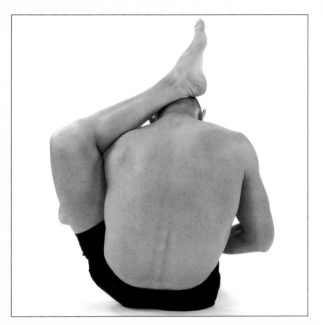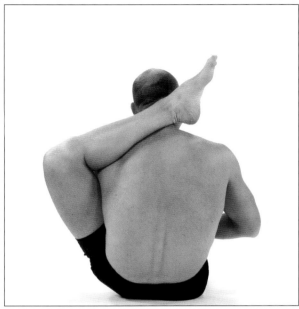

Figure 10.20: *The lower the foot goes behind the head, the more leverage is available from the neck with less effort.*

key places where we need to add tension back into the pose in order to keep it together. We have already mentioned the first one—the back of the neck. It must engage to keep the foot behind the head. Until the rotational forces are reduced, the head and neck have to work harder to keep the leg behind the head. An element of leverage is required, but we also need some strength in the neck. For this reason, it's also a good idea to do preparatory postures that help strengthen these muscles. Otherwise it can be easy to strain the neck while trying to hold the leg behind the head.

Postures that strengthen the back of the neck include those that have you looking forward or up while in a horizontal position. Any of the forward bend variations where you reach the chin towards your straight leg force you to contract the muscles on the back of the neck. Over time, these build up the strength and stamina needed to help keep the leg behind the head later on.

The second place we add tension to the posture is in the hamstrings. Although some of us may

be passively keeping the foot behind the head because we have enough flexibility in the hip joint, the rest of us may need a little help from the leg. If we can engage the hamstrings at about ten or maybe twenty percent of their strength, we will create a downward force that brings the lower leg down the back. For some of us, this additional effort can make the difference between a leg that stays put versus one that flies off the top of our head.

The last place we need to contract is the lower back; we will extend the spine to balance out the amount of pressure we have put in the lower back by flexing it. The key to this is sitting up as much as possible. By engaging the spinal extenders and trying to sit upright, we resist excessive flexion in the lumbar spine, which can potentially compromise the discs and vertebrae.

There is a secondary effect to this. As we sit up from the lumbar spine, we extend it from its already flexed position. As you know by now, the movement of the spine is directly related to the movement of the pelvis and hips. By sitting upright we put more pressure on the hip, as we ask it to externally rotate even further. So the pelvis is forced to move around the head of the femur again, thereby increasing the pressure on the tissues around the hip joint.

Although we are each clearly different, the most variation in anatomy is found around the pelvis and in the hips. Also, proportional issues may show up in a posture like *Eka Pada Sirsasana*. People with long torsos and short femurs may be using their shoulders to keep the foot back behind the head rather than their neck, hamstrings, or low back. Those with long femurs and short torsos may find the foot touches the opposite shoulder. So adapt your posture as needed based on your own anatomy.

ONE SIDE VERSUS TWO SIDES

Just as we have seen in each of the postures building up to this pinnacle, *Eka Pada Sirsasana* has a two-sided version, *Dwi Pada*

Sirsasana. Many of the same dynamics at play in the other poses show up here as well. The adaptations we have seen in the one-sided versions are around the pelvis and hips. And all of these compensations tell us a story, if we are able to observe them. Elements like shortened ribs on one side, the sit bone coming off the floor, and the foreleg placed too high on the back of the head all say something, and they all tie together. The area above the pelvis of the leg we're putting behind the head often gets shortened, either because the ribs move down or the pelvis moves up. In this posture, the pelvis typically moves up. But why?

The pelvis usually lifts after the leg has been drawn back and the foreleg is being brought down behind the head. If we don't take the leg as wide as we can and literally pull it tightly across the side of the body, it will cause the torso to shorten. As we bring the leg down behind the head, it continues to pull the leg across from the hip joint. This will lift the hip even more, exacerbating the patterns. The sit bone comes

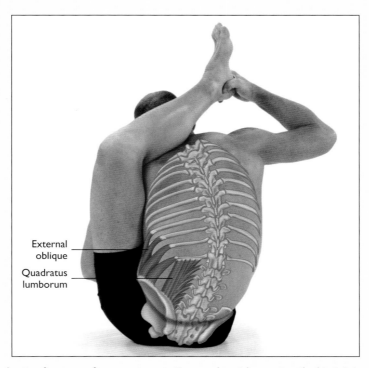

External oblique

Quadratus lumborum

Figure 10.21: *Pulling the leg too far across forces compensations and avoids opening the hip joint.*

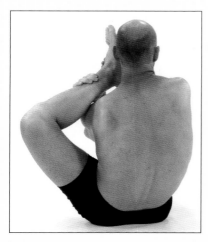 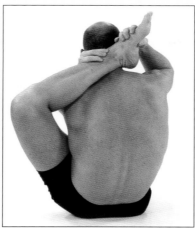 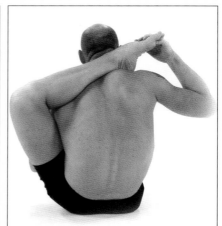

Figure 10.22: *Taking the knee wide helps assure space in the ribs as well as the pressure being placed in the hip joint. It also can help to get the ankle lower on the neck.*

up, the ribs shorten, and the leg will probably sit too high on the back of the head.

If we take advantage of the kinematic chain of joints in the lower leg and move the leg wider as we fold it in, it doesn't need to come across the body as far. (This presumes you do not have proportional issues that require you to keep the thigh tight to the torso.)

When the leg goes back and wide, away from the body first, the pelvis is pressed down into the floor. It is only when the leg is pulled across the body that the pelvis can lift up to create compensations in the pelvis. Remember, this posture is no different than the ones that preceded it. If our left pelvis lifts as we put the left leg behind the head, the real movement happens at the right hip joint.

Two-Sided

Similarly, as we move into the two-sided version of this pose, we see that some of the compensations simply can't happen. For instance, there's no way to lift both sit bones off the floor at the same time. We have to stretch the hips adequately in the one-sided version. When we try to bring the second leg behind the head, it has to go even further than the first

one! The second leg has to go behind the first leg. Not only does it need to be flexible enough for this to happen, but the first leg must be comfortable and there must be enough depth for the leg to stay put. If you have ever tried to do this pose, you know that your hands are busy enough, between keeping you balanced and trying to get that second leg back enough around the first, that they can't be responsible for holding the first leg in place.

If we haven't opened the hips adequately on the way, there will be even more pressure throughout the entire body. It is common for us to tense up when placing that second leg behind the head. This is especially true for those of us who do not have the most flexible hips. Our muscles tighten to help stabilize us, so that we can work on getting the second leg behind the head. It is often at this moment that we feel increased pressure in the lower back. This is a pivotal moment (with the highest potential for injury) if you haven't maximized the depth of external rotation needed to get into the pose.

Common Observations

It is easy to forget how much we use the opposite hip joint to compensate for the one we're really

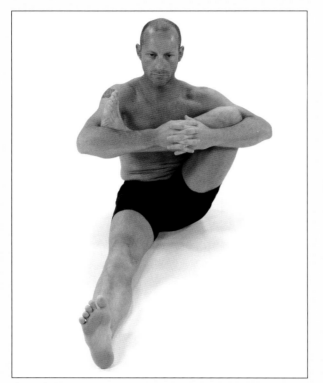 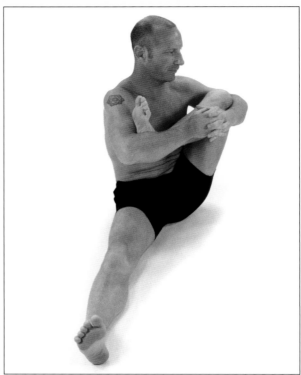

Figure 10.23: *This rocking movement simply moves the pelvis at the right hip joint.*

working with. Sometimes it's a pattern that begins with the common preparatory stretches or warm-ups we do before trying to put our leg behind our head or go into Lotus. Cradle stretch is one of these warm-ups. Maybe the foot sits nicely in the crook of the arm at the elbow, or perhaps we have hugged the leg tightly with both arms. We then begin to twist back and forth in this position in an attempt to "open the hip." The next time you do this, pay close attention to which hip joint you are actually moving. Often when I see students do this as a preparation, they are simply moving the pelvis on the opposite side. This has no bearing at all on the hip they want to work.

To be fair, sitting up and squeezing the leg in does put pressure on the hip we intend to open. But as far as I can tell, swinging the cradled leg from side to side makes hardly any difference at all. Perhaps it satisfies the mind. Instead of rocking the leg back and forth, sit up, focus on getting the pelvis to tilt forward and add pressure to the intended hip joint.

CONCLUSION

We have looked at postures that create and train external rotation at the hip joint, as well as some that actually open these tissues. There is a balance between the two. *Padmasana* and *Eka Pada Sirsasana* ask that the tissues be open already. *Janu Sirsasana* and *Kapotasana*, on the other hand, offer us a way in by putting pressure on the tissues that we need to open, thereby improving the flexibility needed to do more advanced postures. It is also true, however, that sometimes the only thing that will open up the tissues for a particular pose is the pose itself! *Eka Pada Sirsasana* falls into both of these categories.

11
ANATOMICAL PATTERNS IN TWISTS

Twists of all shapes and sizes are extremely beneficial and tie directly back to one of yoga's most basic and central purposes: to maintain suppleness of the spine and general health of the central nervous system. The spine is the epitome of our core. It is our central axis and houses the all-important spinal cord. In one way or another, just about everything we want to accomplish physically requires the spinal cord. This is the "mainline" of our own information highway!

But where do twists really come from? The spine is the obvious answer. But the hips and shoulders play a key role in our ability to work deeper into the spine in twisting postures. This is one reason yoga pays such close attention to these two areas. Many poses force us to open our hips and shoulders so that we can eventually work more deeply into the spine. Tension in one area can have surprising ripple effects.

In twisting postures, tight shoulders and hips can make it difficult to create the posture we want. Let's take *Marichyasana C* and *D* or *Ardha Matsyendrasana* as an example. In these postures, we twist past the bent leg, which requires very flexible hips. In order to wrap our arms into the bind, the shoulders must also be open enough to rotate around the knee and behind the back.

As usual, we'll be working toward a "pinnacle posture" as we explore twists. This seems a

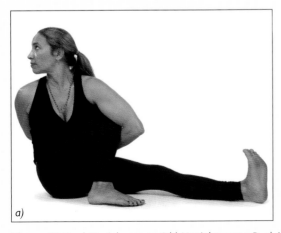
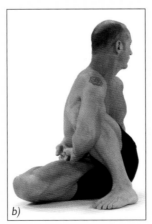
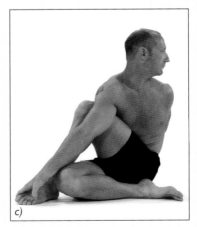

Figure 11.1: *a) Marichyasana C b) Marichyasana D, c) Ardha Matsyendrasana.*

bit tricky because, anatomically, all twists are created the same way in the spine. Since I'm postulating that the hips and the shoulders are common inhibitors in twists, our pinnacle pose requires great range of motion in both of these areas as well. A bound *Marichyasana D* should do the trick. In this posture not only do we have to twist through the spine, but we also need to work through tension in the outer hip of the leg that is bent into Half-Lotus and our shoulders as we rotate the arm around the knee and behind our back. So the question is, what postures prepare us for this? How do the various twists build on one another to enable us to do a pose such as this *Marichyasana D*?

SKELETAL ANATOMY OF A TWIST

In the spine section of this book, we introduced the design of the facet joints. The facet joints are located at the top and bottom of each vertebrae and connect to the vertebrae above and below. The orientation of the facet joints determines the type of movement we find at that part of the spine. You will recall that the orientation of the facet joint in the thoracic spine allows for the greatest amount of spinal rotation.

In addition to the facet joints, the twelve thoracic vertebrae are each associated with a pair of ribs. Anatomically, the ribs are part of the support mechanism of the spine. The ribs and the tissues between them, the intercostals, can restrict our ability to twist. When these tissues are stretched, as they are in a twist, it is much harder for us to breathe. As we inhale, we ask the ribs to separate from one another when the intercostals are already stretched from the twist itself. We're basically asking them to stretch twice as much.

How the Anatomy of the Hips Affects Twisting

The hip joint, the SI joint, and the lumbar spine create a functional chain of joints. This chain is not unlike the kinematic chain of the leg. As a result, the hips influence what happens to both the SI joint and the spine in twisting. We can see this relationship between the hips, the SI joints, and the lumbar spine in both standing and seated twists in our practice. In both standing and seated poses, the hip's movement can allow for more "perceived" twisting through the spine. It can also restrict this perception. When we allow the hips to move along with the twist, the hip joint actually increases the amount of total rotation in the pose. But if we intend to stabilize the pelvis, the twist comes only from the spine. Twists like this can feel limited by comparison. As I've said before, neither is

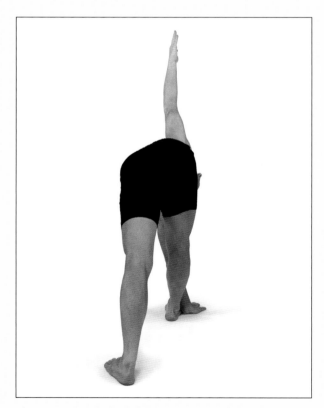

Figure 11.2: *With the pelvis tilting the twist comes from both the spine and the hip joints.*

right or wrong. They simply create different sensations and appearances and put pressure on different tissues.

For instance, in Revolved Triangle, when the hips tilt off of the horizontal plane, the overall twist through the torso can feel deeper. If we prevent this from happening by fixing our hips in the original position, it's harder for the upper body to get as far around; we'll likely feel as though we haven't twisted as far. And this may be the case; however, this variation emphasizes the twist that is happening in the spine itself. This same idea can be applied to all twists, whether standing or seated. If you fix your pelvis as you begin to rotate, then the actual twist will come from the spine alone and not from a combination of the hip joint and spine.

Note that as you stabilize the pelvis, it can actually counter-twist, or move in the opposite direction of the spine. This can create more pressure in the vertebrae and the SI joint, so be careful in all twisting postures if you have SI joint dysfunction or instability. You may have to allow for more hip movement with SI joint dysfunction. That said, one of the benefits of putting more pressure into the vertebrae is that it directly impacts the tissues that restrict our ability to twist.

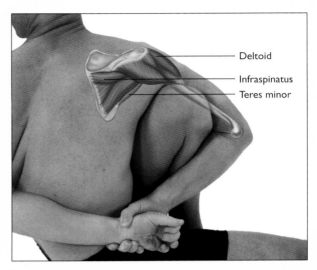

Figure 11.3: *The three muscles that restrict internal rotation of the shoulder joint.*

How the Anatomy of the Shoulder Affects Twisting

Many twists include "binding" the hands or arms. These binds can be as simple as hooking an elbow on the outside of the knee or placing a hand on the floor. No matter how simple, binds create leverage and depth in twists. They also create a foundation of sorts—when you do a twist and feel like you are going to fall backward, binding the hands can help keep you upright and balanced.

In the fullest expression of these twists, most binding has the shoulder internally rotating

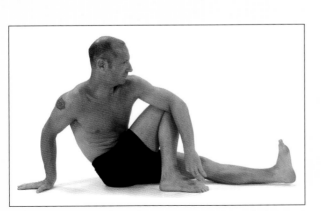
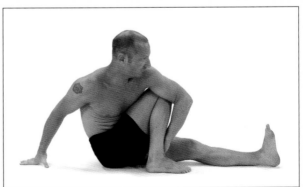

Figure 11.4: *Binding is easier when the torso, and therefore the arm are closer to or past the thigh.*

around the thigh or knee, which allows the arm to reach back for the bind. Therefore, the external rotators of the shoulder joint must be lengthened to allow for this rotation. Only three muscles externally rotate the humerus. Two of these are rotator cuff muscles, the infraspinatus and the teres minor. The third is the posterior portion of the deltoid. These are relatively small muscles, but they have a notable impact on our ability to move the humerus into position for a bind.

Recall that the scapula is mobile. In this type of bind, the scapula must protract and rotate down around the front of the body. As it does, it puts the shoulder joint into a better position to rotate around the knee. If the shoulder doesn't come forward enough, the rotation of the shoulder is restricted by the thigh.

POSTURE EXAMPLES

Revolved Triangle Pose

We first looked at Revolved Triangle in the section on forward bending. Now let's look at this pose in reference to it being a twist. When I think of twisting, I think of the spine; so when I twist, I focus specifically on the spine, trying to squeeze out as much movement as possible. By focusing on the spine and not allowing the hips to provide the illusion of rotation, we will increase the spine's range of motion.

A tilted pelvis in *Parivrtta Trikonasana* is not right or wrong. It simply illustrates that we have used all the twisting possibility in our spine and that we are now relying on the hip joints to deepen the twist via the pelvis. As always, it's your choice whether to allow this to happen in your own practice or with your students.

When the pelvis tilts, it is technically abducting horizontally at one joint and adducting horizontally at the other. The pelvis has already moved into a forward-bending position, so the hip joints are flexed. When the pelvis tilts, it increases the space between the femur and pelvis on the side you are twisting away from and lessens the space on the other side.

I have often asked myself, how much tilting should I allow a student to do? What are the benefits of allowing or not allowing some of the twist to come from the pelvis and hips? If we allow the pelvis to tilt at the hip joints, the student achieves a larger overall twist. That's a good thing. If the person has a cranky SI joint, then allowing the pelvis to tilt may be crucial in avoiding inflammation or aggravation of that joint. Also good.

But there are downsides as well. I tend to think of the practice as a refinement of physical patterns, right? Well, if a tilted pelvis were the pattern that the body goes into naturally, then wouldn't it be meaningful to play with the edges of our ability to control these patterns? Can we stabilize the pelvis and keep the twist in the spine? Can we separate these two actions from one another?

If we do not allow the pelvis to tilt, we are forced to look at our true range of motion (ROM) in the spine. Without stabilizing the pelvis, we never really know what our true spinal ROM is. In addition, because we allow the pelvis to move and become part of the twist, we might unconsciously miss an opportunity to actually bring more movement to the spine. Not allowing the hips to move should increase the ROM of our spine over time.

I hope it is now clear how the spine is fundamental to twisting postures. But the question remains, to what extent should we play with our innate physicality? It is here that change can happen. If you remain at a place where twists are easy, change is less likely to occur.

Revolved Side Angle Pose

There are many lessons to learn from *Parivrtta Parsvakonasana*. In fact, not only do the modifications to this posture build one on each other towards the full posture, but because each stage is so rich, the full expression can be seen as a "pinnacle" in and of itself.

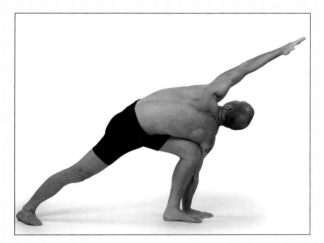

Figure 11.5: *Parivrtta Parsvakonasana.*

We will take several lessons from this pose and apply them to the other twists. In a complete Revolved Side Angle, the back foot is rotated in a position similar to that found in Warrior 2. At the front, the torso is twisted, and the palm is firmly planted on the floor. Binding under the leg is an option and illustrates how there are two possibilities for binding in twists. The first one is similar to *Ardha Matsyendrasana*, while the second is closer to a bound *Marichyasana C* or *D*. (See why no yoga pose should be considered in isolation?)

For the purposes of breaking down the elements of Revolved Side Angle Pose, let's start with the back knee on the mat. I often have new students begin in this way to aid in balancing. As well, it reduces tension through the hip flexors in the back leg, which allows the pelvis to move and adapt to the twist.

Now, let's start on the left side. This means the left leg is in front, the right leg is in back, and the right arm is working its way onto the outside of that left leg. So how do we anchor our torso in the twist? The simplest bind is one seen in many yoga classes. The hands are in a prayer position with the lower elbow on top of or outside of the left thigh/knee. This makes for a nice twist. In fact, it might be all that is available to us when we first start out. But how do we go further if we want to? What has to change?

I remember teaching a class many years ago. When I got to this posture, everyone went into the pose with their hands in prayer position, as I just described. That's when I made a very obvious and, at the same time, seemingly profound statement. It was something like "If you never try to put your hand on the floor, then you will never put your hand on the floor." It begs the question, "How will you go further if you do not try?"

After I said this, about half the class put their hand on the floor. Perhaps not all of them had their palm completely flat, but they tried, they experienced a new depth in the pose, and they felt new sensations. Remember, difficulties in practice are opportunities; nothing will change if we don't play the edge.

Let's get back to the pose. We have the right knee on the floor facing forward and the left knee bent at 90 degrees. The first thing we must do is lean forward and deepen the flexion at our left hip joint. The flexibility of our hips will partly determine how close the abdomen or chest will be to the front thigh. Two anatomical actions are happening at this point. As we fold, we're not moving forward in a straight line. We're actually moving off the midline to bring the arm outside of the leg. This happens in the spine as well as in the hip joints. In anatomical

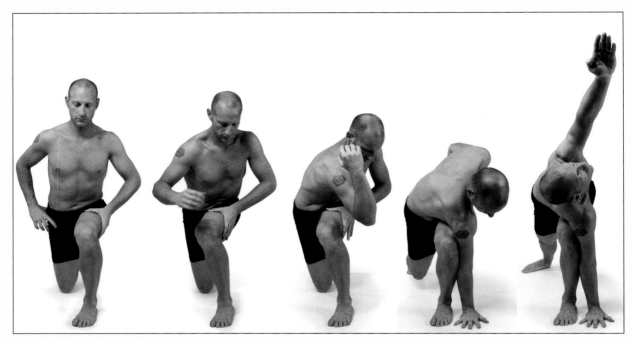

Figure 11.6: *Stages of adducting and flexing the hip to get the hand to the floor.*

terms, this would be adduction of the left hip joint as the pelvis moves, combined with lateral flexion of the spine.

The moment we start reaching the arm to the outside of the leg, we begin to mix in spinal rotation. To successfully combine these three movements, we need openness in some key places. The spine has to be free enough to twist. But for me, the real key to deepening this pose comes from the hip on the same side that we are trying to bind (the left hip in our example). If the outer part of the hip (namely, the gluteals) is not open enough, the leg won't adduct at the hip joint enough to allow a deep twist. To rephrase, if the leg itself isn't adducting enough, it is harder to get the torso (and thus our shoulder and arm) to the outside of the leg. If we can't get the torso across this line, then the only thing we can do is place the elbow on top of or just barely outside of the leg. This is why I encourage students to use their left hand to physically adduct the leg (push it across the midline) while folding forward and working into the twist.

In the beginning, placing the knee on the floor can make a significant difference in our ability to adduct the front leg at the hip joint, first by helping us balance easier, and second because of the effect a straight leg (knee off the floor) can have on the tension around the pelvis. With our left leg in front of us, the quadriceps will work to prevent too much flexion at the knee. In other words, they resist flexion by contracting. A similar thing happens with the gluteals in the same leg—they resist the downward motion of the hips. We could say that they resist flexion by engaging enough to keep the hips from dropping towards the floor.

With our back knee on the floor, these muscles do not tighten the way they do with the knee off the floor. When the back knee comes up, there is more weight to manage, so the muscles must engage more strongly. When the muscles are strongly engaged, it is more difficult to move or lengthen them. As a result, placing the knee on the floor means that the abductors of the front leg, the gluteus minimus and medius, don't need to contract as much. Because they are more relaxed, they will not restrict our ability to adduct to the same degree as they would if they were engaged in holding us up.

Simply put, if we can more easily adduct the leg at the hip joint, it's that much easier to bend forward, adduct the leg, and twist at the same time. For those of us with tight hips, this small change can make a world of difference.

The Shoulder Relationship

Now that we understand a little more about the hip, let's explore the shoulder. Then we can put it all together.

To take the bind around the outside of the leg to the next level, we need to work the armpit as close to the thigh as possible, with the arm on the outside of the leg. This helps to establish the connection between the arm and leg at the root of the arm first. If you think about it, the further away the armpit is from the knee or thigh, the further away that hand will be from the floor.

To shift our focus away from the hand, we just bend the elbow so that it leads the way to the floor. This helps establish the relationship

between the armpit and the thigh. Once the armpit is pressing into the thigh, the elbow can straighten out and we may, just may, find that our anatomy allows us to lower the hand to the floor (or at least closer to the floor than it ever has been).

Tying it Back Together

Now that we have covered the basics in the hips and upper body, let's look at how these two areas work together anatomically. Let's assume that you have "bound" your hand to the floor or you have placed a block on the floor and are "binding" to it.

Whether we recognize it or not, the work in this pose goes beyond just twisting the spine. The hips play a key role. Therefore, we still want to keep our attention on the hip. Opening the hips allows us to work with the spine more easily so that the posture can deepen. For me, deepening the pose means increasing the flexibility of the outer hip, deepening the bind (if necessary) and thereby deepening the twist. The simplest way to deepen the stretch of the hips is to deepen the bend in the front knee, sending it further forward. How *much* further depends on the individual.

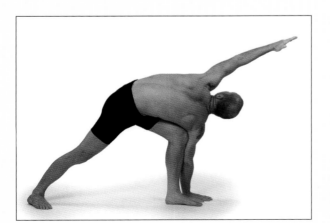 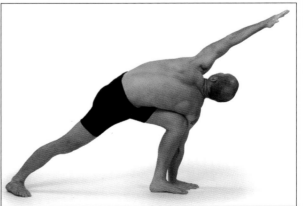

Figure 11.7: *The binding of the arm on the outside of the knee is more precarious the higher the hips are and the straighter the knee is.*

At the hip joint, deepening the bend in the knee increases the amount of pressure on the gluteals, because it causes us to go deeper into flexion at the hip joint, which part of the gluteals restrict. The placement of the arm creates more pressure in the hip by keeping the hip adducted.

Often this "binding" falls apart because the knee goes from an 80-degree angle to a 120-degree angle. This straightens the knee more, which allows the arm to slip around the front of the knee. Thus sending the knee forward a bit and lowering the hips not only deepens the pressure in the hip but also strengthens the bind.

With these pieces in place, the twist is finally set on a firm foundation. Once the hand is on the floor (or on a block) it can create some resistance to draw you into a deeper spinal twist. Pressing the hand into the floor creates movement at the shoulder joint that also deepens the twist. In addition, the leg presses outwards on the shoulder, as the knee naturally wants to abduct. This, too, helps to deepen the spinal twist.

Lifting the Back Knee

Now we have to get the back knee off the floor. Some of you can probably bring the palm to the floor without even putting the back knee down. But if you pay attention as you go into this pose, or watch someone as they do, you might notice something interesting.

Often we bend the back knee as we twist to get the shoulder or armpit to the thigh and then bind. This tells us something. It tells us that we need a little slack in the back hip flexor. Putting slack in those tissues makes it easier to adduct the opposite hip. The more taught the hip flexors are, the more they can potentially restrict movements of the pelvis. Softening the hip flexors allows the front leg to come forward more easily. For some students, just moving the back knee forward a few inches can be of great assistance in trying to bind.

Either way, once the back knee is off the floor, we have some decisions to make. First, do we rotate the back leg to place the heel of the foot on the floor, or do we keep the heel lifted off the floor? The other is whether or not we give up the binding in the front for the sake of putting the back heel on the floor. These choices are intimately tied together anatomically.

When the heel of the back foot is up, it's much easier for the pelvis to stay straight, forward, and low so the bind stays in place more easily.

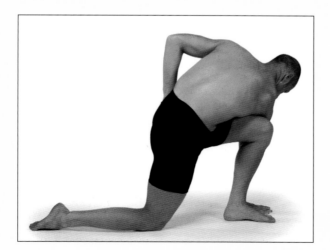
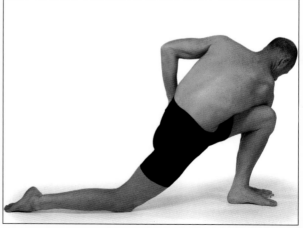

Figure 11.8: *By pulling the back knee in, we slacken the hip flexors and allow a little more ease in binding the arm.*

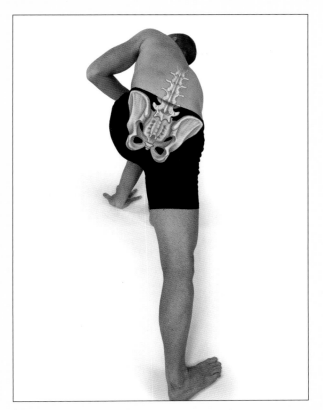

Figure 11.9: *The pelvis is at a strong angle and the back foot has crossed the line created by the front foot.*

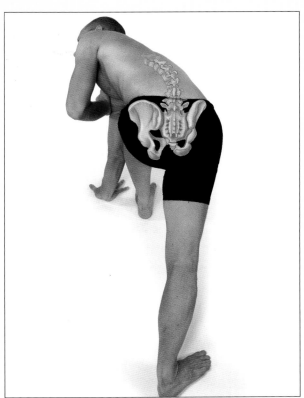

Figure 11.10: *Here the pelvis is more in line and you can see the front foot and that the back heel is just wide of the front foot.*

But as the back foot rotates, the opposite side of the pelvis tends to lift back and up to compensate. Because the pelvis has rotated with the foot and leg, it is no longer facing forward, but is at an angle.

As the side of the pelvis opposite the back foot lifts higher, the front knee starts to straighten. This often causes our bind to slip off or undo itself. This can be avoided. First we want to pay attention to where we placed the back foot from the beginning and where it ends up when we rotate it to bring the heel to the floor. When we lower the heel, if the alignment (relative to the front foot) crosses through the arch of the back foot, we often find that the hips will be more "out of whack," or rotated. If, on the other hand, we rotate the back foot for heel-to-heel alignment, or possibly a little wider for some people, the pelvis typically will not angle out to the same degree.

Seeing how all these components of the postures fit together, we may decide to emphasize different parts. Many students I see do not give enough attention to establishing the depth of the arm across the thigh, or how well they connect their hand to the ground. This is often exemplified by the hips being high or pushed out to the side.

Another common scenario is planting the back foot too soon. If the foot is planted firmly for a student who does not already have the right openings, it works against their depth of the pose. I would even go as far as saying that they often never evolve the depth of this posture.

Simple Twist—*Marichyasana* C

We will look at three anatomical aspects to this twist. They are the pelvis, the binding, and the twist. All three must come together for the posture to happen. The same elements that we discussed in the Revolved Side Angle apply to the Seated Twist.

In this particular seated posture, while both legs are flexed at the hip joint, one is flexed at both the hip and the knee (the leg we are going to bind). This tends to pull the pelvis under in a posterior tilt on the side of the bent knee. This is usually obvious in people with tight hamstrings. With this added tension, the pelvis might also tilt slightly, so that the sit bone on the side of the bent leg lifts off the floor. There's another reason why this can happen. Sometimes the sit bone lifts off the floor because of the relative proportions of the upper and lower leg. If your foreleg is shorter than the femur, your sit bone will either be on the floor or closer to it. If your foreleg is longer than the femur, the opposite will occur. Your sit bone will lift higher off the floor.

Oftentimes tight hamstrings will prevent beginners from just being able to sit upright. The hamstrings pull the sitting bone under, which causes a posterior tilt, and the spine flexes. As a result, their weight moves behind

the center of gravity and they start to fall back. Because gravity draws them back, their foundation is unstable. If they can't sit up, how can they possibly bind?

The importance of taking the pelvis into an anterior tilt for seated postures should not be overlooked. The solution to this pattern is pretty simple: place the hand on the floor behind you. Initially, a beginner does this to keep from falling back, as well as to help sit up straight. But we should know what we're trying to achieve and what the hand on the floor tells us about the anatomy.

First we need to look at the hips and the role they play in this aspect of the pose. There are two choices: either the knee moves across the midline, or the individual moves around the knee. The second is often done quite dramatically with a big lean back (gravity will take us back that way anyhow). This takes the twist as low as possible in the spine, which can be aggravating for students with lower back issues and SI joint problems.

In order to move the knee across the midline, we need length in the outer line of the hip

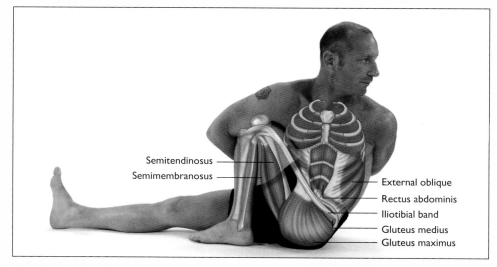

Figure 11.11: *We often find that the pelvis drops into this posterior tilt when the hamstring and hip joint muscles are tight. This forces the abdominals to hold us up.*

and thigh, namely the glutes. If we are flexible enough, this allows the knee to adduct across the midline from the hip joint. Once this happens, further flexion at the hip and spine are needed to take the chest towards the thigh where the arm will reach forward to begin its required rotation.

The rotation of the arm into the bind requires certain actions at the shoulder complex. First, as it reaches forward, the torso flexes. The scapula moves around the front of the torso in protraction, the humerus internally rotates in the shoulder joint itself, and the scapula rotates downward and elevates at the same time. When the scapula moves, so does the clavicle. In this case, the clavicle does its little known rotation along its axis. Finally, the elbow bends or flexes to finish the movement. Keep in mind that all of these actions together have naturally created a twist in the spine simply by moving the leg across the midline and flexing the torso. These actions pull the pelvis in such a way that the spine ends up twisted relative to it.

For these movements to occur as easily as possible, all elements of the twist should be seen as a chain from the bottom up. This includes the hip joint, pelvis, and lumbar and thoracic vertebrae. The hamstrings must have enough length to allow us to sit up and move forward at both the hip and the spine. This vertical posture allows the armpit to get as close to the knee as possible, which in turn puts the rest of the arm in a position to rotate and bind around the knee.

If any muscles that are involved in the twist are tight enough to restrict the internal rotation required, then something else will compensate. Often it will be the scapula, which lifts up in elevation. You see this often when a student is trying to bind and their shoulder ends up scrunched up by his or her ear. This might suggest restriction in the arm or shoulder, but it could just as easily be any of the elements down below. This is what happens when all of the components of an *asana* do not add up.

Finally we come to the twist. To be honest, if you have gotten to this point in the pose, you're already in a twist! What lies ahead is just deepening the rotation through the spine. There are a couple of anatomical pieces to add here.

The spine is designed to twist in the thoracic section. That said, a twist happens relative to the position of the pelvis. In other words, from anatomical position with the pelvis in neutral, the spine rotates in either direction relative to its base, the pelvis. If the pelvis moves with the spine, it is not a spinal twist. It is movement at the hip joints. Normally, in any twisting *asana* we see a combination of movement in the hips and spine.

Let's go back to *Marichyasana* C. With the pelvis in neutral, moving the leg across the midline tends to pull that side of the pelvis forward. If the left leg is bent and the knee moves towards the right, the left side of the pelvis will be pulled forward during a twist to the left. You could say that the pelvis (or lower part of the spine) moves in the opposite direction of the upper torso, which automatically creates or increases the depth of the twist.

If, however, the pelvis moves in the same direction as the twist, it does exactly the opposite. It reduces the twist in the spine, right? If you look at someone who is already in a twist and you see that their pelvis is at an angle (that is, not parallel to the front of the mat), it will almost definitely be turned in the direction of the twist. This pelvic movement is not necessarily wrong, but it does reduce the overall twist in the spine. This may be

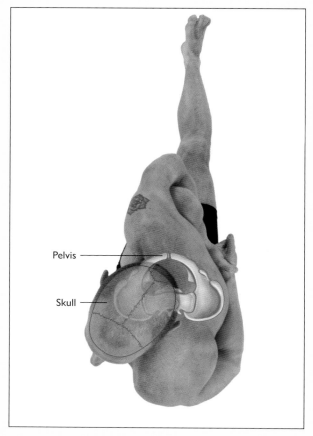

Figure 11.12: *When the pelvis is square to the front, the twist is more purely in the spine.*

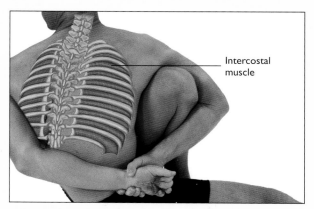

Figure 11.13: *We forget how significant the tension from the ribs and intercostals can be in a twist.*

necessary for some individuals, depending on the condition of their sacroiliac joint or even their spine.

If the pelvis is square, it is in a neutral position and all the restriction comes from the elements more directly related to the spine itself. Potential restrictors of a spinal twist are the abdominal muscles (the obliques, specifically) and the small muscles surrounding the facet joints in the spine. But perhaps the most significant and most obvious restrictors of twists are the ribs and intercostal muscles. Unfortunately, they are frequently overlooked.

The intercostals are three layers of muscles between the ribs. When we twist, we put pressure on the ribs as well as the tissues between them. This is one of the most obvious inhibitors of twists. We can observe the impact

of tension in these tissues by observing the breath. It is harder to breathe in twists because the ribs have a hard time moving relative to one another, making space for the incoming air. What prevents them from moving? The change in the position of the ribs relative to the vertebrae they attach onto and articulate with. The twisting loads the tissues and ribs with tension, making it both harder to twist further and harder to breathe. The flip side is that twisting also stretches the tissues, which increases our ability to deepen the twist and breathe more easily in the pose.

Each of these elements—the pelvis, the arm and shoulder, and the ribs and spine, can limit your ability to bind in a twist. The body is good about working around one restriction, but working around two or three restrictions becomes more difficult. I am hopeful that by deconstructing a posture this way you will more clearly see which parts you can emphasize in your practice. The long-term result will be a more integrated posture, a deeper twist, and perhaps even a binding!

Ardha Matsyendrasana

Let's look at *Ardha Matsyendrasana*. The most advanced version of this pose requires us to wrap the arm around the outer thigh and grasp

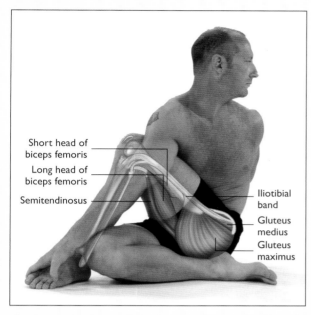

Short head of
biceps femoris

Long head of
biceps femoris

Semitendinosus

Iliotibial
band

Gluteus
medius

Gluteus
maximus

Figure 11.14: *The restrictions are similar as we adduct the hip and get the armpit as close to the thigh and knee as possible.*

the foot on the floor outside the knee. This is a very deep twist.

More than any other, this twist shows the direct relationship between the twist of the spine itself and the hip joint. The set up alone can be challenging. We'll use the left side again for our example. So the right leg is folded in with the heel right in front of the opposite hip. The leg is lying on its side and the hip is externally rotated. Because the right leg is simply folded and rotated, the right side of the pelvis is (quite naturally) on the floor.

The left leg is flexed at both the knee and the hip, with the foot placed on the outside of the left knee. If your hips are tight, then the left side of the pelvis is likely to lift off the floor as you enter this position. In order to bring the left leg across the right and place the foot on the floor near the folded knee, we must adduct the left hip joint as it crosses the midline and our other leg. Just taking the leg across and getting the foot in the right place can be challenging for some of us. The tighter the hip is, the higher

the left side of the pelvis and sit bone will be from the floor as the leg comes across.

Once we have set up the legs, it is time to work towards binding the hand. In order to get the arm to reach the foot, we will take a similar approach to what we did in Revolved Side Angle with the hand bound to the floor.

First things first. We have to be able to sit upright. The inability to do so is primarily due to tight hips; that is, the pelvis cannot move around the head of the femurs. Once we can sit up straight, our next task is to get the armpit as close to the thigh as possible to initiate the binding. As in Revolved Side Angle Pose, a combination of movements must happen here. We must flex and adduct the left hip as well as rotate the spine.

If the gluteals and outer hip muscles on the left side are tight, it will be extremely difficult to bring the armpit to the thigh because the leg's ability to adduct is restricted by the hip. Without sufficient adduction, we will not be able to get the upper arm around enough to reach for the foot. When we can't bind to the foot, we lose the opportunity that a posture like this provides in opening the tissues of the outer leg and between the ribs. In other words, this bind is key to holding the pose and deepening the stretch.

The same technique we applied to Revolved Side Angle and all of its restrictions applies here. Although the twists seem very different, the restrictions are the same: the hip. Rather than repeat the restrictions, let's compare the two *asanas*.

The first thing that is obviously different is that we are seated on the floor in *Ardha Matsyendrasana*. This makes it harder to get leverage to move forward towards the thigh.

In the standing pose, our body weight and gravity help take us towards the thigh. In the case of a seated twist, we have to sit up to move in that direction. This is generally more difficult for those of us with tighter hips, which reinforces the importance of the preparatory work of standing twists with an intense focus on the hips.

When we have gotten far enough forward, we must press the arm back against the thigh in order for the hand to reach its destination on the foot. The reciprocal relationship between the back of the arm and the outside of the leg is at the heart of the bind. We need to push the leg across so that the arm can make a straighter line towards the foot. At the same time, the thigh pushes back on the arm, encouraging and (especially in the beginning) helping to create and deepen the spinal twist.

As we press the arm back and the hand moves towards the foot, we're ready to tackle the bind. Often in the beginning, the elbow can feel stress or strain. This can be another revelation that we have tension in the hip! The tighter the hip, the more pressure it creates between the leg and the arm (as the leg tries to move out of its adducted position). This pressure often manifests as hyperextension of the elbow. The binding creates a force that pushes in both directions. You can rotate the arm to avoid elbow problems at this point, but don't avoid this for too long. Instead, use it to focus your efforts on opening the hips more to reduce the pressure you find at the elbow.

Marichyasana D

Although I chose *Marichyasana D* as our "pinnacle pose," it could easily have been *Ardha Matsyendrasana*. The two postures offer different bindings, which make them difficult in different ways. Both offer a deep twist. The most significant difference between them, other than the binding, is the position of the legs.

In *Marichyasana D*, the leg that we are not trying to bind is in a Half-Lotus position. This adds a new level of restriction. Is the restriction in the actual spine? No. The restriction here brings us back to the hips. Let's say we want the right leg in Half-Lotus and we will bind around the left knee. We're already familiar with several of the components and movements required by this *asana* (*Marichyasana D*): Lotus, hip adduction, and binding our right arm around our knee. However, we have the additional element of moving the torso towards the left knee. To make this happen, the pelvis must move around the head of the femur, creating an even deeper hip flexion. With the right knee folded in Half-Lotus, we also need the hip joint to have plenty of external rotation available. The knee is already in a more vulnerable position here, but now we're adding more rotation. Due to the position of the Half-Lotus leg, these movements can compress the knee by way of the foot being on the inside of the left thigh.

Think about it: as you move forward towards the left knee and flex, adduct, and twist, the opposite hip must also change or adapt. In this case, it will try to adapt to the pressure coming into it from both ends (from the hip end and the foot/ankle end). By sitting up, we are asking the hip to allow for even more rotation. If the hip is tight, tension gets sent down into the knee because the femur rotates at the knee end instead of at the hip joint at the pelvis. And by adducting the left leg, we are pressing the foot into the abdomen and pelvis. This creates even more pressure in the knee. What's the bottom line? *Marichyasana D* creates increased pressure in the Lotus knee. Proceed with awareness.

On top of all that, *Marichyasana D* requires that the shoulder internally rotates as we bind to the hand behind our back. The binding also adds its own tension to an already pressurized posture.

Taking the Bind

As we journey towards the full bind, I would like to offer an intermediary version. I always try to create adaptations or modifications of a pose that lead to the fullest expression of it. So I consider the patterns of the full posture and then take into account why they are not happening. I thereby determine a modification that will get the body headed in the right direction.

Assuming a Half-Lotus position, we can draw the left knee towards the chest. This allows us to explore the sensations in the hip, knee, ankle,

and possibly the spine. As we approach the twist step by step, we can assess the sensations we feel and determine how to proceed. There are a few options for what I would call intermediary bindings. You can hold onto the outer edge of your foot, slip your hand just inside the foot, or simply hug your knee in.

Now let's assume we are ready to try for the bind. The same techniques from *Marichyasana C* apply here. We need to get far enough forward that the armpit is close to or resting on the thigh. If the torso is too far away, the rotation of the shoulder joint is limited and the elbow will not be able to bend in the way that it needs to. There is no way to bind if the elbow isn't past the thigh and knee.

I tell students that the first goal is to get the binding arm as deep as possible. Only after the first arm is bound is it time for the second arm to swing around the back. If you do not get the first arm as deep as possible at first, then there is nothing for the second hand to bind to.

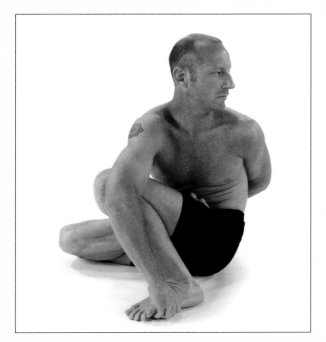 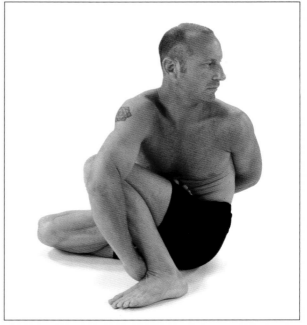

Figure 11.15: *The intermediary binding both adds pressure to the hip and helps us control the amount in the lotus knee.*

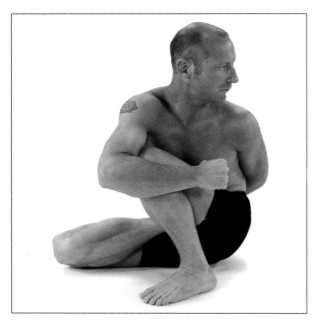

Figure 11.16: *If we're even further away from the binding, this may be enough to keep us upright and heading in the right direction.*

CHALLENGES IN TWISTS

Proportions

Proportions do matter. Perhaps nowhere does it matter more than in postures that require us to bind the way these twists do. The proportion that matters most in this case is femur length relative to torso length. If you have a long torso and short femurs, it will be more difficult to bind because, as you fold forward, your armpit is situated above your knee. How do we bind and make it stay?

There are different options depending on the pose. For a general seated twist, you either have to reduce the length of your torso or lengthen the femur. Lengthening the femur itself is impossible, but temporarily shortening the torso can be done. This is not that difficult, but it does go against your natural inclination to lengthen the spine. Generally speaking, our goal is to lengthen the spine in twists. However, this might be one instance where we can make an exception. To shorten the torso, you will

have to specifically flex the spine—basically hunching over a bit. When you do this, you reduce the distance between the shoulder and the pelvis. Now that the shoulder is lower, the bind might be possible. Although not ideal, it can work.

In the Revolved Side Angle, there's another option. While you will probably have to shorten the torso, you can also use the knee to assist in binding. Although you cannot literally lengthen the femur, by deepening the bend in the front knee, you can increase the pressure between the outside of the leg and the arm, which helps to hold the bind in place.

Binding the Hands

Some people say their arms are not long enough to bind their hands behind their back. This is another case where proportions matter. If you have relatively short arms compared to the rest of your body, you will have a harder time binding. (Grasping a wrist might forever elude you!) This, however, is not the most common problem in binding. More often than not, I find that the correct technique is missing.

A common problem is that people rush into an unsuccessful bind. They don't take advantage of each element of the pose that is needed to create the whole. If you are having trouble binding, look at each of the pieces we have discussed individually to see which is not contributing to the overall success of the twist and the bind. Then you will know where to work.

Another common error is when students sit back and twist too soon. This is often a leftover pattern from a beginner's twist. Starting out, it may be necessary to put your hand behind you on the floor to stay upright. However, in so doing, chances are that you will lean back, which takes the torso away from the thigh that you're trying to bind.

The posture should be attempted using the following sequence: First, move your torso in front of the thigh, so that the armpit is nice and tight against the leg. If you have proportion issues, make yourself smaller here as well. Second, try to bind. Get the first arm in as deeply as possible first. If your arm doesn't internally rotate very well, then focus on other postures that lengthen these tissues or take advantage of any intermediary bindings that are possible. Once you have gotten this arm in as deep as it will go, then—and only then—begin to lengthen and swing that second arm around your back. This is the bind.

The final part of the pose requires opening up in the twist. The order is important. Well, it isn't important to those who are flexible enough to do the twist without thinking about it, but for the rest of us, it matters! Once we are in the pose, the anatomy starts to understand its place in the posture, and it becomes easier.

Trying to Breathe

Breathing is one of the most difficult things to do while in a twist. I'm sure many of you have experienced this in your own practice. This reveals how intimately connected the breath is to our twists; more specifically, it says something about how the ribs connect to the spine, and how the tissues between the ribs are related to movement between the ribs and our ability to breathe.

When we breathe, the ribs lift and separate from one another. This is especially true if the stomach is restricted, as it is in a twist. Even if you are not using *bandhas* in your practice,

everyone's abdomen is more compressed in twisting postures. When the breath cannot move outwards through a soft abdomen, it is naturally directed upwards into the chest.

Keep in mind that while the ribs are trying to lift, they are also under the pressure of the twist. Twisting increases the amount of force on the rib cage. It also increases the amount of tension found in the intercostal muscles between the ribs. Both the ribs and the muscles between them are getting stretched, and stretching increases tension. While under this extra tension from twisting, the ribs are also trying to move away from one another so that the lungs can expand. As the lungs expand they add even more tension to the already stretched tissues. Thus we need to lengthen the tissues between the ribs—the intercostal muscles.

So the question becomes, how do we lengthen these tissues so that we can actually breathe in a bound twist? The answer is in the question. We have to put ourselves in a position where it is difficult to breathe and try to breathe more deeply. What better way to stretch these tissues than from the inside, using our own breath? Postures that stretch the sides of the body, such as Triangle or Side Angle can be helpful, but in this case, breathing in the very pose itself is the best means to stretch the tissues that are causing the restriction.

It seems silly to answer a question with the question itself, but this speaks to the larger truth about our body and our practice. We should put a little more effort into what we cannot do well, as opposed to playing to our strengths. To improve at anything (in this case, a yoga pose), we must do more of that same thing and focus on the elements that assist in making the overall posture work.

Sit Bone Up or Down?

There are some postures where the sit bone is intended to be up (off the floor), and others where it is intended to be down (on the floor). Many postures may begin with the sit bone up and evolve to a place where it is down. First off, we need to distinguish what kind of posture it is. We also need to consider our intention to create length or space through an area of the body. On a personal level, we might ask the question, "Does my body allow me to put my sit bone down, or will it ever allow that?"

Twists are one place where we can argue for or against the sitting bone being grounded. We may need to acknowledge that there is a difference between anatomical possibility and our intention. Trying to get the sit bone to the floor is different from actually putting it there. *Trying* to do it creates intention. Putting it there will lead to actual physical changes in the posture.

Our pinnacle pose provides a great example. For most people, the sitting bone will be lifted in *Marichyasana D*. If they put the sit bone down on the floor, then the knee that is folded into Half-Lotus will often lift up off the floor. Why is the sit bone up? Why is the knee up? The answer to both of these questions comes back to the hips.

There is nothing wrong with intending the sit bone towards the floor. This might create a number of counter intentions, including lengthening the spine and sitting upright. However, when it is actually done and the knee is in the air, we may be putting ourselves in a more vulnerable position. Why? Because the knee is already in a vulnerable position due to being folded and rotated. When the knee floats in the air, we naturally try to draw it back down towards the floor. By pressing it down, we send more pressure into the knee joint. (You can refer to the anatomy section on the knee for a refresher on this.)

There are exceptions. As noted, proportions do matter in twists, not just for binding, but also for having the sit bone down. If you have a particular proportion of foreleg (tibia) relative to the upper leg (femur) and the hips are open enough, then the sit bone can be down without the knee of the Lotus leg lifting up. This however does not make it right or wrong. It is about what you are trying to create for yourself in the moment and how that ties into your long-term progress in this posture. We must decide how to do the pose in a way that adds pressure in the right areas without increasing pressure in undesirable places.

You might ask yourself, "Am I capable of working towards having both the sit bone and the knee down without potentially causing injury?" "Will my proportions even allow that to happen?" "Am I creating vulnerability at the knee joint by forcing this variation of this pose?" Our body has the answers.

CONCLUSION

Although this section is about twisting, it is just as much about the hips and shoulders, as well. As in all *asanas*, we must look at the individual parts that add up to the whole. It's easy to fall into the trap of saying, "I don't have a good twist." The bigger truth is that we probably don't have adequate flexibility in the hips or shoulders for the twist. This might also prevent us from working more deeply and specifically with the spine. All that remains is to practice! We will gradually work our way through the postures in this family as the body opens over time.

12
ANATOMICAL PATTERNS IN ARM BALANCES

Who wouldn't want to be able to lift up lightly into Handstand? That would be a great party trick, right? Not to mention how good it feels! If Handstand is not the perfect representation of the physical grace, strength, balance, and flexibility that we cultivate on the mat, I don't know what is. It's no surprise that so many practitioners aspire to do Handstands. And they're fun! They are also challenging physically and mentally. They require strength and the ability to control your center of gravity. Mentally, they can bring up instinctive fears of falling and of losing control (to a degree). Handstands challenge our perceived limitations.

You can approach Handstand in a number of ways. Naturally I take the anatomical perspective. That said, I also recognize that the mental component is sometimes just as important, or even more important, than the technique applied. Overcoming the fear of falling over is one lesson that can be carried off the yoga mat and directly into your daily life.

It is critical in a posture such as this to create the foundations of physical strength and to slowly change or adapt one's mental patterns around perceived abilities and fears. Doing so will ultimately support the destination we have in mind. The idea is to build the physical and

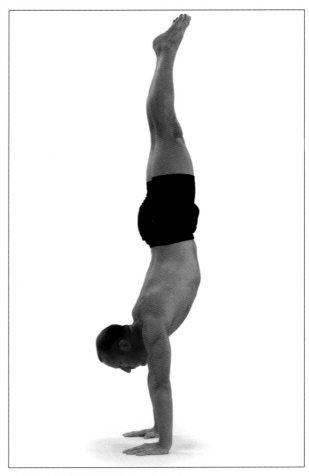

Figure 12.1: *Handstand.*

mental strength while creating the appropriate neuromuscular patterning in the body. And if you don't already practice Handstand, I have some good news. You can create the strength and skills needed to turn upside down, a little bit at a time, using *asanas* you're already familiar with.

Now, understanding and theorizing about all of this is great, but in the end you must be willing to actually *do* the work. You have to be disciplined enough to practice over and over again if you want to see the fruits of your labor. This applies to anything we wish to learn, both in and out of our *asana* practice. It's another life lesson to be gained from our work on the mat.

I learned Handstands from my teacher, John Scott, and I use the same method that he showed me to teach others. Few students are truly patient enough to work on Handstand one step at a time. It requires absolute trust and faith in your teacher and in yourself.

His method was simple enough and is conveniently broken down into small steps. First, he insisted we don't use the wall. Thus my fear of falling over immediately entered the picture. I found myself in the middle of the room on my mat jumping. Luckily, I was not trying to go all the way into a Handstand. I was only trying to get to the point where I would place my hands on the floor, lean into them, then bend my knees and spring to an Up-*Bakasana* position.

John wanted me to be able to enter this position on an inhalation and then hold it for one full exhale and inhale, before coming down on an exhale. It took about two months of daily practice before I could do this with control. For a long time I would inhale up and exhale back down. There was no holding. I needed more time to be able to hold Up-*Bakasana*, and I wasn't even straightening my legs yet. It wasn't until I returned to my teacher approximately three months later that I moved on to the next stage.

When I started working with John again three months later, he taught me to move from that

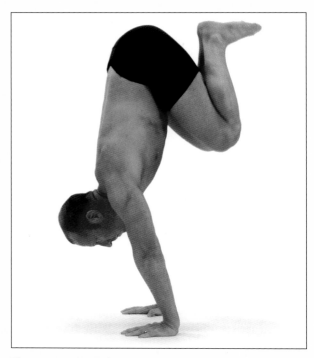

Figure 12.2: *Up-Bakasana.*

Up-*Bakasana* position to a Full Handstand. To do this, I had to inhale as I brought my legs all the way up and straightened them above me. I can't recall exactly how long it took to figure this out, but it was nowhere near the amount of time I needed to accomplish the first stage. Even more importantly, I started to understand the relationship between my work in Handstand and a number of other postures I was either doing or trying to do.

I believe that every one of you, with the right technique and enough time to practice, can do a Handstand. But few students are ready and willing to do the work required. Many of us just are not patient enough. We get caught up with reaching our goal before taking the steps that will get us there successfully. In essence, we want a short cut, a secret trick that will make it happen in the blink of an eye. Good luck with that!

What's that? I can almost hear you … You say you have been working on Handstand for six years and still can't hold it for any length of time in the middle of the room? Really. Let's think about this for a moment. If you have been doing the same thing over and over for the last six years and still haven't reached your goal, it may be time to look at your approach.

Has your mind convinced you that Handstand is not possible for you? Could it be the methodology you are using is holding you back? I'll take a guess: You've been training yourself with the wall, right? Kick up on the wall, any way you can, right? Uh huh. It's not the wall's fault that you aren't advancing in this pose. Let's take a step back (away from the wall) and look at the scenario in terms of creating a neuromuscular pattern. Think about it. What kind of pattern are you creating when you kick your legs up on the wall? What kind of pattern is *not* created when you kick up on the wall?

For the most part, kicking up onto a wall builds a lot of momentum. This pattern of momentum usually doesn't serve people when they head to the middle of the room. Usually it shows itself as a Handstand that ends up in a backbend. What's *not* created is even more important and relevant to the conversation. I typically see two things in students who kick up onto the wall. First, they lack core strength and an ability to control their center of gravity as it goes up above their hands. Second, their shoulders are not quite far enough forward relative to the hands. As a result, the students either backbend too much in order to get their feet to touch the wall, or they fall quickly to their feet once they leave the wall.

Having said all that, I will admit that there is a way to use the wall, successfully build strength in the arms and create a pattern that will support you in the middle of the room. If I am going to use the wall to help someone, I have a particular effect I want to have. In the beginning, the most important component is where the shoulders need to be relative to the hands. Quite naturally, people are afraid of falling forward and therefore never get their shoulders to move far enough forward relative to their wrists.

In order to get comfortable with this and to train the muscles, you have to set yourself up correctly from the beginning. Get your hands close enough to the wall so that if you were to lean forward into your hands, the top of your head would touch it; in other words, you'll be looking forward. As you bring weight into your hands, the top of the head touches the wall. If we were to drop a line down from the edge of your shoulder it would land a few inches in front of your wrist.

The next step is to pull your head back from the wall and at this point, kick your feet up onto the wall. Then look forward and take the top of your head towards the wall. If the set-up is correct, the alignment should allow you to easily take your feet from the wall. That doesn't mean take them away quickly, but if you take them away slowly, you should be able to take advantage of your head on the wall for added stability.

Press your hands firmly into the floor, as you'll soon see this is going to activate a very important muscle related to Handstands. Squeeze your legs together and think about both of your legs acting like one leg. Last, you may have to add extra tension to the abdominal muscles to help stabilize your core.

There are two caveats. First, don't overdo this. Too much can start creating wrist problems. The second thing is to not over strain the back of your neck. Even though you're lifting your head up, do not over tighten it.

In sum, there is a certain freedom that comes from holding yourself upside down on your hands. There is a natural joy to this posture, possibly connected to childhood aspirations—who knows? But it does feel good and can be extremely empowering. And it's accessible to anyone with patience, dedication, and the right approach.

TWO TYPES OF ARM BALANCES

Many more accessible *asanas* contain the building blocks of Handstand. In this chapter we explore arm-balancing postures that will lead you to become comfortable upside down on your hands. Many variations of poses fit into the arm balancing category. For our purposes, we will look at two types. I divide them in this way because each requires a different function at the "core" of the upper body. Just as there is the "core" that we are familiar with related to the spine and the center of gravity around the top of the sacrum, there is also one located near the center of the chest when we start working with arm balancing postures.

The first type of arm balance has the pelvis sitting above an imaginary horizontal line that passes through the shoulder. Handstand is an example of this. In the second type, the pelvis is below this same imaginary line. In *Tittibhasana*, for example, the pelvis is well below the shoulders and the feet are pointed upwards. For the most part, both of these postures are static or in the "state of the *asana*."

Sometimes, though, we are in an arm balance while moving from one posture to another. One common transition is the movement from *Tittibhasana* to either *Bakasana* or a Full Handstand. These between postures or transitions complicate the muscular functions, but fundamentally rely on the same muscles as the static pose.

The muscle that most closely aligns itself with the stability of the core of the upper body is the

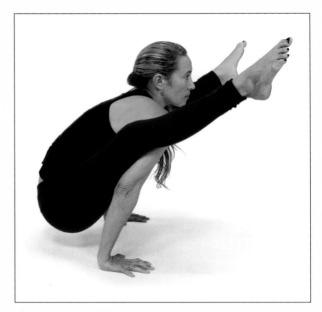

Figure 12.3: *Tittibhasana.*

serratus anterior. To activate it in the postures that we are about to discuss, we must use the hand and its relationship to the floor. The serratus anterior is both a powerful mover and stabilizer of the shoulder blade in arm balances. (Refer back to the psoas of the upper body for more detail.) However, before we dive further into specific muscles and actions used in arm balancing, let's establish our foundation—the hands.

THE FOUNDATION

At the base of any arm balancing postures are the hands (sometimes the forearms). When we're upside down, the hands play the role of the feet as they support all of our body weight. If you thought the surface area of the feet was a ridiculous size relative to the rest of the body, what about the hands? The boney orientations of the hands are different, as well. In the foot, the bones themselves line up in such a way that the weight coming down from the body through the tibia gets dispersed evenly across the feet. About 50 percent of your body weight goes into the heel of the foot and the other fifty percent is distributed forward of the line of the tibia.

This isn't the case in the bony structure of the hand. First, there is no heel sticking back from the line of the bones in the forearm. This means that almost all of our body weight lands under the forearm bones (in the heel of the hand); just a tiny bit is carried by the fingers up front. This also means that most of our weight will be taken by the heel of the hands, secondarily by the palm. Thus the fingertips can help control our balance rather than being consumed by weight-bearing. Because of how weight passes through the arms in inversions, the wrist takes the brunt of the pressure in the hands.

Some postures allow the elbows to bend and move backwards, reducing the angle at the wrist. This minimizes potential compression at the top of the wrist. Other postures ask us to straighten the elbows, which tends to put more stress on the top of the wrist. Without establishing a balance of strength and flexibility, this can be a source of pain and discomfort.

You may recall that the flexors of the hand and wrist are stronger when in a hyperextended position. This is the position of the wrist when doing an arm balancing position. In an arm balance, these flexors resist hyperextension, at the same time helping us to balance in the pose. The fingers, which are controlled by these very muscles, are quite active both when moving into and holding a balanced position on the hands.

In this sense, the fingers act like toes, gripping as weight moves into them or lifting as weight is pulled away from them. Our fingers don't just *feel* the floor. They increase our awareness of how to press into the floor, as well as how to root down through the palm of the hand. This awareness allows us to better build the pose above. (Note the images of B.K.S. Iyengar in *Light on Yoga* that show him using his fingers in arm balancing postures.)

WORKING THE ARMPIT

When the hands press into the floor in an arm balancing pose, they have to be pressing from somewhere. It's an important concept to remember! This shifts our focus of strength and stability from the hands upwards to the shoulder girdle.

It is the combined movements and actions of the scapula, clavicle, and humerus at the shoulder joint that really create the strength and stability needed to work with a variety of arm balances. The "psoas of the upper body," as I've already described, is at the heart of this. Let's review: two muscles comprise the psoas of the upper body—the serratus anterior and the latissimus dorsi. The serratus protracts and upwardly rotates the scapula, helping to bring the scapula and humerus forward and overhead beyond what the muscles of the shoulder joint can do. Once the arm is in this position, the strongest shoulder extender, the latissimus, can then help stabilize the shoulder joint.

When your hands are on the floor in a pose like High Plank, the serratus anterior stabilizes the scapula (separate from the literal shoulder joint). It helps to keep the shoulder blade pinned down to the rib cage by lifting the rib cage between the two scapulae. The serratus anterior is key to establishing the pattern that is needed both to get into (movement) and to stay in (stability) arm balancing postures. These movements often require protracted scapulae.

In addition, in arm balances we need to consider both the stabilization and movement of the shoulder joint itself. The deltoids, pectoralis major, and rotator cuff muscles do this two-pronged work. Finding our way into arm balances and then staying there requires finesse and coordination of several muscles of the upper body.

CREATING THE PATTERN

In addition to considering the muscles that need to contract or release in an arm balance, we should also consider neuromuscular patterns. We can focus on these patterns as we practice to strengthen the muscles we will eventually use in Full Handstand. Where does this work start? Ask yourself what other postures require you to protract and upwardly rotate the shoulder blades. You might have to go back further in your sequencing than you think! Which postures take the arm into this position? Go ahead: put your arms up as though you were doing a Handstand, even if you're sitting down. Now think. What yoga postures put your upper arms and scapulae in this position? How about Down Dog? Backbending? Bend your elbows and you will see a forearm balance and even

a Headstand. All of these postures rely on the serratus to protract, upwardly rotate, and help stabilize the scapula. Ah ha!

The Very First Piece

Let's go way back in our sequencing for a moment. There is a moment in each Sun Salutation that provides an opportunity to train these very muscles. It is directly after the hands go to the floor in the first forward bend. There is a divergence of opinion as to how one should look up from this position. It is common to keep the back as straight as possible and lift up onto the fingertips. This does create a certain type of pattern that can be positive, but it's not the pattern we want to strengthen the upper body for arm balances and Handstands.

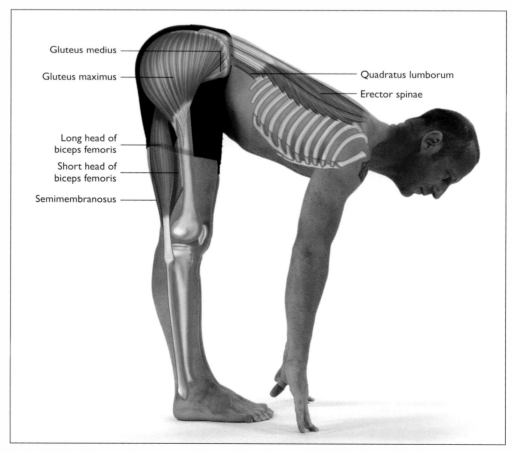

Gluteus medius
Gluteus maximus
Long head of biceps femoris
Short head of biceps femoris
Semimembranosus
Quadratus lumborum
Erector spinae

Figure 12.4: *In order to lift up in this way, your lower back muscles and hamstrings must contract.*

On the positive side, lifting up with a straight spine creates a long, flat back. This reduces the flexion in the lumbar spine, which can be important for students with disc problems. So the question is, what would help a particular individual create a particular pattern at a particular time in their development of a pose? What is this student trying to learn from this movement?

This extended way of looking up requires the back muscles to tighten to partially lift and straighten the spine.

It also requires that the hamstrings contract to rotate the pelvis around the heads of the femurs. Therefore, this pattern may be appropriate for students with disc issues, students who are trying to figure out how to move their pelvis, and students who are learning the nuances of working with their hamstrings. It might also

be appropriate for practitioners who have already established the relationship between their hands, the floor, and the work involved that leads to doing Handstand. But for those working towards arm balancing, there is an alternative. Unfortunately, this is more difficult and requires more effort, in a different way.

In this pattern, the hands go flat on the floor, just as they would for an arm balance. Placing the hands in line with the toes is ideal, but not necessary for someone just beginning. Some students may need to put their hands flat on the floor in front of the line of their toes. (Everyone should plant their hands shoulder distance apart). You may need to bend the knees to reach the floor.

Next, put the appropriate amount of weight into the hands and lean forward. A series of things occur as you lean forward into the

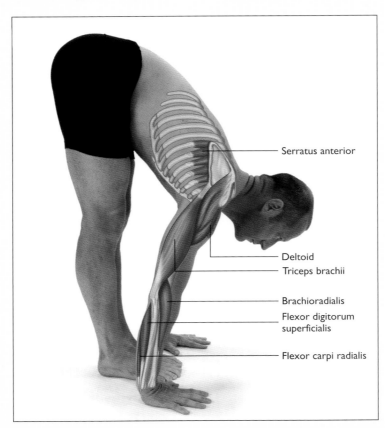

Figure 12.5: *By taking weight in the hands the stabilizing muscles needed for a handstand will activate.*

hands. First, your fingertips will start to feel the floor and will strengthen over time. Second, you will begin to push back into the floor as the weight goes into the hands. When we do this, we start to use the shoulder girdle muscles. The other shoulder muscles that stabilize you in an arm balance are trained to contract in a synchronized way with the rest of the tissues.

At this stage of the pattern, we add another element that is outside of the shoulder girdle: the hamstrings. As we transfer weight from our feet into the hands, the hamstrings don't have the same need to contract for balance. Our hands have taken some of that responsibility. In other words, with this new pattern, the hamstrings can relax somewhat. They no longer need to lengthen and contract at the same time.

With all of this in place, we look up from the hands. This shift in gaze triggers the very muscles we're trying to engage. It subtly teaches us how to bring our weight into the hands and be comfortable with that sensation. It also establishes a particular relationship between the alignment of the shoulders relative to the hands that is recreated in many arm balances. If we set ourselves up in Handstand and look at it from the side, we would normally find that the shoulders are just in front of the wrists. In other words, if we dropped a string down from the front edge of the shoulders, that string would hit the hand somewhere in front of the wrist and behind the fingertips. Although you can see this alignment from the images in the book, you'll find the same pattern in nearly all arm balancing postures in any other yoga book or magazine. Look for yourself!

Why is all of this potential pattern training located here in the Sun Salutation? And why is it located at this very spot within that sequence? Perhaps because our first Handstand is in the next movement of the Sun Salutation; when we jump back (assuming we do) all of our weight

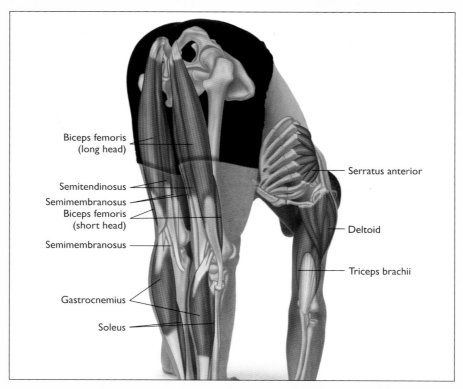

Figure 12.6: *In addition, as weight transfers into your hands, the hamstrings are able to relax more.*

is briefly on the hands. At this stage of the practice, we aren't sustaining any part of this pattern for more than an inhale or exhale, so we can build the strength needed for sustained arm balancing over a period of time—not just within one practice, but over many practices and many, many Sun Salutations. Perhaps this is a simple definition of a Handstand, but it is one nonetheless. The real question is if you treat it like one?

Chaturanga Dandasana

Let's take a look at *Chaturanga*, our landing point for stepping or jumping back. It is also a great place to find and activate the serratus anterior muscle.

If we start out in High Plank before lowering down, the scapulae protract. Well, they *should protract*, which leads us to my point. Spend a moment in High Plank, pressing the hands firmly into the floor to activate the serratus

anterior. Continue this action, and then try not to move the scapulae while you lower down into *Chaturanga Dandasana*. They will move, but see if you can keep the serratus anterior engaged while lowering (isotonic contraction). This will assist in strengthening the serratus anterior, which we discuss at length in the arm-balance section.

Being in *Bakasana*

Now let's consider a static arm balancing position from an anatomical perspective. Then we can discuss how to transition into and beyond a static *Bakasana* to see the muscles in action. We'll build this pose up from the floor. The hands are flat on the mat and the wrists are hyperextended. Whether you do the pose with bent or straight elbows, the shoulders are always out in front of the wrists. With bent elbows, there is less hyperextension in the wrists. This clues us into how important it is for the shoulders to be in front of our point

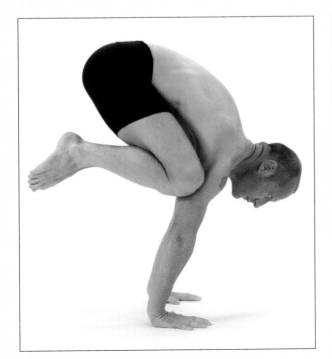 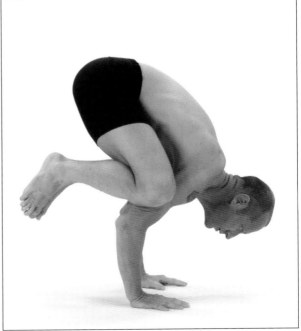

Figure 12.7: *With elbows bent or straight, the torso is at least perpendicular to the arms, the shoulders are forward of the hands, the head is up.*

of balance, the hands, to help balance out the weight on the other side of the hands (the lower extremities). The head also shares the work of counterbalancing our weight. Head position in *Bakasana* and other arm balancing poses is crucial! It needs to be up.

Note: the torso is almost perpendicular to the angle created by the arms. Our center of gravity, the pelvis, is way back behind our foundation, the hands, and gravity is pulling it down towards the floor. Our head and shoulder positions counterbalance this downward pull.

When we position ourselves for *Bakasana* we bend (flex) the knees and hips. The knees end up either on the elbows or higher up on the arms. As we lean forward into the hands, we have to hold the legs up with our hip and knee flexors as well as core strength. By drawing the legs in, we bring the weight of the lower

body closer to our center of gravity and our center of gravity closer to the balance point of the *asana*.

Tight quadriceps muscles can reduce the amount of knee flexion that is possible. Tight hamstrings can reduce the amount of hip flexion (how far up the knees can get above the elbows) available. If the hips are generally tight, it will be harder to get the lower extremity into a ball shape. This could lead to other challenges in doing the pose.

Once in *Bakasana*, the stabilizers must all kick in. We could try to boil it down to one muscle, but that's not realistic.

Remember, everything in the body is connected and functions as such. In this pose, however, the shoulders must be strongly stabilized to maintain the torso at that improbable angle.

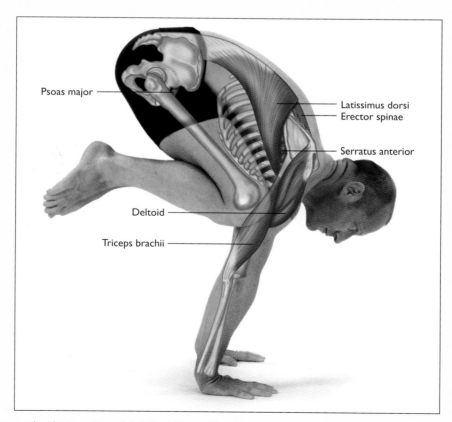

Figure 12.8: *The muscles that create and stabilize this position.*

Helping this stabilization is an unlikely group of muscles in the back—the paraspinal muscles (the erector spinae group). These muscles contract to keep the pelvis from falling down and help to maintain a rigid spine.

The paraspinal muscles only work on the back, though. Their effort must be balanced, which brings us to our core. The psoas and abdominal muscles are also active in controlling our center of gravity in *Bakasana*.

Moving from *Tittibhasana* to *Bakasana*

I realize that most people have a hard time transitioning from *Tittibhasana* to *Bakasana*. But it is worth mentioning here, because it brings us to the heart of the strength and stabilization needed to develop a Handstand.

A transition like this requires two key places of control. The legs have to swing around, but not as much as people think. The leg movement

between *Tittibhasana* and *Bakasana* isn't really that large. Really, we're just bending the knees.

The real work in this transition is getting the pelvis to move from below the line of the shoulders to become even with or above the line of the shoulders. Let's think about this. The pelvis has to move up in space. How can this happen? I mean, the pelvis itself can tilt forward or back. But in order for it to lift upwards, doesn't the torso have to move as well? How do we move the torso to shift the pelvis in such a way? Look at the image of *Tittibhasana* and then moving into *Bakasana*.

In the first, the torso is angled down and back. In the second, the torso is angled up and back. What has changed from one image to the next? The most dramatic change happens at the shoulder girdle. This shift leads to a change in angle between the arm and the torso.

In *Tittibhasana*, the torso is almost parallel to the angle of the arms. In *Bakasana*, it is perpendicular or beyond! Thus the movement required to go

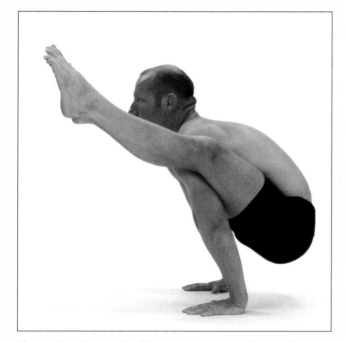
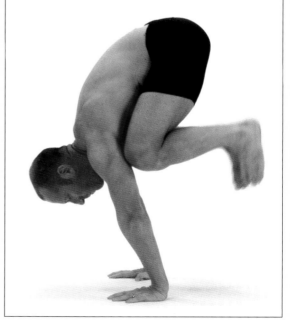

Figure 12.9: *The angle of the torso changes at the shoulder girdle to move from one position to the next.*

from *Tittibhasana* to *Bakasana* is at the shoulder girdle and scapulae. Which movements have we been talking about that could move you from one position to the next? Flexion of the shoulder and upward rotation of the scapula.

Note: This same action allows someone to lift up and jump back. Although this requires some other complex components, essentially a shoulder action moves the torso through the arms and back to *Chaturanga*.

Moving from *Bakasana* Upwards

To continue from *Bakasana* upwards to Handstand is just a more dramatic expression of the same movement. I will add another layer and tie in a concept from the first half of the book. When we think about upward rotation of the scapula and flexion of the shoulder, we think about either the scapula or the humerus moving. When we move from *Bakasana* to Handstand, we have reversed the origin and insertion of a few muscles. This means that the head of the humerus stays in place. It is the scapula that rotates around the humerus if more flexion at the shoulder joint needs to happen. It is then left to the upward rotators of the scapula to move the torso upwards within the scapulae.

Two groups of muscles have to work in this movement: the upward rotators of the scapula and flexors of the humerus. The upward rotators of the scapula (the serratus anterior and trapezius) lift the torso between the scapulae. The strongest flexors of the humerus (the deltoids, pectoralis major, and even the rotator cuff muscles) are crucial in moving and stabilizing the shoulder joint.

The movement from *Bakasana* upwards is not just about the shoulders. Control of our

center of gravity is intimately related to this movement. In this case, the center of gravity (the pelvis) is constantly being pulled back to the ground because of its weight. This means we must overcome gravity to move the pelvis higher than in *Bakasana*.

This is a great place to mention the *bandhas* and their relationship with our center of gravity. Your bandhas can create more than the energetic aspects of support and lightness. They can also add physical strength, technique, and focus.

From an experiential point of view, firmly pressing the hands into the floor initiates this upward pelvic movement. This is how the hands, shoulders, and pelvis become interrelated. The shoulder muscles work to move the torso, and the paraspinal muscles work to prevent too much flexion of the spine, actually beginning to extend the spine. As the spine extends, the pelvis begins an anterior tilt. The hip flexors, which generally create this anterior tilt, are also activated at this point because they squeeze the upper legs into the torso in *Bakasana*.

As the pelvis moves higher, all of these elements work together and it reaches a point of balance. At this point, there is a counterbalance created with the shoulders, head and hand position relative to the pelvis.

JUMP BACK, JUMP THROUGH

As mentioned earlier, the jump back in the Sun Salutations is another place to practice and experience this lifting work. We could argue whether or not it should come before Handstands. I would rather just point out the relationship between the Handstand and the jump back and let you worry about when it is appropriate to work on for yourself or for a student.

Vinyasa Yoga practitioners are often concerned with lifting up and jumping back. I remember when I was focused on it. While it certainly helps with the flow of practice, it doesn't make you a better person, much less a worse person if you can't!

A common complaint is that, "My arms are too short!" To be fair, proportions can make a difference in how you perform certain *asanas* or what those postures will ultimately look like. However, in terms of being able to lift up, short arms won't stop you. That said, they will make it difficult to pull the legs through if you also have a long torso. (Just think: challenges are opportunities.)

How do you know if you have short arms? Sit on the floor with your legs out in front of you. Reach your hands towards the floor on either side. If they are an inch or two off the floor, it's true. You have short arms relative to your torso. However, this doesn't mean you can't lift up off the floor, nor does it mean you will never be able to jump your legs back and through the arms.

First of all, most people find that their hands barely reach the floor in this position. If they do touch the ground, there is hardly any bend in the elbows. And it is the bend in the

elbows that we want to see because as the arm straightens, our bottom lifts. When I sit on the floor in this position my hands do reach the floor, but only with a slight bend in the elbows. I can barely lift up off the floor with my hands in this position.

Let me point out a very simple and obvious element. In order to lift up with the legs still in front of us, we need some bend in the elbows. How do we do that? Simple, we bring the shoulders closer to the floor. This allows us to bend the elbows. How do we get the shoulders closer to the floor? We fold at the waist far enough to either touch or get close to touching the toes.

Once you have done this, move the hands along the floor somewhere between the hips and your knees (about mid-point between the two). You should now have a decent bend in the elbows. This bend is the minimum you need to be able to lift your bottom off of the floor assuming everything else works. (By "everything else," I mean stabilizing the legs to the pelvis and having the necessary strength in the shoulders.)

By leaning forward, we put the torso in a position where the chest is almost facing the floor. In addition, the shoulders are most

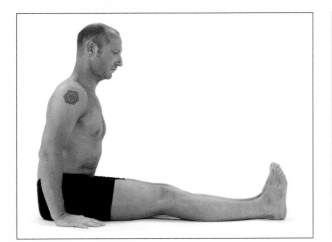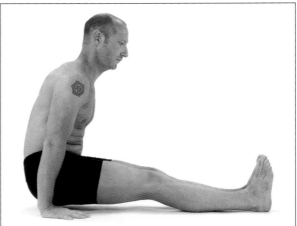

Figure 12.10: *With my hands this far back, I have a hard time lifting very far off the floor.*

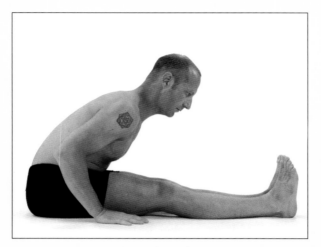
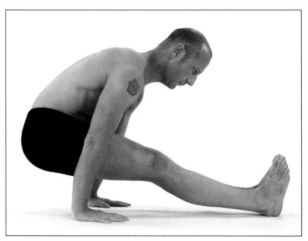

Figure 12.11: *In the first image you see that my shoulders are now closer to the floor and there is more bend in the elbow. I am now able to lift up off the floor.*

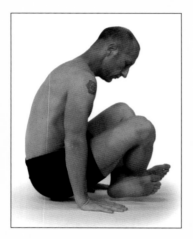
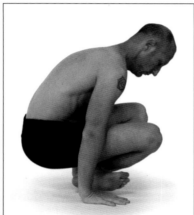
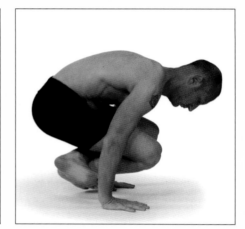

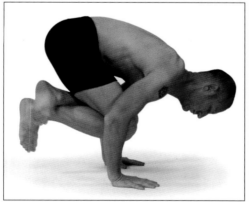
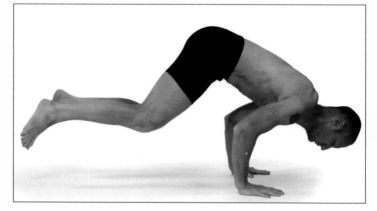

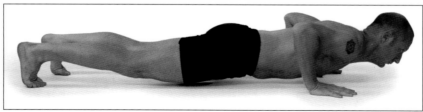

Figure 12.12: *The movements and positions of the shoulders, head, and torso are all similar to what we've been talking about.*

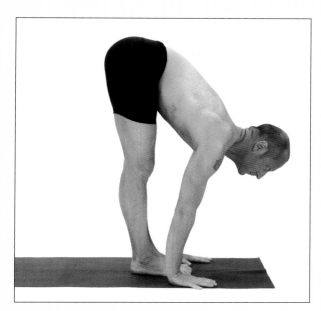

Figure 12.13: *The shoulders are in the same position here as they are in Bakasana and Titthibasana.*

likely in front of the hands and the scapulae are pointing in a direction where, if they protracted, it would help lift the torso up.

Note: All of these elements are related to our arm-balancing pattern.

To turn this from a lift-up to a jump back, there are other things to consider. First, we cross the legs. The smaller and tighter you can make your legs and torso the better. After doing this, you have to place your hands in front of your hips, just like we did with the legs straight. Then, you lean forward to take the weight into the hands and set the shoulders up in front of the hands. This is not dissimilar from the hand-to-shoulder relationship of the "look up" in the Sun Salutation.

After lifting up in this position, the next step is to swing the torso back through the arms. The actual movement to get the torso (and thus the legs) behind the arms requires movement at the shoulders. Swinging back through the arms is a combination of upward rotation of the scapulae and flexion of the shoulder joints.

This is much like the movement we explored when we moved from *Tittibhasana* to *Bakasana* and then into Handstand.

At a certain point, the hips get high enough and you can throw or release your legs back until you land in a *Chaturanga Dandasana*. See, it's simple! Actually, it took me a long time to be able to do this the first time. Perhaps a shift in perspective of what actually creates the movement will help you move to the next stage.

From the beginning, as you lean forward and push your hands into the floor, your core muscles will have to engage. When these muscles contract, they help to stimulate (or are stimulated by) the energetic quality of the *bandhas*. (Refer back to the chapter on these topics for more detail.) *Bandhas* and core are an important part of lifting up and jumping back.

TAKING IT UPSIDE DOWN

There are two additional postures that I would like to connect to our Handstand. *Pincha Mayurasana* (Forearm Balance) and *Sirsasana* (Headstand) utilize a similar shoulder action or pattern that we have seen in all these arm balances. It is helpful to think of Headstand as a Forearm Balance with your head lightly touching. The term *Headstand* can lead us to think, even if only subconsciously, of putting a lot of weight on our head.

Pincha Mayurasana and *Sirsasana* use the strength of the serratus anterior and the other arm muscles we have been talking about. They both require the scapula to be upwardly rotated and protracted—two key functions of the serratus anterior. All of this is going on while the arms are flexed, which recruits the deltoids and other muscles.

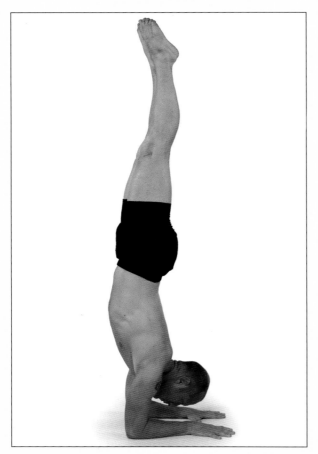

Figure 12.14: *Pincha Mayurasana.*

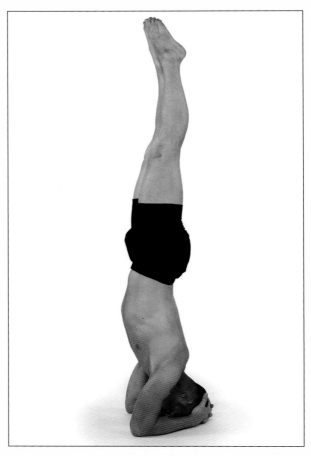

Figure 12.15: *Sirsasana.*

As with the other inversions, without the foundation of strength and patterning in these muscles, these postures are going to be difficult. I have seen many students who have struggled with Headstand and Forearm Balance for long periods of time. They are also postures that bring up the fear of falling over and potential injury to the head and neck.

In both of these postures, pressing the elbows firmly into the floor activates the right muscles. We can often see this lacking in students as scapulae that are too close to the ears, or occasionally even sticking up off the back. The next time you do either of these two poses, notice the scapular movement created by pressing the elbows more firmly into your mat.

The Pelvis

In order to balance in *Pincha Mayurasana*, *Sirsasana*, or Handstand, the pelvis must align with our foundation. In all of these postures, a pelvic tilting pattern helps to create this alignment.

When we get upside down as in Handstand, Headstand, or Forearm Balance we have to tilt the pelvis when it arrives over its foundation. Technically we're looking for an anterior tilt (this can be hard to imagine when upside down). This tilt creates a small curve in the lower back. Too much curve can lead to a collapse of the posture.

Remember, the center of gravity is located somewhere near the top of the sacrum.

Therefore, movements of the pelvis and its position say a lot about whether we are balanced over our hands or forearms in postures like these. If the pelvis doesn't tilt in the appropriate way, we won't get all the way up, or we'll constantly feel as though we're being dragged back down to the floor by gravity.

If we take the spinal curve too far, we could go crashing down in precisely the direction we're always trying to avoid: over on our backs. Of course, there are other reasons we could be falling over, including a faulty foundation or leaning back rather than tilting our pelvis. (This is what I most commonly see in Headstands.)

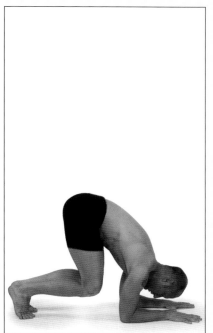 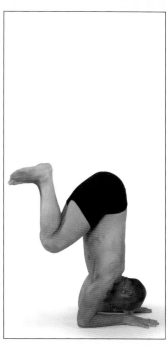 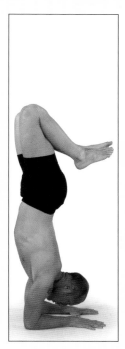 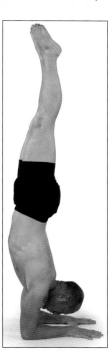

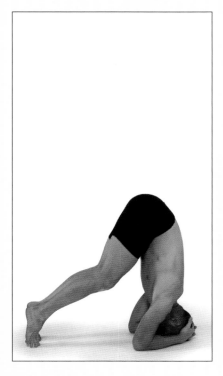 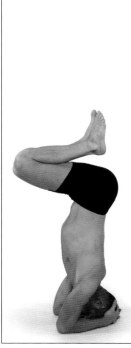 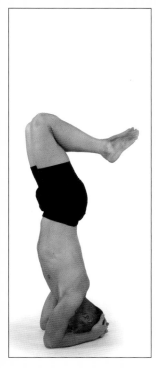 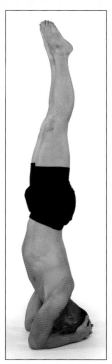

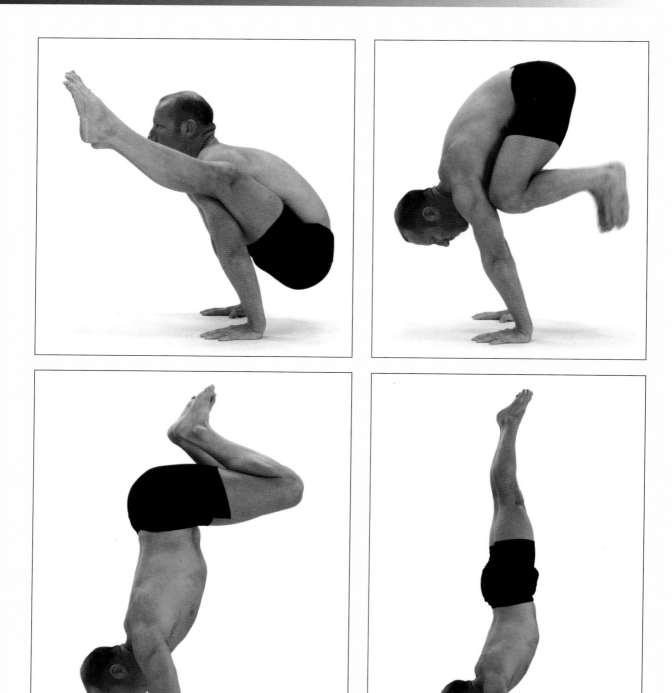

Figure 12.16: *Look at the similarity of shoulders, head, and finally pelvic movement.*

This anterior pelvic tilt is also used to get from a *Bakasana* to an Up-*Bakasana* position or even beyond to a Handstand position. There is an interesting anatomical lesson here as we see how muscles can switch their normal origin and insertion. In this case, the paraspinal muscles, which normally maintain the spine in an upright or erect position, relative to a stable pelvis (i.e., standing), have been flipped upside down. They now act to pull the pelvis into a little backbend when upside down.

There are many moving parts when doing different *asanas*. In these three last postures things easily become confused by virtue of simply being upside down. Hence the need to establish good patterns for the foundation first. The important part for us right now is to see the relationship between these postures. This awareness is the first (big) step towards further developing your arm balancing *asanas*.

The first part is the foundation, whether it is the hands on the floor in a *Bakasana* or the forearms on the floor in *Sirsasana* and *Pincha Mayurasana*. The action created is pressing into the floor to activate the serratus anterior and other shoulder muscles. The second part is stabilizing the core through the abdominals as well as the paraspinal muscles. These work to get us to the third part, which involves not only tilting the pelvis but aligning it over the foundation of the hands or forearms. The actions in all of these postures are similar.

WORKING WITH LIMITATIONS

The most common limitation in a basic arm-balancing posture is strength. While some poses do require a certain amount of flexibility in addition to strength (for instance *Tittibhasana* requires that the hamstrings and adductors be open enough for the legs to be

behind the arms), mostly these poses are about upper body strength.

Difficulties are opportunities. If I think back to what I couldn't do when I started and what I can do now, it is much easier to see what can change. I am not just talking about physical changes, either, but the regular questioning of what you believe is possible. Going from not being able to touch your toes to being able to touch your toes is a great feeling. But that's just the tip of the iceberg.

If you have been working on Handstand for a long time with no success, don't just keep trying in the same manner. Do not think that it is not possible. I am sure you have experienced enough change over time for you to know that everything can and will change, as long as it has direction. Work with building strength over a long period of time and look for the theme or pattern that you may be lacking in your practice. You may find these same shoulder muscles show up in a few other postures that may surprise you. As you make these discoveries, it will all add to a mental intention that will lead you to doing Handstand.

Caveats

Perhaps you have had some realizations and made some new connections that leave you excited to get started. If this is the case, please keep in mind that you have to create a process that will work for you. In other words, don't try to make all the changes you think you need in one day. Instead, add in pieces and concepts over time, or at least over a few months.

If you don't take this long-term perspective, you might overwork all of the elements we have been talking about. In particular, working with arm balances can create a lot of strain on the wrists. Work slowly over time with the larger muscles of the shoulders and armpits to create the correct pattern. Let the forearm muscles around the wrists strengthen as the shoulders and serratus anterior muscles get more comfortable with their new role.

ESTABLISHING HANDSTAND PATTERNS

When I meet someone who wants to do Handstands, or who has been trying to do Handstands, I look at their entire practice. I observe how they have established their hand foundation throughout the practice, whether they press their hands into the mat as well as other patterns we have been discussing, such as looking up from *Uttanasana*, how they lower into *Chaturanga*, what their *Bakasana* and Headstand look like, or more basic observations like focusing on pressing into the hands and engaging the serratus. How the student "looks up" and jumps back in Sun Salutations reveals a lot. This same quality or relationship between the hands and the floor shows up in many standing postures, as well. Whenever the hand goes to the floor, I look to see that it is actually pressing into the floor. It doesn't have to root down with maximum strength, just enough that it's obvious to me, the observer.

If that is not in place, I start there. Making the connection between that basic pattern and Handstand is a powerful motivator. Once my student understands the relationship, they do the work.

Setting up the Shoulders

Getting the shoulders into the right place relative to the hands can be a challenging thing to teach. If a student has not been doing this as they "look up," then it is likely to be stressful to their shoulders. (When I use the word *stress* I mean more work or effort than the shoulders are accustomed to.)

The shoulders need to be almost in line with the fingertips to get the movement started in the next step. Sometimes just bringing the shoulders out this far will evoke a student's fear of falling on their face, or they might realize they don't have enough strength to support themselves. This is a good teaching moment: as a teacher you can connect this position with other places in the practice, such as looking up from *Uttanasana* and *Bakasana*. There is no way around it. Your shoulders must be strong to do Handstand.

The Beginnings of Handstand

Once the shoulders are in the right spot relative to the hands, we begin the hop to the Up-*Bakasana* position. Oftentimes when students begin to jump up, they bring their shoulders back either to the line of their wrists or further. This brings the weight of their body behind the line of gravity, so they don't go up at all. Lining the shoulders up directly over the wrists is not a bad thing, but it is something that you work towards, not start at.

Another common pattern I see is students who have their feet so far behind their hands (almost as far as a Down Dog) that they have to jump forward more than they have to jump up. This creates a forward momentum that must be stopped by something. If there's no wall (which is quite possibly where this pattern was learned), the shoulders not only have to support the body weight, they also have to work like a braking mechanism to stop the forward momentum. Although this is possible, it's really quite an advanced skill.

We want to create a pattern where the body goes up more than it goes forward. When the student places their hands on the floor, I set their feet up only a foot or so behind their hands. Then I have them lean forward into their hands until I see their shoulders come to the desired position (just in front of the line of the wrist). When that's in place, the knees can bend to bring the bottom down towards the floor and they can hop up rather than forward.

At first, I ask students not to hold the Up-*Bakasana* position for any length of time. I like them to inhale up and exhale down. By doing this, I start with a small and achievable piece of the pattern. I add in verbal cues to press firmly into the floor, and/or keep the shoulders forward. I usually stand close to and on one side of the student, with my hand approximately where their sacrum should end up. If I see them going too far, I push the sacrum back in the direction they came from.

Remember, I did nearly two months of daily practice before I could hold the Up-*Bakasana* position. Be patient with yourself and with your students.

Using the Wall

If you want to use the wall, you can do so appropriately. Use it in a way that begins to create the patterns we're after, while avoiding the patterns we don't want to encourage. After all, being upside down is still fun, and it helps build strength in the arms and shoulders.

The key is to set yourself up on the wall so that your shoulders are far enough forward.

If the shoulders are in line with the wrists, it's unlikely that you will be able to hold Handstand with your feet off the wall. (This may be a worthwhile goal long term, but I've never seen anyone who can do this from the beginning.)

As you set up your Handstand on the wall, I suggest you use your head; literally. I set a student up so that when they are up on the wall, if they were to move forward with their shoulders and look up, the top of their head would be touching the wall. Then the wall prevents them from being too far forward in their shoulders and at the same time prevents collapse.

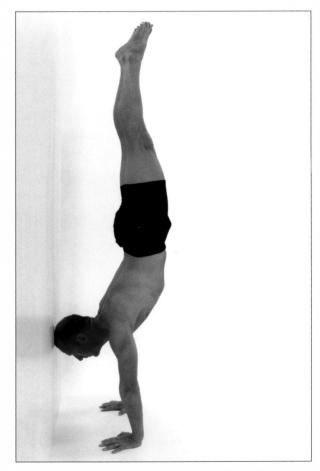

Figure 12.17: *Using your head against the wall and then bringing your feet off of it will help you get used to the shoulders being in the right place.*

Initially, I allow students to just throw their legs up on the wall for a basic understanding of how to set up their shoulders and head. Then after a few sessions, I use the same hop into Up-*Bakasana* to have them focus a little more on their core. Once the student is up on the wall with their shoulders forward and their head touching, it is time to slowly bring the feet off the wall.

This is where the most amount of gain happens. All of the tissues in the shoulders are in the "right" place for developing the strength they need to be in Handstand. Because the legs are off the wall, we must use our core muscles to correct and stabilize the torso and pelvis to maintain a well-balanced line through gravity and our foundation.

13
ANATOMICAL PATTERNS
IN BACKBENDS

Backbends have been a long and slow process for me. I wasn't born with a super bendy spine, and I always feel there is more work to do in these postures. The work of *asana* is never done! But my own struggles in this category of poses have provided an opportunity to use my body as a laboratory to figure out the anatomical pieces that interrelate. Once I figure them out, I can work with different elements to impact and change my own body.

This process forced me to look at how my Upward Dog related to my backbends and how tension around various joints was preventing me from being in a comfortable place while backbending. Was that pinching feeling in my lower back really necessary in Full Wheel? As it turns out, it wasn't necessary and I really appreciated the journey that brought me to that realization.

For conversation's sake, let's say that a Full Wheel or *Urdhva Dhanurasana* is the pinnacle of backbending. There are deeper, more dramatic backbends, such as *Kapotasana*, where one is on their knees in a backbend and holding onto their feet or heels. You can even drop back into a backbend as part of this

family. That being said, *Urdhva Dhanurasana* is universal enough for our conversation.

It is easy to classify certain postures as backbending poses based simply on the position of the spine. I take it a step further to create two basic groups. In the first we are in a prone or face down position. From here we lift into a backbend. These postures include *Salabhasana*, *Bhujangasana*, *Urdhva Mukha Svanasana*, and *Dhanurasana*. In the second we are face up in a supine position. In these postures the limbs often support the backbend in some way. They include *Ustrasana*, *Kapotasana*, *Setu Bandhasana*, and *Urdhva Dhanurasana*. I make this division because each type requires different muscular actions, and they feel quite different as well. For instance, the prone type does not typically take us beyond our unassisted range of motion. The supine type uses the leverage of the limbs to deepen the backbend. One exception is Upward Facing Dog, which is a prone backbend that is supported by the hands and feet. The more important element to all of the backbending postures, regardless of how we classify them, is that they all rely on the interrelationship between multiple joints. Seeing this bigger picture is pivotal to creating the right patterns of strength and flexibility in the necessary tissues.

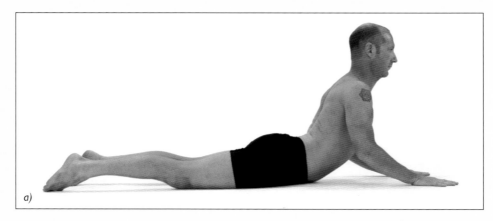

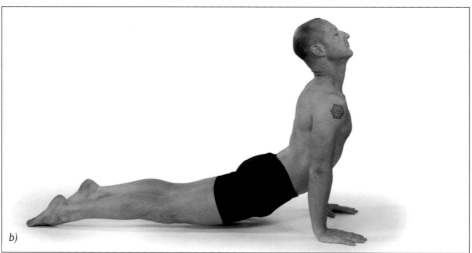

Figure 13.1: *a) Bhujangasana, b) Urdhva Mukha Svanasana.*

TAKING IN THE WHOLE

In keeping with this idea of making connections between postures and anatomical function, the backbending family gives us a lot to work with. As always, we need to remember our theme of integration. Backbends not only teach us to integrate movement between all sections of the spine, but also to integrate the surrounding limbs into the movement of the posture as much as possible. Doing so helps us avoid over-using our most flexible parts (if we have them) and take advantage of the backbend as a whole.

Students, and sometimes even teachers, can overlook the fact that backbends involve more than just the spine. People tend to think that we need to increase the bend in the spine for backbending postures. I'd like to talk about the tissues that allow or restrict the totality of a backbend. Therefore, as I make my way through the various postures on the journey to wheel, not all will necessarily be backbending postures. In other words, because we are exploring the role of the arms and the legs in a backbend, some of the postures in this chapter will be focused on that component of our pinnacle posture, *Urdhva Dhanurasana.*

ON THE WAY TO BACKBEND

Before getting too engrossed in the more traditional supported backbend, let's look at the prone postures for a moment. These postures reveal our unassisted range of motion.

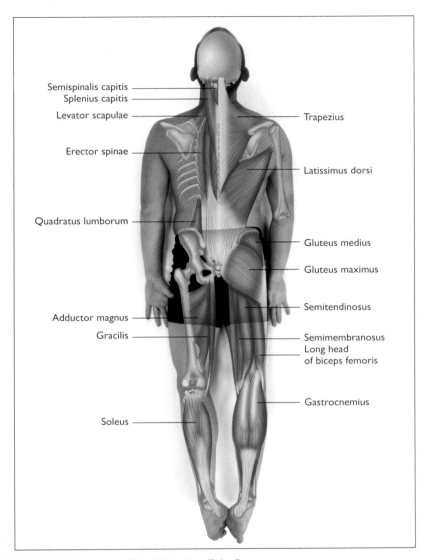

Semispinalis capitis

Splenius capitis

Levator scapulae

Trapezius

Erector spinae

Latissimus dorsi

Quadratus lumborum

Gluteus medius

Gluteus maximus

Semitendinosus

Adductor magnus

Gracilis

Semimembranosus
Long head
of biceps femoris

Gastrocnemius

Soleus

Figure 13.2: *The entire back body assists in lifting the body off the floor.*

When we do postures such as *Salabhasana* and *Bhujangasana* (Cobra Pose), we use muscular effort against muscular tension.

As we begin to lift ourselves up in *Salabhasana*, for instance, all of the muscles on our posterior body contract—the calf muscles, hamstrings, gluteals, and paraspinals, all the way up into the back of the neck. What are they working against? They are working against the resistance of the anterior side of the body and gravity. The shins, quadriceps, hip flexors, and abdominals all provide tension that the posterior part of the body must work through.

Here we see the strength of the posterior tissues working against the resistance of gravity and the anterior tissues. When we add assistance to our posterior tissues we are using an assisted range of motion. *Dhanurasana* and Up Dog offer us this help, taking the unassisted range of motion further while still using the strength of the posterior muscles. The muscles do not shut off when we add assistance.

Dhanurasana

When we move into *Dhanurasana*, we move beyond our unassisted range of motion.

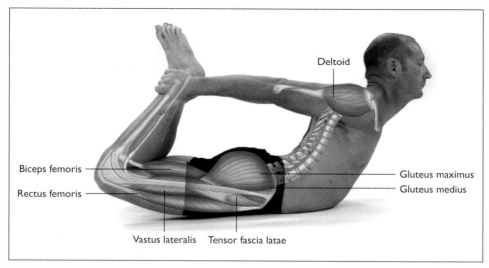

Figure 13.3: *The quadriceps engaging against resistance assists us in lifting higher.*

Our hands reach back to grab onto the feet or ankles-and then something interesting happens. We create tension between the hands pulling and the feet pushing that initiates the lifting action in the pose. The relationship between the hands and feet brings the posture to a deeper place. Without this relationship, we would be limited to the same height as our *Salabhasana*. The co-contraction of the buttocks and paraspinal muscles combined with the tension created by holding onto the feet allows us to lift higher and keeps us lifted up!

Pulling the feet against the hands lifts our chest higher and usually rocks us back towards the pubic bone. The dynamic between the push and pull and how this manifests movement in the body is intriguing. Creating tension in the lower leg, or rather, by straightening the lower legs against the resistance of the hands, allows us to move in the opposite direction at the hip joints. This creates extension at the hips, allowing for a deeper backbend.

Up Dog

This is often the first backbend we arrive at in our practice. Many classes begin with some

variation of Sun Salutations, often including Upward Facing Dog sandwiched between *Chaturanga Dandasana* and *Adho Mukha Svanasana* (Down Dog). In fact, when these two postures are sequenced up against Upward Dog, they also relate to our backbend.

Remember, the path to *Urdhva Dhanurasana* is comprised of other backbending postures. These other postures begin the neuromuscular training in our bodies. Since Up Dog is often done early in one's practice, it is likely where the patterns of backbending take root.

It's not uncommon in the development of our practice to focus exclusively on bending the spine in Upward Dog. While this is the essence of the pose, it is not where the real teaching of it lies. Upward Dog teaches us where the energy of the backbend comes from. It also teaches how to create the dynamic of a full-body backbend. This reveals patterns that lead us to a deeper and more comfortable *Urdhva Dhanurasana*.

Let's take a step back before going any further into Up Dog. We often arrive at this pose via *Chaturanga Dandasana*, thus here we establish the placement of our hands and feet,

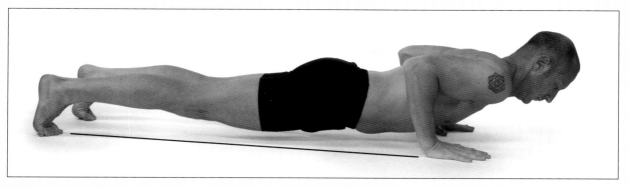

Figure 13.4: *The distance between your toes and hand in Chaturanga is crucial for understanding our Up Dog.*

the points of leverage required to deepen this backbend.

Chaturanga

The distance between the hands and feet in *Chaturanga* directly impacts our transition into Up Dog. Visualize a line connecting the heel of your hands together across the mat. Then draw a line connecting the big toes in the same way. The distance between these two lines, between the hands and feet, is extremely important in determining what our Up Dog looks (and feels) like. In essence, the backbend of Upward Dog must fit between

the foundation that we give it in *Chaturanga*. This is where the compensations in Up Dog can begin.

Creating the Foundation

The foundation set in *Chaturanga* literally rolls over into Upward Dog. It is critical that you observe the way in which you or your students make this transition, especially when shoulder or back pain is involved. We know that *Chaturanga* always gets blamed for shoulder pain, but remember, no pose lives in a vacuum; it is connected to the postures that surround it.

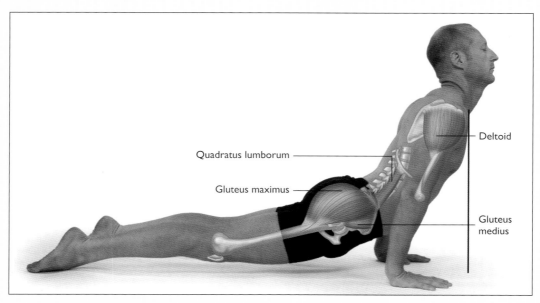

Figure 13.5: *The shortened distance from Chaturanga now causes us stress and strain in the shoulder, wrist, and lower back.*

If the distance between the hands and feet is too short in *Chaturanga*, the same will probably be true of Up Dog, causing our shoulders to be too far forward of the hands. If you dropped a plumb line from the front edge of the shoulder, it would pass somewhere in front of the fingertips to the floor. It's ok if the shoulders are slightly beyond the wrists here, as it is when doing a Handstand or its related postures. But if the shoulders jut out too far, there can definitely be painful consequences.

Rolling Over the Toes

There are at least four factors that lead to the shoulders being too far forward: 1) the foundation of *Chaturanga*, that is, the distance between the hands and the feet; 2) alignment of the hands, elbows, and shoulders; 3) rolling over the toes; and 4) flexibility of the spine. Let's review some of what we have already discussed regarding *Chaturanga*. Remember that we

talked about the position of the hands, wrists, and elbows. When the elbows are over the wrists, the wrists bend at a stronger angle and the mass of the upper body juts out over the foundation of the hands. With the hands under the elbows, they are also closer to the feet.

When students shift from *Chaturanga* to Up Dog, it is common to push forward when rolling over the toes. This causes the feet to move even closer to the hands. If you have a flexible spine, this might be fine. If, however, your spine doesn't bend very well, then let the compensations begin! One of the most common compensations happens at the feet. You may be familiar with this already.

The Foot Compensation

If your spine is less flexible, after you have rolled over the toes into Up Dog, your feet may pull

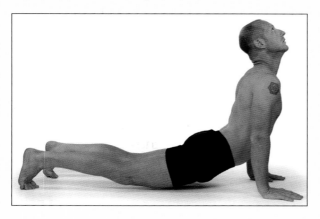
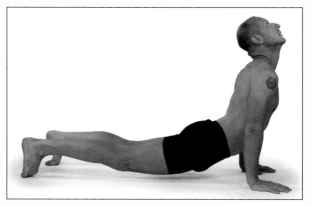
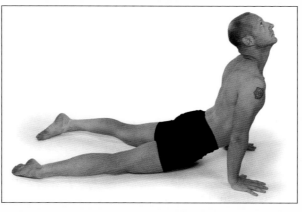

Figure 13.6: *These three variations are all saying that the distance between the hands and the feet is not correct.*

back. This can manifest in a variety of ways. Your feet may be set up on the tops of the toes, as in *Chaturanga*. Your weight may rest on the "knuckles" of the toes with the heels pointed up. There's even a chance that your feet will pivot out with your heels pointing outwards.

Although these can seem like minor technicalities, they tell a story. They are an indication that the body is compensating for inadequate distance between the hands and feet. Each of these three actions brings the torso and shoulders back in space. Sometimes they shift us far enough back to avoid strain and sometimes not. Surprisingly, the strain of this shortened foundation can go unnoticed. I have corrected this one detail many times to the relief of my students' shoulders and backs.

Whether or not discomfort is felt, when the shoulders are out in front of the fingertips, strain is caused. The shoulders bear the brunt of the strain because the weight and force of the upper body is too far out over its foundation. I am willing to bet that this has caused as much trouble to people's shoulders as *Chaturanga* itself.

When the shoulders are forward of the hands, the wrists are under a lot of pressure (see Figure 13.5). The further out the shoulders go, the more hyperextended the wrists. The more hyperextend the wrists, the more pressure that is felt at this joint. You can imagine where this goes. Long-term compression of the wrist can easily lead to pain.

At this point, any adjustments to how far or close the feet are from the hands affects more than the shoulders and wrists. Imagine seeing someone from the side while they are in Up Dog. If someone picked up their feet and moved them either forward or back (while their hands remain fixed), you'd see a shift in the position of the shoulders and wrists. However, that movement would also impact their back.

How the Back Reacts

When the shoulders are too far forward, the back muscles tighten. This contraction maintains integrity in the spine and prevents collapse of the whole structure. The shoulders can only handle so much weight. Even though this is a backbending pose, your back muscles naturally shorten and contract. If this happens because of an overly short foundation, it will make the spine more rigid, rather than more flexible.

In addition to tightening the back muscles, we also run the risk of over-tightening the gluteals. The gluteals actually have no choice in the matter, because this shortened Up Dog has morphed into something between a Locust Pose (*Salabhasana*) and an Up Dog. (In *Salabhasana*, the spinal muscles have to engage because you do not have the leverage of the hands/arms and feet/legs.)

All these factors spin off into a series of compensations. They reveal themselves in different ways, depending on the individual and their patterns of movement, strength, and flexibility. Compensations can include tight buttocks, squeezed shoulders, a scrunched neck, and a pinched lower back. It can take some serious sleuthing to find our way back to the root cause of the issues—the placement of the feet!

COMMON PATTERNS IN UP DOG

To Squeeze or Not To Squeeze

There is a great debate in Upward Facing Dog. Should you squeeze or not squeeze your buttocks? Before I tell you where I land in this debate, let's discuss both sides.

Why Squeeze?

My guess is that most people squeeze their buttocks in Up Dog unconsciously. The body's neuromuscular system dictates the movement and contraction of the muscles in such a way to bring about the end result—a backbend. When you squeeze the buttocks (the gluteus maximus in particular), you extend the hip joint, which helps to create the backbend. The gluteus maximus is a powerful hip extender. Of course, you could argue that if it is a backbend you are looking for, then you should use the muscles that deepen it. Why avoid using them? It's a good argument.

Some people feel compression in the lower back or at the sacroiliac joint when they squeeze their buttocks. This is truly on a case-by-case basis, and I can't say what type of person will or will not run into trouble. In addition, others actually relieve pain or compression in different areas by squeezing their buttocks. Confusing, right?

It helps clear things up if we look at the action of squeezing the buttocks relative to the pattern that it creates. This pattern tends to fully show itself in the more evolved backbend, *Urdhva Dhanurasana* or Wheel. Here the neuromuscular patterns we used in Up Dog are clear. To get up into Full Wheel, it makes perfect sense to use the gluteus maximus. However, there is a consequence of this. In addition to being a powerful hip extender, the gluteus maximus also externally rotates the hip. In Wheel Pose, the external rotation created by this strong muscle pulls the knees apart.

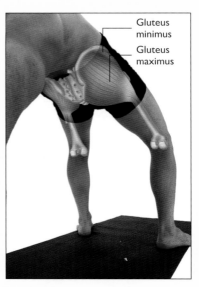

Figure 13.7: *The gluteus maximus although helpful in creating hip extension, may also cause too much external rotation and send the knees wide.*

The question then becomes whether we can access the extension that gluteus maximus creates without using the rotational strength of this muscle. The answer is, yes, we can, but this involves advanced levels of control. This may be why folks argue against clenching the butt in Up Dog. Another reason to avoid clenching the buttocks is the potential compression of the SI joint and the lower back.

Why Not Squeeze?

Then there are those who would have us relax the buttocks in Upward Facing Dog. By default, this is often the harder of the two actions. It is difficult to cease squeezing. It takes more effort. The effort, however, is in letting go rather than in doing. This is a fantastic neuromuscular lesson, as it breaks the normal, unconscious patterns in the body.

When we stop contracting the bottom in Up Dog, the posture must come from somewhere else. Other hip extensors have to pick up the lost work of the large gluteus maximus.

Relaxing the buttocks also creates a reliance on the hands and feet, as both are the driving force in creating the backbend. The resulting posture can feel passive and may not feel "right" for some people.

Releasing the gluteus maximus in Up Dog can also undo the pattern that arises in Full Wheel when we flip ourselves upside down. In theory, if we have trained ourselves to relax the buttocks in Up Dog, it should be much easier to do the same in Full Wheel if we want to. If we pull this off, it could solve the problem of the knees falling out to the sides.

I don't see the harm in some contraction of the buttocks in Up Dog. If it causes pain in a student's SI joint or lower back, then you need to work with them on an individual basis. Bottom line: use the buttocks enough to assist in the extension of the hip joint, but not so much that it replaces the hands and feet as the foundation of the pose.

Overdoing the gluteals in Up Dog could spill over into other non-backbending postures. A common connection I make with students is with poses that require openness in the hips to rotate externally. For some this might be as simple as Lotus. For others it might be connected to putting a leg behind their head. Every time these students contract their buttocks in Up Dog, they reinforce a neuromuscular pattern that is not serving them in these other postures. Tight gluteals restrict our ability to externally rotate the hip joint.

Over-Doing the Lower Back

The lower back is the primary place that we backbend. There, I said it. I am not in denial. As we already know from the anatomy sections of this book, the lumbar spine is designed for forward and backward bending. We shouldn't deny this function or try not to bend from here. We're designed this way. We have no choice. That said, the ease with which we bend in the lower back can lead to an ignorance of weakness or an overemphasis of strength, which can in turn lead to further imbalances causing problems or pain.

Our goal is to have the spine integrated in its movement and bending. We do not want to see the lower back bend without the upper back bending. When this happens, the lower back can become a place of added stress and tension.

If we aren't moving mindfully, the body will simply do what it can to achieve the intention of the pose—to hyperextend the spine. If your spine is not naturally flexible, common compensations in the buttocks, spine, and shoulders are likely to arise.

Lack of Bend in the Upper Back

A lack of upper back bend may simply be due to anatomy. It is naturally the part of the spine that bends the least in a backbend. In my mind, this makes it a place to focus on more. As hard as it might be, adding intention and pressure into the upper back in a backbend can relieve some pressure from the lower back. It also causes all parts of the spine to be included in the action of the pose.

How do we make the upper back bend? This is not so easy and requires intention and focus. It is helpful to slow it down for a while. Give yourself time to become aware of what you are already doing and to create new patterns. As the upper back takes more pressure, we can take advantage of those 12 vertebrae and their corresponding joints. With time, pressure, and intention, your upper back will change.

Let me ask you a question. Where do we first connect our hands to the floor and translate pressure into the upper back? Tic tock, tic tock. That's right! In the "look up" movement we spoke about and its related patterns. Some of this will depend on what stage of development you are at when you work on the "look up" in your Sun Salutations. I remember when I was forced by my teacher to maintain my hands flat on the floor and do the look up. I didn't move, except for my head a little bit. But that was just the beginning of the process; it revealed where I wasn't moving in my spine. Hold this thought. I'll take it a step further at the end of this section.

Neck Scrunching

Another common pattern in Up Dog is people throwing the head back as far as possible. I relate this to tightening the buttocks before going into Up Dog. They likely go together. Again, this reveals a certain lack of integration between the parts of the spine. Yes, the head and neck are more or less all the way back in the full expression of the pose. The question is how you get there and why.

Throwing the head back is another unconscious way of giving us the feeling that our back is bending more than it really may be, even if it is just the cervical spine that's doing most of the bending. The body is unconsciously focused on the ultimate destination of the pose.

How far back the head actually goes is often debated. There is a fear that taking the head too far back can injure vertebrae or cause a grinding of the joints in the cervical spine. I don't buy that. Clearly, there are exceptions with certain conditions or even age groups, but most people should have absolutely no problem taking their head straight back. Can it compress the back of the neck? Of course. So we have to come back to the "how" we do it part. If you lengthen the neck it is unlikely to be a problem. In fact, I can make a good argument for actually taking your neck back more often. You are sitting there reading this book. Without moving, notice the position of your neck. It's probably in this position a lot. Replace the book with a laptop, iPhone, or other device. Having the neck in this position (as many people do for several hours a day) can lead to shortness in the tissues in the front of the neck, just as sitting can lead to shortness of the hip flexors.

Up Dog is an opportunity to undo this. Can you overdo it? Yes. Should some people not do it? Yes,

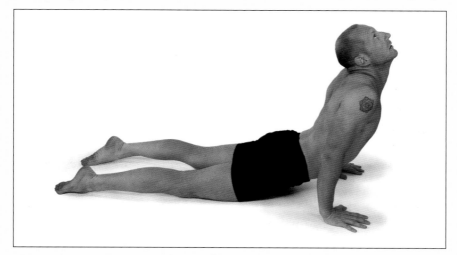

Figure 13.8: *Scrunching the neck and throwing the head back give the feeling that the backbend is deeper than it really is.*

but they're probably the exception. At the same time, do not encourage people to tighten the back of their neck; just help them create length in their neck before taking it back and ultimately creating length in the front of the neck.

Squeezing the Shoulders

Another common pattern in Upward Facing Dog is over-squeezing the shoulder blades. I realize this is sometimes taught as a technique for opening into the pose, but I disagree with this. I do not want to make a big deal out of it being right or wrong. I am sure people find benefit or they wouldn't be doing it. If it is appropriate for the practitioner at their stage of development and exploration, I can't argue with that. I just don't teach it this way and I'll give you my reasons. My opinion is that squeezing the shoulder blades teaches certain patterns in the realm of backbending that I don't want to see later on. It's associated with three things that I find disadvantageous; neck scrunching, over-rotation of the humerus externally, and difficulty inhaling in Up Dog.

The Squeeze and the Neck

In order to squeeze the scapulae together, we use two muscles, the rhomboids and the trapezius. The rhomboids are a relatively thin muscle that has no direct connection to the neck. It retracts and assists in elevating the scapula. The trapezius directly connects to the neck via the base of the occiput (the bottom of the skull). The trapezius' other actions are elevation and upward rotation of the scapula.

When the rhomboids and trapezius contract strongly, it is easy for their other functions to get mixed into the movement. In other words, strongly squeezing the scapulae towards each

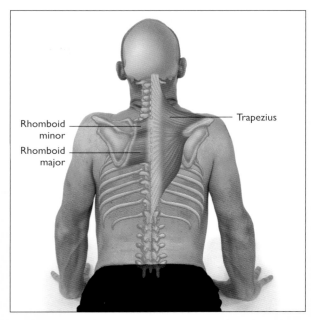

Figure 13.9: *Squeezing the shoulder blades can potentially, overdo the neck, unground the hands, and restrict breathing.*

other in retraction can take the neck back. I'm not suggesting that this squeeze by itself will create this action, but it is a secondary action of the trapezius.

Elevation (shoulders towards the ears), which is created by both the rhomboid and the trapezius muscles, is also undesirable in Up Dog. Will squeezing the shoulder blades together necessarily mean that someone will squeeze their shoulders into their ears? No. But for a beginner, or for someone who has not had this broken down for them, these actions are likely to be mixed together, whereas it may be easy for an advanced practitioner to isolate these actions.

Over-Rotating the Humerus

Over-rotation of the humerus externally is another undesirable action. In this case, because the scapula is retracting, the humerus moves back in space, and due to the angle at which the humerus fits into the scapula, it naturally rotates externally when we squeeze the scapulae together. Unless this is consciously

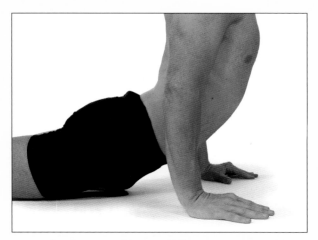

Figure 13.10: *Squeezing the shoulder blades and rotating the humerus can potentially unground the hands.*

controlled, with a pattern in place, it can lead to un-grounding of the hands. The rotation naturally makes us want to lift the thumb side of the hand off the floor.

Breath and Scapulae

The final piece is the breath. As an Ashtanga Vinyasa practitioner, I place a huge amount of importance on the ability to inhale. I also know that Up Dog is a common place for people to give the breath short shrift. The breath is more restricted in any hyperextension of the spine because of the pressure placed on the rib cage. Squeezing the shoulder blades together adds more pressure and tension into the ribs. You can feel this easily enough. Just take a deep breath with your scapulae in neutral, and then squeeze them together and take another deep breath. I realize all of these effects are not the intention of squeezing the shoulder blades, but they do happen.

Tying the Habits Together

The most moveable parts in Upward Facing Dog are typically the lower back, the scapulae, and the head and neck. When all of these move

together, the feeling of doing a deep backbend is obtained. Students with relatively inflexible lower backs will be even more inclined to take advantage of the relatively moveable scapulae and neck. That said, all things can change with time and I've seen this happen time and again with Up Dog.

It is possible to do all of these movements and bend the entire spine deeply. Most people don't do this. Beginners especially have difficulty creating all of these movements. So which part should you teach first? How can we organize someone in their Up Dog so that they are working the parts that need to work and not taking advantage of their most moveable ones?

How to Do Upward Facing Dog

The idea of putting that title above these words concerns me. Although my way of doing Up Dog is right for me and for the students I attract and work with, I cannot be certain that this method is right or will work for you. But since we just heavily ripped apart Up Dog, it makes sense that we put it back together.

All of the descriptions below are really just suggestions. As I stated way back in the introduction of this book, it is not my intention to teach you how to practice or how to teach. My goal is to get you to think about what you are doing and why. Ultimately you have to teach or practice from your own experiences. Hopefully these suggestions will have a positive influence.

Upward Facing Dog is entirely reliant on its foundation—the hands and feet. This is why I spent so much time talking about *Chaturanga* and the transition into Up Dog. To figure out the right distance between the hands and feet, I offer students a few options.

Dealing with the Hand-to-Foot Distance

If you find your shoulders out too far from your hands and wrists in Up Dog and think your feet may be too close, you have some options. Before that, however, I recommend working with just Up Dog. I have my students place their feet in the correct position relative to their hands. If the shoulders are too far forward, which is often the case, I have them move their feet back until I see the front edge of their shoulder just in front of the crease of the wrist.

By feeling this correct position, they learn kinesthetically what their destination is. When we add the transition from *Chaturanga* back in, there are a few options. One option is to reorient *Chaturanga* so that the feet are further away from the hands. When we do this, my students' feet end up closer to the right place for their shoulders after they roll over their toes.

Another option (this is what I do) is to slide the toes back slightly before moving forward and over the toes. I go back before going forward. This is a little more complicated and has some other potential risks. It can cause the skin on the big toe to get ripped up, for instance. It is a way to create the right distance though!

Finally, you can simply flip each foot individually so that the tops of the feet are on the floor. This is the method I commonly teach beginners. This brings the feet further away from the hands than they would be if the student rolled over their toes. If I find that the distance is then too far, which could happen, I have them pull their feet forward, in essence dragging their feet across the mat slightly to find the right spot.

Establish a Strong Foundation

In Up Dog, we want the legs off the floor completely. For this to happen we need to work the foundation of the pose. Both the hands and feet should be pressing into the floor. The energy for this action comes from further up the chain of joints.

Many teachers cue Up Dog by saying, "Push your hands into the floor." But the pushing shouldn't and can't come from just the hands alone. Once again we find ourselves working with the muscles in the armpit, in this case, the muscles that depress the scapulae (the pectoralis minor and the lower portion of the trapezius). Interestingly, the scapula itself doesn't move if we do this action correctly. Instead, the rib cage is lifted up between the shoulder blades.

As for the feet, the energy originates in the hip joint. When I take Up Dog, my intention is to use the leg as one long piece. I imagine that it is not in segments for the moment. I initiate a little hip flexion to press the top of the foot into the floor. Because I am working to keep the knees straight, the quadriceps are already engaged in this action. In fact, it is natural that the rectus femoris (the quadriceps that crosses the hip joint) will create a little hip flexion here.

The Buttocks

The combination of squeezing the thighs and the general backbending nature of the pose can easily force the buttocks to engage. I only work with people and their tight bottom if I see the tension showing up from the beginning or I sense that they are "over-doing" the posture generally.

In order to undo the pattern, I've taken people all the way to the point of having them lie on their stomach and relax. Next, I have them place their hands on the floor where they would have them for their Up Dog. Sometimes just this movement of the arms causes the glutes to contract. If it does, I make them aware of it and have them start over again. In the next stage, their hands are on the floor and they begin to lift into Up Dog without contracting the buttocks. Sometimes I'll have them contract and relax repeatedly to put the kinesthetic sensation into their system.

I continue to build this up and stay focused on the student until they are moving from *Chaturanga* into Up Dog, verbally reminding them to relax their bottom until they are

toward the end of the Up Dog. When they reach this point, it seems reasonable that a bit of squeezing will only deepen the pose. What I try to stop is an unconscious squeeze initiating the movement into Up Dog.

A Trick to Working into the Upper Back

When my teacher brought it to my attention that I was not bending in my upper back, I felt like I was entering a ridiculous mission. That was in 2001, and what seemed unobtainable then has proven to be rewarding and enjoyable work. It was a long time, one or two years, before I had any sense that I might actually be moving the vertebrae in my upper back.

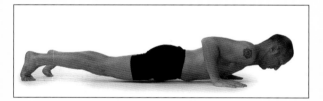
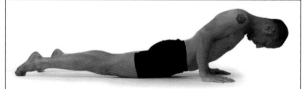
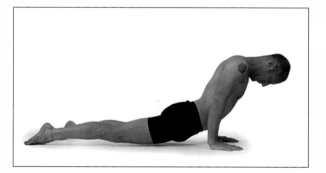
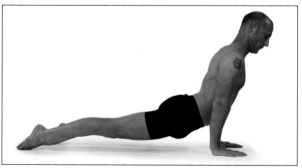
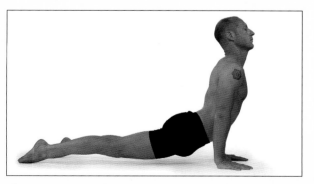
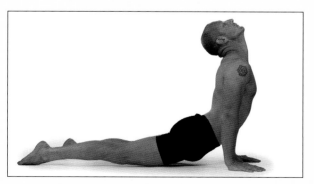

Figure 13.11: *This technique may help you find space and focus in your upper back.*

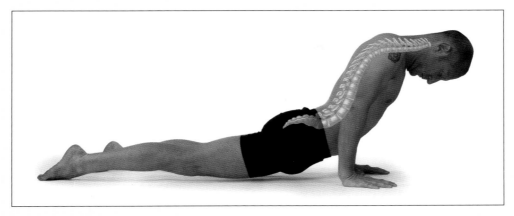

Figure 13.12: *The vertebrae separate to help us find the movement toward extension.*

John Scott planted the seed in an interesting way. It is not the traditional way to move from *Chaturanga* to Up Dog. Over the years, though, I have come to realize how it worked for me and why. The technique is simple enough. If you try it, you will see how obviously entrained your body is to move through this transition. As soon as you're ready to move from *Chaturanga* to Up Dog, drop your head so that the chin moves towards the chest. Don't force the movement, just let it relax. Then as you make your way into Up Dog, slowly undo your head and neck so that it is synchronized with the breath and the movement of your body. Do as much backbending as you can without including your head and neck until the very end. The destination remains the same, but this technique forces you to move through all parts of the spine.

I've made up a story to support this technique. As we drop the head and drag it along into Up Dog, we take the vertebrae of the neck and upper back into flexion. This is the exact opposite direction they are ultimately going in. By taking the vertebrae into a flexed position from "neutral," we have to extend to get these same vertebrae to move back to neutral again.

By initiating the movement from flexed to neutral, we use the same muscles used to further extend the spine. In this way, we set up a neuromuscular pattern that teaches these muscles to engage while going into Up Dog. This will never be a huge amount of movement; however, it does create the intention of moving in the thoracic spine.

What to Do With Your Shoulders

Working with the shoulders continues the work of moving the upper back. I've already said that, for many people, squeezing the scapulae together gives the impression that the upper back is bending more. I have a simple way of working with the shoulders: keep them as neutral as possible. By doing so, you remove the most moveable part from the sensation of bending the upper back. This way, shoulder and spine movements aren't blended together, providing better control over the movements of Up Dog.

I have students imagine a bar running across their back perpendicular to the spine. I usually touch them right between their scapulae to make a kinesthetic connection to where I want them to bend. I will also sometimes put my arm across the same area to mimic the feeling of a bar being across their back. By not moving the scapulae, we can more easily access the thoracic vertebrae in the upper back.

COMMON PATTERNS IN *URDHVA DHANURASANA*

Several common patterns show up as we move into *Urdhva Dhanurasana*. We all have our own strengths and weaknesses. Our work is to decide how to bring these into balance. While our goal may be the backbend itself, we need to think more holistically about the postures and patterns that comprise, and/or lead to a balanced *Urdhva Dhanurasana*.

There are many variables to consider in creating a backbend. If we simplify things a bit, it mostly comes down to the flexibility and strength of three main areas. These are the shoulder complex, the spine, and the hips. Just taking these three parts and holding them in your head will help broaden your understanding of the backbend. You will also start to see how the restrictions relate to the limitations you may see in other postures.

The Psoas of the Upper Body in *Urdhva Dhanurasana*

We covered the anatomy of the shoulder in the first part of the book. Here I want to apply that information directly to *Urdhva Dhanurasana*. The psoas of the upper body plays an important role in the backbend. Recall that two muscles create the psoas of the upper body—the serratus anterior and latissimus dorsi. The latissimus dorsi comes to the forefront in backbending as it can restrict how deeply we get into the shoulders. This then impacts the spine.

What Restricts the Actions We Want?

In what position do we find our scapulae when we set up the backbend? As we lie on our back and place our hands on the floor near the shoulders, we would generally like the arms and elbows parallel to one another. With our hands in this position, the scapulae are protracted and upwardly rotated. As we lift into the backbend, we need the scapulae to continue rotating in that direction. As they do, the shoulder joint flexes and rotates externally. It is harder to discern what the actual movements are when we're on our back and upside down. External rotation, in this case, means that the elbows are pointing in the same direction we are facing and not pointed out to the side (internal rotation). Take a moment to close your eyes and visualize the movement as if you were setting up and then moving into the backbend.

This means the action we are trying to create is resisted by the downward rotators of the scapula, and the extenders and internal rotators of the shoulder joint. Do you know which muscles do all of this?

The Muscles Themselves

The downward rotators are the pectoralis minor, rhomboids, and levator scapula. None of these are particularly big, powerful muscles. The extenders of the shoulder are a portion of the pectoralis major, the latissimus dorsi, the teres major, and the long head of the triceps brachii. Lastly, the internal rotators are the pectoralis major, the latissimus dorsi, the teres major, and the anterior portion of the deltoid. You may notice there is an overlap and relationship between the muscles that are extenders and internal rotators. These are the strongest restrictors to the shoulders in a backbend. At the center of this restriction is the latissimus, along with its little helper, the teres major.

This is exactly why I chose this muscle as part of the psoas of the upper body. It closely

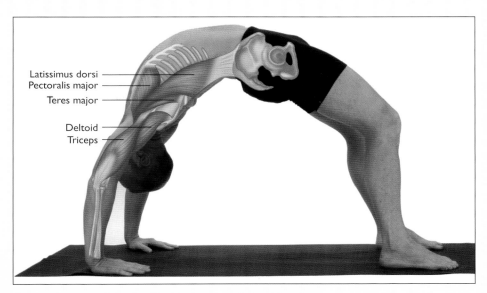

Figure 13.13: *The muscles around the shoulder that can restrict backbending.*

mirrors what we see when the real psoas muscle restricts hip flexion. You can go back and read the comparison of the upper and lower body for more details on how these movements and muscles mirror one another. For the moment, it is sufficient to remember that the real psoas restricts hip extension and internal rotation.

For the shoulders, this means that as we move into the backbend, the psoas of the upper body can restrict our ability to flex and rotate the shoulder the way we want. This restriction is one of the most common patterns we come across. The latissimus in particular is the heart of the challenge in getting the elbows to point straight up with the arms parallel to one another. It is one of the main reasons we see the elbows point out and the arms not straightening in the backbend.

Stretching the Psoas of the Upper Body

The question becomes how do we undo enough tension in these tissues to allow for more comfortable, deeper movement through the shoulders? In the backbending pattern, we need the latissimus to lengthen. It takes some subtle attention to detail to engage the serratus so that it upwardly rotates the scapula and aligns the latissimus and other muscles so that they are properly lengthened.

Down Dog and *Urdhva Dhanurasana*

Interestingly, Down Dog can help open the shoulders for backbends. Let us think about what our ideal is for Down Dog and the shoulders. Do we want the shoulder blades heading towards one another on the back? No. Do we want the elbows pointing out while we're in Down Dog? No. Do we want space between the shoulder blades? Yes. What action is this at the scapula? It is protraction and upward rotation; the serratus anterior contracts to correctly position the scapulae.

In Down Dog, we bring the scapulae around our rib cage. We rotate the upper arms so the elbows are not pointing out to the sides, but are, instead, heading more towards the floor. This sets us up to place pressure on the latissimus dorsi and teres major. Because of the position of the scapulae and the way gravity is working,

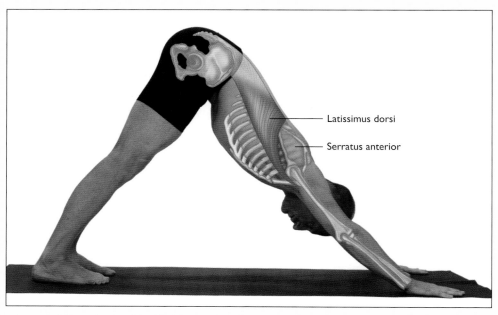

Figure 13.14: *Serratus brings the shoulder blade around the front and helps align latissimus in a way that it can be lengthened in this posture.*

this is an opportunity to lengthen the same shoulder extenders we're after in a backbend. This is different than simply arching the back and watching the scapulae squeeze together.

We can have this same experience if we put in some extra effort while working on our backbends. As we go up or are up in the backbend itself, if we create arms similar to what we talked about in Down Dog, the pressure from the feet pressing into the floor will put pressure into the latissimus and other shoulder extenders. This helps to undo the

"elbow pointing out" pattern that is so common in backbends and Down Dog.

A Technique

I believe that the arms should be more or less the same in Down Dog and the backbend. If you disagree, then this technique isn't for you. When you do use this position, you will take advantage of the kinematic chain of the arm to release the shoulder joint and then get it to rotate the way we want. Want to give it a try?

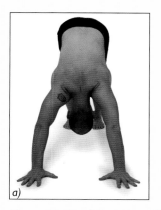 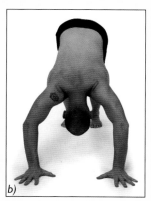 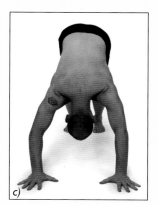 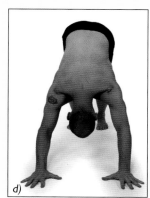

Figure 13.15: *a) Scapulae retracted, shoulders internally rotated, b) elbows bend to open the chain of joints, c) scapulae now moving around the front with elbows still bent, d) shoulder blades are wide and around the front, the arms are rotating externally. The same technique can be used when upside down and in a backbend.*

In Downward Dog, bend the elbows slightly. This assures us that the shoulder joint and scapulae will move in the next step. Once the elbows are bent, rotate the arms so that the elbows are squeezing an imaginary ball in front of your face. Notice how the scapulae start to come around the front of the chest. Then slowly start to straighten the arms. Most people will notice more pressure on the outer edge of their armpits, which is right where the latissimus dorsi and teres major muscles are.

To take this into the backbend, repeat the same instructions once you are up in the pose. That is, bend the elbows slightly, rotate them so that the elbows are heading towards one another in front of your face, and slowly start to straighten. A main difference here is that if you now push with your feet, you will feel the pressure come into the shoulder area. DO NOT squeeze or push with all of your strength! Just work with about 20 percent of your strength to feel it out first.

Taking it Further—*Kapotasana* Arms

I want to take the arms a step further using *Kapotasana* as an example. Why? Because they take us even deeper into the amount of shoulder opening one needs. This work will help tie in another common pattern that we see in backbending—inability to get the hands on the floor or yourself off the floor if you *do* get the hands flat.

All of the elements we just spoke about for the shoulders in backbending apply here as well. But I would also like to add the triceps brachii. Why the triceps brachii? Because it is a two-joint muscle. Why is that important? Because the position of one joint affects the position and tension surrounding the other.

You may recall that we spoke about other two-joint muscles such as the hamstrings and quadriceps in the anatomy section. The triceps brachii is the quadriceps of the arm. This means that when the elbow bends, it is restricted by the tension of the triceps brachii. In anatomical position, you won't notice this restriction. But the triceps brachii long head crosses the shoulder joint and is known as an extender of the shoulder. If you flex the shoulder with a bent (flexed) elbow, you will notice how much more restricted it is.

Do this. Stand up, or stay seated if you like, but have enough space that you can flex your arm at the shoulder joint with your arms straight. When you have gone into flexion as far as you can, notice the angle of the upper arm. It is probably close to vertical. Now, bring your arm down and bend the elbow completely; keep it bent while you flex the shoulder joint again. Do you notice a change in tension? Can you see a different angle?

Put this into *Kapotasana*, as done in the Ashtanga Vinyasa system or perhaps an even more familiar Raja *Kapotasana*. When those arms reach back and the elbow bends to take the ankles or a single foot, it becomes much more difficult to extend the shoulder. It is also quite common for the elbows to go wide. This happens for the same reason that it does in the backbend. Tight hip flexors and tight shoulders can even mirror one another in either a backbend or *Kapotasana*. The elbows and knees go wider to avoid the triceps brachii tension in the arm and the hip flexor (let's say the quardriceps) tension in the legs.

Let us relate this to our backbend, specifically for those who have a hard time getting their hands to the floor (when setting up for the backbend), or for those who get their hands to the floor but have a hard time lifting

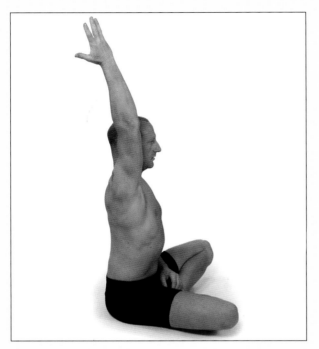 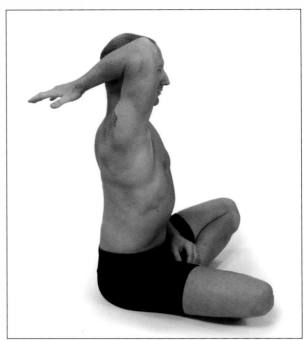

Figure 13.16: *You can see that as the elbow bends, no matter how hard I was trying, the elbow moves forward because of the tension and dynamics of the triceps.*

themselves up. The difficulty in getting the hands nicely planted on the ground can be a flexibility issue. An inability to get off the floor can also be a strength issue that results from the muscle being in a lengthened position.

Because of the arm's position, the bent elbow, and the flexed humerus, there is more tension and thus more length in the triceps. We need the strength of the triceps brachii to help us straighten the elbow. In fact, it is the only muscle that creates that action. When it is maximally lengthened, it is weaker. As the muscle fibers get pulled apart from one another, they have a harder time contracting.

Other parts play into this as well. You may recall the story I told about the student who did the hip preps prior to a backbend and was then able to get her head off the floor for the first time? In this case, the hip flexors needed a bit more length in them to help get the pelvis higher and to change the angle at which the shoulder was sitting on the other end. This is

a good example of how all the parts have a relationship with and affect one another.

HIP ANATOMY IN *URDHVA DHANURASANA*

I'll let you in on a secret to backbending: think "front opening" more than "backbending." If the tissues on the front of the body are not flexible, they restrict our backbend. In particular we're talking about the hip flexors and how they restrict our ability to get the hips higher to allow the pelvis to float comfortably in the tension of the tissues surrounding it. When the hips go higher, the spine and shoulders are also affected.

When the hips are restricted and sit low relative to the spine, we see a familiar pattern. With the pelvis lower, the knees usually have to bend more to compensate. It is not that the knees aren't allowed to bend at all, they are. They can't straighten because the added

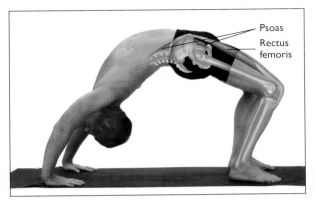 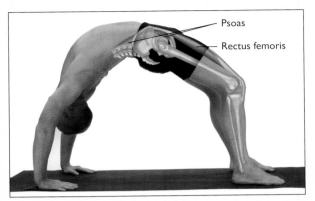

Psoas
Rectus femoris

Psoas
Rectus femoris

Figure 13.17: *In the first image, the hip flexors are tight and restrict the pelvis ability to lift and rotate. In the second image, hip flexors have been released allowing the knees to straighten, pelvis to lift and rotate appropriately.*

pressure from the knees straightening would likely cause compression in the lower back. This happens because the hip flexors prevent the pelvis from tilting (posterior tilt) in the direction of the backbend. The arms may be bent or straight. If the arms were straight, the angle of the arms would be far from vertical. They might be as much as 45 degrees heading in the direction of the knees. This pattern leads to a strong compression of the wrist joint.

In this same pattern, if we are able to release the hip flexors, the knees can straighten more. If the knees straighten more, the pelvis moves in the direction of the shoulders. When this happens, the shoulders get closer to lining up with the hands. And when this happens, the pressure in the wrist is reduced. It's all connected.

Wide Knees in *Urdhva Dhanurasana*

Wide knees in a backbend are often corrected in class. There are a number of ways to work with this. What is the anatomical reason that the knees fall out? We could talk about the strength of the adductors versus the flexibility of the abductors and external rotators of the hip. Both can and should be worked with.

In order to get up into our backbend, we most likely need our gluteus maximus to contract.

This is exactly the kind of movement this muscle was designed for. Although the buttocks may be needed to initiate the movement into a backbend, over-contracting it can cause other patterns we don't necessarily want.

The big gluteus maximus muscle serves two functions in our body in terms of pure movement or action. It extends the hip (which is what we're doing in a backbend) and externally rotates it. If we over-contract the gluteus maximus, it not only lifts our hips up in the air but also emphasizes external rotation at the hip joint. This is commonly seen in a backbend as the knees pointing outwards, and the feet usually go along with them.

There are two ways to remedy this that I am aware of: 1) reduce the contraction of the glutes or 2) even more subtle, reduce the glutes' function as an external rotator of the hip joint. To do this, engage the adductors. This will help shut off the external rotation function of the gluteus maximus, as well as any abductors that might be contributing to the knees sticking out. Which muscles are these? The deep gluteus minimus and medius are the primary abductors of the hip joint.

There is another reason why the knees go out that's a bit more unconscious. It is to avoid the hip flexors. This is another example of the body doing whatever it has to in order to reach its goal. When the knees go wide, they reduce the amount of tension running through the hip flexors (like the elbows bowing out to avoid the shoulder extenders). One of the keys is the quadriceps group, especially the rectus femoris that crosses the hip joint. Keep in mind that the tighter the hip flexors are, the more the gluteals need to work to create hip extension against their resistance. This makes it harder to shut them off, sometimes impossible.

When the knees are closer together, this quadricep places a nice clean line of tension on the pelvis. When the knees go wide, the angle changes and the amount of tension is reduced. When the tension increases in the hip flexors, it tends to pull the pelvis down and forward. A common consequence of this, especially in a backbend, is a shortening and possible compression in the lower back.

This same thing happens in Reclined Hero Pose (*Supta Virasana*). We want the knees together, but as they come together, we usually see an increased arch in the lower back. As tension in the hip flexors increases, they pull on the front of the pelvis and rotate it downwards. This makes the back arch more. We can counter-rotate the pelvis to resist the pull of the hip flexors and reduce the amount of arch.

There are always exceptions to the knee position in a backbend or in *Supta Virasana*. There is more variety in the hip than in any other joint, and the size and shape of the pelvis also varies from person to person. If you want to see how much hip flexor tension you have, try bringing the knees together in a backbend or in *Supta Virasana*. Notice if that space increases or even decreases the amount of pressure in your lower back or SI joint.

I have met some people who position their knees quite wide for their backbend. I ask them to bring their feet together and do another. Some of them have a hard time getting off the floor with their feet and knees in this position. To me, this shows how much tension is in their hip flexors and that their pattern of taking the knees wide avoids this tension. It is time for them to change the

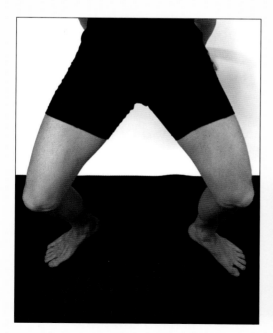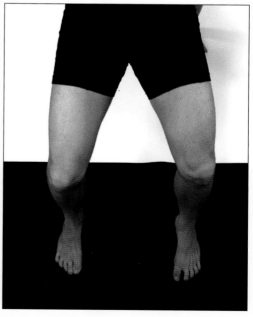

Figure 13.18: *With the knees wider, the distance between the pelvis and the end of the knee is reduced. The closer the knees are, the longer the hip flexors would have to be.*

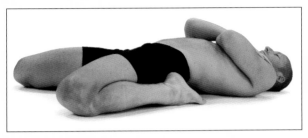
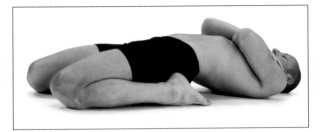

Figure 13.19: *With the knees wide, my back flattens. When I squeeze my knees, the back arches. This is saying that the tension from my hip flexors pulls my pelvis into a stronger anterior tilt as the knees come together.*

pattern and the anatomy that goes along with it.

Remember, we want to work with the postures that add up to the stated goal, *Urdhva Dhanurasana.* As the hip flexors open and the buttocks soften in their rotational component, the knees naturally move closer together and are more easily held there.

CONCLUSION

Once we have gotten the shoulders and hips out of the way, all that's left is the spine itself. It is certainly possible that your spine doesn't like to bend. That said, if there is no known anatomical dysfunction going on (like fused vertebrae or disc dysfunction, etc.), everyone should be able to bend his or her spine to a certain extent. The good news is that the amount of natural bend in any spine can and will change with a regular yoga practice.

The deepest of backbends are definitely impressive. When I see someone who is in a

backbend but looks like they're in a forward bend, I am impressed and in awe of the anatomy at work. Some people are simply born able to do this; others have worked hard to obtain it. Both are inspiring.

These bendy types are comprised of the same stuff as the rest of us. They do not have extra vertebrae or a lack of them. What they have is a combination of good genetics, open connective tissue, really open hip flexors, a flexible spine, and open shoulders. Each part plays a role in allowing a deep backbend. Whether or not bendiness like this is good for you remains to be seen. The yoga experiment is in progress.

Backbending is an excellent place to work on your skills and ability to see the interrelationship and integrated function of the body. Each piece of the backbend plays its role, and if one is blocked, it usually affects the other parts. See if you can read the messages revealed by the knees or elbows splaying out or reduced angles in certain places, and consider how this relates back to how you or your students attempt backbending poses.

CONCLUSION

The journey of yoga goes far beyond the anatomy of the body and far beyond the pages of this book. And this book has been a journey, not just for you, but for me as well. The subject of anatomy is vast and there are many perspectives from which it can be studied. I have simply offered mine and have tried my best to make this journey one that you can follow and understand. I've tried to be your narrator on a ride through your body's functional anatomy, helping to connect it to yoga for you along the way. It was my intention to point out the similarities between different aspects of the postures and their relationship to anatomical functioning. I hope this has given you a different perspective, a new way to look at the interrelatedness of yoga postures.

The journey for all of us is not finished. If there is one thing I would like for you to have gained from this book, it is that our anatomy and its function and form are wondrous. From the subtle aspects to the more gross physiological functions, we are truly integrated beings. There is no doubt about this and if you leave these pages with a sense of just how integrated we are, I am happy.

In the first half of the book, we saw the convergence and integration of anatomy itself. It was almost painful to separate the body into its parts and pieces and then bring it back together in a meaningful way. When you intersect the complicated physical nature of *asana* with anatomy, things become more complicated and potentially convoluted.

It has always been my desire to have both my anatomy students and yoga students become free thinkers, to question what they *think* they know, and not just for the sake of questioning, but for the sake of diving deeply enough to obtain experiential knowledge of the subject. The journey should continue from here.

If I have caused you to question what you think you know, then I am happy. If I have caused you to experiment with your own body, I have succeeded. Even if you return to the exact same view you had before reading this book, that's okay with me! That you were open enough to hear another perspective is important to avoiding a dogmatic response to the difficult problems we may be faced with as students and teachers.

There was no possible way for me to cover every piece of anatomy or every single *asana*. It was not my desire to spoon feed you my way of describing things. Instead I hoped to show you the relationships between parts of the anatomy, between different *asanas*, and between anatomy and *asana*. I hope I have succeeded.

These pages are far from my final words on yoga and anatomy. In an effort to not get stuck in what I think I know, I reserve the right to contradict myself and to change my mind in the future. It is with this openness that I offer these words to the conversation around yoga today.

Namasté,

David Keil

TERMS TO DESCRIBE POSITION AND DIRECTION

The anatomical position provides a standard reference point for an individual: the body is upright, with the head, eyes and toes all facing forwards, and the arms and hands are hanging by the sides, palms turned to the front.

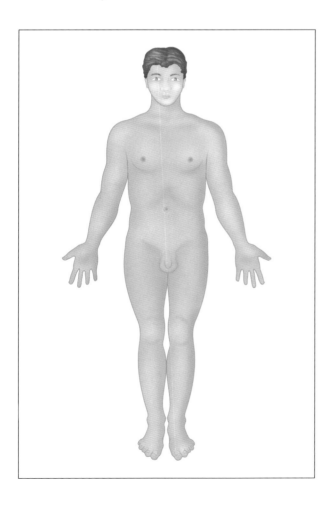

Afferent	Directed inwards to an organ or a part of the body, e.g. spinal cord.
Anterior	Situated at or towards the front of the body. Also called *ventral*. A term prefixed with antero signifies 'before'.
Deep	Situated far away from the body surface.
Distal	Remote or away from any point of origin of a structure. From Latin *distans*, meaning 'distant'.
Dorsum	The back or posterior surface of something, e.g. back of the hand, or upper surface of the foot.
Efferent	Directed away from an organ or a part of the body.
Inferior	Situated below, or directed down, away from the head. Also known as *caudal*.
Lateral	Towards the side, or located away from the midline of the body or organ.
Medial	Towards the midline of the body or organ.

Palmar   Relating to the anterior surface (palm) of the hand.

Peripheral   Towards the outer surface of the body or organ.

Plantar   Relating to the posterior surface (sole) of the foot.

Posterior   Situated at or towards the back of the body. Also called *dorsal*. *Postero* is a combining form, denoting a relationship to the posterior part, e.g. posterolateral.

Prone   Position of the body in which the ventral (anterior) surface faces down.

Proximal   Nearest or closer to any point of origin of a structure. From Latin *proximus*, meaning 'next'.

Superficial   Situated near or at the body surface.

Superior   Situated above, towards the head. Also known as *cephalic*.

Supine   Position of the body in which the ventral (anterior) surface faces up.

REFERENCES

1. Wilson, F.R., *The Hand*. (Vintage Books, 1998)

2. Levangie, P.K. & Norkin, C.C., *Joint Structure and Function, Third Edition*. (F.A. Davis Company, 2001) (p. 369)

3. Zihlman, A.L., *The Human Evolution Coloring Book*. (Harper Collins, 2000)

4. Zihlman, A.L., *The Human Evolution Coloring Book*. (Harper Collins, 2000)

5. Werner, R. & Benjamin, B.E., *A Massage Therapist's Guide to Pathology*. (Williams & Wilkins, 1998) (p. 102)

6. Werner, R. & Benjamin, B.E., *A Massage Therapist's Guide to Pathology*. (Williams & Wilkins, 1998) (p. 101)

7. Werner, R. & Benjamin, B.E., *A Massage Therapist's Guide to Pathology*. (Williams & Wilkins, 1998) (p. 94)

8. Levangie, P.K. & Norkin, C.C., *Joint Structure and Function, Third Edition*. (F.A. Davis Company, 2001) (p. 328)

9. Zihlman, A.L., *The Human Evolution Coloring Book*. (Harper Collins, 2000)

10. Levangie, P.K. & Norkin, C.C., *Joint Structure and Function, Third Edition*. (F.A. Davis Company, 2001) (p. 336)

11. Levangie, P.K. & Norkin, C.C., *Joint Structure and Function, Third Edition*. (F.A. Davis Company, 2001) (p. 331)

12. Cailliet, R., *Knee Pain and Disability, Edition 3*. (F.A. David Company, 1992) (p. 12)

13. Levangie, P.K. & Norkin, C.C., *Joint Structure and Function, Third Edition*. (F.A. Davis Company, 2001) (p. 298)

14. Levangie, P.K. & Norkin, C.C., *Joint Structure and Function, Third Edition*. (F.A. Davis Company, 2001) (p. 292)

15. Levangie, P.K. & Norkin, C.C., *Joint Structure and Function, Third Edition*. (F.A. Davis Company, 2001) (p. 292)

16. Levangie, P.K. & Norkin, C.C., *Joint Structure and Function, Third Edition*. (F.A. Davis Company, 2001) (p. 293)

17. Levangie, P.K. & Norkin, C.C., *Joint Structure and Function, Third Edition*. (F.A. Davis Company, 2001) (p. 294)

18. Kapandji, I.A., *The Physiology of the Joints, Second Edition, Volume Two, Lower Limb*. (Longman Group Ltd., 1980)

19. Kapandji, I.A., *The Physiology of the Joints, Second Edition, Volume Two, Lower Limb*. (Longman Group Ltd., 1980)

20. Myers, T., Fans of the hip joint. (*Massage Magazine*, January/February 1998).

21. Travell, J. & Simon, D., *Myofascial Pain and Dysfunction – The Trigger Point Manual, Volume Two*. (Williams and Wilkin) (p. 92)

22. Myers, T., Psoas-piriformis balance. (*Massage Magazine*, March/April 1998)

23. Walker, J.M., The sacroiliac joint: A critical review. *Phys. Ther.* 72:903, 1992

24. Kapandji, I.A., *The Physiology of the Joints, Second Edition, Volume Three, The Trunk and the Vertebral Column*. (Longman Group Ltd., 1980)

25. Levangie, P.K. & Norkin, C.C., *Joint Structure and Function, Third Edition*. (F.A. Davis Company, 2001) (p. 120)

26. Gorman, D., *The Body Moveable*. (Ampersand Press, 1981)

27. Bigliani, L.U., Morrison, D.S. & April, E.W., The morphology of the acromion and its relationship to rotator cuff tears. *Orthop. Trans.* 1986;10:228

Other Resources

Cailliet, R., *Low Back Pain Syndrome, Edition 5*. (F.A. David Company, 1992)

Cailliet, R., *Shoulder Pain, Edition 3*, (F.A. David Company, 1991)

Kapandji, I.A., *The Physiology of the Joints, Second Edition, Volume One, The Upper Limb*. (Longman Group Ltd., 1980)

Myers, T., *Anatomy Trains: Myofascial Meridians for Manual and Movement Therapists*. (Elsevier Health Sciences, 2001)

INDEX